Early Praise for
The Savvy Insomniac

"A compelling book of remarkable breadth and uncommon insight. Maharg brings a deft touch and a deep understanding to the problem of insomnia in modern America."

–A. Roger Ekirch, author of *At Day's Close: Night in Times Past*

"In *The Savvy Insomniac,* Maharg explores the science and treatments for insomnia throughout history up to the current day: an investigation seamlessly woven into her personal experiences. This well-researched book will not only provide perspective for individuals with insomnia, but also for clinicians seeking to help their patients."

–Deirdre A. Conroy, Ph.D., Clinical Associate Professor, University of Michigan Department of Psychiatry

THE SAVVY INSOMNIAC

THE SAVVY
INSOMNIAC

A Personal Journey
through Science to Better Sleep

LOIS MAHARG

Fine Fettle Books

Printed in the United States of America

First Printing, 2013

ISBN 978-0-9894837-1-1

Fine Fettle Books
4730 Midway Drive
Ann Arbor, MI 48103

www.thesavvyinsomniac.com

10 9 8 7 6 5 4 3 2 1

For all who lie awake at night
wondering why

Contents

Sizing Up the Beast

*There is a gulf fixed between those who can
sleep and those who cannot. It is one of the great
divisions of the human race.*

Iris Murdoch, *Nuns and Soldiers*

Mention trouble sleeping, and you'll get an earful of advice. "Have you tried melatonin?" "It could be your mattress." "My mother swears by chamomile tea." If you're a bona fide insomniac like me, or even if you only tangle with the sleep demon in bouts, you've probably tried these things and more. But you may as well take baby aspirin for a migraine. None of these common cures for sleeplessness remotely touches what you're grappling with.

Advice from sleep experts, available in lists of do's and don'ts on the web and in magazines, may be more useful—or not. The idea of going to bed and getting up at the same time every day may strike you as fine for the office computer, but too rigid for yourself. Setting your bed and wake time according to the clock may also be incompatible with the demands of family and job. Daily exercise, another item in the do column, confers plenty of health benefits. But it may or may not help your sleep. And among the insomniac's thou-shalt-nots—do not read or watch television or movies in bed— are activities that you may have discovered sometimes court rather than sabotage sleep.

Less helpful yet are the assumptions about insomnia that drift like dust motes in the air, exposed when normal sleepers decide it's time to shine a ray of light on your predicament. "Can't sleep? There must be something bothering you." "You've got to find ways to cut down on stress." "Maybe it's time to give up coffee." "Have you considered psychotherapy? You've got to tackle the problem at its *source*." Maybe you agree with some of these common beliefs. Or maybe you're a skeptic, like me. Maybe this sort of chatter is something you tune out.

What's real is the struggle going on in your life, which, if you've picked up this book, you may be waging on your own, with or without the assistance of pills. And for many insomniacs that struggle is harder than commonly supposed.

Bouts of insomnia leave Abby, a stay-at-home mom, feeling angry all the time, and concerned about her ability to do what needs to be done. "I just can't *function*," she said. "I have no patience with my children. I tend to be very reactive, and anything can set me off. I go into crying spells. It's a lot like PMS."

Kay, a full-time student, experiences mixed-up sensations day and night: "I feel like I'm sort of in the mud, I'm constantly trying to get through the mud. I spend so much energy in my day trying to function on no sleep that by the time it's time for sleep the next night, I'm just wired."

Concern with functioning is a feature of many insomniacs' lives. Your nights and days get weirdly scrambled, your body thrums with energy at night and feels depleted during the daytime. Like chronic pain or depression, insomnia can affect you 24/7.

For other insomniacs, the problem goes beyond functioning to surviving: "When I'm going through a bad stretch," said Julie, whose children and part-time job keep her feeling constantly behind, "there are times when I feel that all I'm doing is surviving, that my life is passing me by and I'm not really enjoying it."

"I was starting to survive on two or three hours a night," Liz, a medical librarian, said. "I wasn't getting to sleep till five in the morning, and then getting back up again at seven to get to work. And I thought, 'I can't keep doing this. This is insane.'"

Function and survive: These words, which crop up time and time again in the narratives of insomniacs I interviewed, speak of adversity and struggle. They suggest a deprivation as basic as lack of food, shelter, clothing, or air. Yet for much of the twentieth century the affliction was dismissed as trivial and "all in the head."

"Of course there is *something* the matter with these people," said Woods Hutchinson, a physician writing in *Good Housekeeping* magazine, about insomnia sufferers nearly a hundred years ago. "Perfectly healthy, normal human beings don't imagine themselves sick, nor do people who are 'all there' become utter fools gratuitously. For even the vagaries of imaginary disease there is a reason, but to cure many of these cases would mean taking the whole nervous system to pieces and putting it together again differently, and the results would hardly be worth the trouble, even if it could be done."[1]

Hardly worth the trouble? Fortunately, many sleep researchers today disagree. But the insomniac's cup remains less than full. Nearly a century has passed since Hutchinson registered his views, and scientists are still endeavoring to take the nervous system to pieces to discover what the matter is.

Progress has been made. Some scientific studies suggest that compared to normal sleepers, insomniacs are more physiologically aroused. We tend to have elevated metabolic rates and, at night, lower heart rate variability, suggesting greater activity of the sympathetic nervous system (which is associated with stress and the fight-or-flight response). Some research shows we have higher-than-normal levels of alerting hormones in our blood and urine.[2]

Other research highlights differences in the brain. Sleep studies show that during non-REM (quiet) sleep, characterized by reduced metabolic activity and an absence of dreaming, insomniacs' brains are prone to high-frequency waveforms more typically associated with being awake. Investigators have used neuroimaging technologies to enlarge this finding. While good sleepers' brains are mostly quiet during non-REM sleep, key areas of insomniacs' brains are busy metabolizing glucose. This excessive neural activity may reflect a low-level sensory processing that is occurring even as we sleep.[3]

But the picture gleaned from measurements of bodily and brain functions is incomplete. More is known about environmental, behavioral, and psychological factors contributing to insomnia. Thus the big insomnia story, which may one day include an explanation of its genetic underpinnings and the mechanistic pathways by which it develops, is a work in progress. Insomnia is still treated as a subjective complaint that exists because we feel its effects.

For decades my insomnia was something I did my best to ignore. It was a fairly steady nemesis at night, keeping my body achy and tense, and unleashing a jumble of negative thoughts. But by day, though I might feel fatigued and dull, I strove to put it behind me and plunge into my activities. There was nothing to gain by doing otherwise. My wakeful nights were unpleasant enough; why let the sleep demon wreck my days? There were ways to manage insomnia and I'd tried them all. I'd used antihistamines. I'd listened to audiotapes and done relaxation exercises. I'd consulted doctors; I'd taken sleeping pills. And grudgingly, I observed many of the do's and don'ts I read about in advice columns for the sleepless. I felt I was managing as best I could. Besides, I asked myself, how much attention did insomnia really deserve? One didn't die of it. Problems like schizophrenia, major depression, and chronic pain were surely more debilitating. If insomnia had a place on the menu of chronic health disorders, was it not "lite" fare? From any perspective, it made no sense to dwell on it, especially when thinking about insomnia only seemed to make it worse.

Over the years insomnia became an elephant in my bedroom: something massively encroaching on my space, and yet something whose impact I strove, at least in the light of day, to shut my eyes to. The strategy worked pretty well into my late forties. But then something changed. It wasn't that my insomnia grew worse. My bouts of wakefulness had always occurred for stretches of three or four weeks, broken by occasional "catch-up" nights in which I slept hungrily and desperately as though my life depended on it. That pattern remained fixed. But I simply couldn't continue pretending I was leading the kind of life I wanted. Insomnia *was* making me miserable at night, and it *was* diminishing the quality of my days. And the only way I could think to change that was to confront what for so long I had dismissed. I decided both to search inside myself for answers and to immerse myself in scientific research in hopes of finally gaining the upper hand.

I saw from the start that the scientific research held promise. My first trip to a medical library acquainted me with no fewer than seven academic journals dedicated exclusively to studies on sleep and sleep disorders. A cursory inspection of their contents revealed vast quantities of information I'd never heard about in the popular press. Often insomnia was described as a disorder of "hyperarousal," suggesting much study of the brain and the nervous system lay ahead. My plan was also to investigate insomnia therapies of all sorts: homegrown and experimental, as well as the drugs and cognitive-behavioral treatments approved by the medical establishment. So, armed with two college syllabuses on sleep, and with access to a top-tier medical library and help from sleep experts, I set out on my quest.

But my attempts to explore my own insomnia were initially less encouraging. I had spent decades playing down its impact. No sooner did I set out to confront it than I balked. There was something unsettling about my insomnia, something that warned me away. I wanted to look at it squarely in the face but felt apprehensive about what I'd find.

These weren't the only challenges ahead. Before I could evaluate what science had to say about insomnia, I needed to know how people *experienced* the affliction. I knew about my own experience, and I'd talked to my brother and my sister-in-law about theirs. I'd heard about the "fair to middling" sleep of my father, a stoic when it came to enduring health problems, who reported that a doctor once assured him that "rest was as good as sleep." Some 30 million Americans supposedly suffered insomnia just as we did, but apart from these few insomnia sufferers in my extended family, I didn't know a single one. I would need to hear their stories somehow.

I dipped into the world of story and myth on the chance that literary figures might enlarge my understanding of insomnia. There, sleeplessness was often connected to heightened emotional states. Lovesickness was one. Medea, when she first laid eyes on Jason in his quest for the Golden Fleece, was so inflamed with passion that she could not sleep. Queen Dido was smitten with Aeneas; she too could not sleep. Her grief at his departure was so overwhelming that it destroyed her sleep and eventually cost her her life.

Sleeplessness was one of the main signs of courtly love. In Chaucer's "The Knight's Tale," young Arcite, exiled from the land of his ladylove, was "bereft" of sleep, and his eyes were "hollow, and grisly to behold." The Black Knight in the *Book of the Duchess* suffered a similar fate: grief over the death of his lady left him in a state where "my day is night" and "my sleep [is] waking." Don Quixote, too, was famously sleepless pining for Dulcinea.

Another emotion that interfered with sleep in Biblical and literary narratives was guilt. In the Old Testament, King Darius's "sleep fled from him" after he threw Daniel into the lions' den. King Ahasuerus could not sleep at the thought of having failed to reward Mordecai for saving his life. Shakespeare's Macbeth, in murdering Duncan, was so consumed with guilt that he "murdered" sleep (his own). In *Crime and Punishment*, Raskolnikov murdered an old pawnbroker and her sister and felt so much guilt that he could not sleep. In myth and literature, powerful emotion led to the ruin of sleep.

These narratives were certainly compelling, yet not very enlightening when it came to helping me understand persistent insomnia. Plenty of people I knew lost sleep over love troubles or a guilty conscience. But eventually they recovered their equilibrium and went back to sleeping as they had before. The insomnia sufferers whose stories I wanted to hear were those who, like me, were afflicted with trouble sleeping even when life was moving along on an even keel. They might feel exhausted, their muscles tired and their minds dull—just the ingredients you'd imagine would lead to a good night's sleep—yet they had problems getting to sleep, staying asleep, or waking early.

Authors writing about their own sleepless nights have not always found insomnia to be disagreeable. The Romanian writer Emil Cioran acknowledged his insomnia was probably harmful to his health, yet it also forced him to confront the "dangerous, harmful truths" that became his life's work to set down in prose. "When I was about twenty I stopped sleeping and I consider that the grandest tragedy that could occur." He embraced "the melancholy of insomniac nights," which drove him to phantom-like wanderings through the streets of Paris at all hours, as proof of a superior intellect. "True knowledge comes down to vigils in the darkness," he wrote. "The sum of our insomnias alone distinguishes us from the animals and from our kind. What rich or strange idea was ever the work of a sleeper?"[4]

Joyce Carol Oates has expressed similar sentiments. Insomnia may result in anguish and discomfort, she said, yet keeping vigil at night, when one's defenses are down and one's rational powers are at low ebb, may also summon visions. "Unable to sleep, one suddenly grasps the profound meaning of *being awake:* a revelation that shades subtly into horror, or into instruction. Sartre imagines Hell as a region in which one's eyelids have vanished—perpetual consciousness. Yet this wakefulness is also a region of profound revelations."[5]

"I've come to regard my insomnia as something very positive," Oates said elsewhere. "I've written a lot of gothic and horror, and I think the insomnia allows me to tap into something that might otherwise be missing."[6]

How I envy people whose insomnia is a portal to revelation and difficult truths! Who doesn't long to find a silver lining in the cloud? To discover some creative use for wakefulness would make it much more tolerable. Yet people who do that are tapping into resources I haven't found inside myself. There is nothing remotely "grand" about the insomnia I have lived with, or, I suspect, the insomnia of those whose complaints drive a $2 billion sleeping pill industry.

The kind of insomnia that gives rise to complaints is classified in medical lingo as a "disorder," or an abnormality of function. And while lots of people experience occasional nocturnal wakefulness, fewer experience it on a continuing or recurring basis, as I do, in which case it's said to be a chronic disorder.

Estimates of the number of people with chronic insomnia vary, but 10 percent is a figure often cited in print. It affects more women than men, older people more often than younger, the poor more often than the well-to-do.[7] No test can confirm that you've got chronic insomnia. But you know it when you've got it. And if you're reading this book, I'll wager your insomnia is a pretty steady adversary (or perhaps it is for someone you know).

The medical definition of insomnia differs somewhat among the three systems used to classify sleep disorders.[8] Yet these systems are mostly in agreement about the main symptoms: difficulty initiating or maintaining sleep, awakening too early, or sleep that is nonrestorative or poor in quality; and distress or impairment in important areas of functioning. The diagnosis of chronic insomnia turns on the duration and severity of the symptoms.[9] A separate diagnostic category exists for circadian rhythm disorders, in which the sole problem is a mismatch between the timing of daylight and darkness and the time your body clock says you're ready for sleep. (We'll sort out the diagnostic distinctions later.) When insomnia is a regular nighttime companion, something is functioning in a less-than-optimal way.

When I conceived of this project near the end of 2003, there weren't many stories about insomnia circulating in the popular press. Accounts of people with other disorders—depression, bipolar disorder, anorexia, Asperger syndrome—were all over the TV, and in movies and magazines. But except for *Sleep Demons,* a memoir by Bill Hayes, and a few short stories, the only place I found insomniacs talking freely about their lives was on the web in anonymous, sound-bite-sized posts. Since 2003, a few more insomnia sufferers have come forward with their stories. *Insomniac,* by Gayle Greene, and *Wide Awake*, by Patricia Morrisroe, have helped to humanize and increase awareness about an affliction often dismissed as just a normal part of everyday life. Yet experiential accounts of insomnia remain few and far between.

Why have insomniacs kept such a low profile? In what ways has unwanted wakefulness affected their lives? How do they feel about it, what are they doing about it, what kind of help are they looking for? These questions could only be answered by some of the 30 million insomnia sufferers who remained anonymous to me. So by word of mouth and through the web, by posting fliers and advertising in the newspaper, I began to make contact with the members of my tribe.

☾

Brandie was one of the first insomnia sufferers I met. She talked to me about her sleep one afternoon in her home. Shy at first, she warmed to the topic.

Brandie told me she's never been able to sleep at night. She's "too wound up, too hyped up to sleep." When she does sleep (she may go a few days without any sleep at all, she said), it's usually from 6 a.m. to 11 or 11:30 a.m. Fortunately, this doesn't interfere much with her work as a personal assistant for a woman in a wheelchair. If Brandie is needed at a time when she's asleep, she's able to get up, do her work, and go back to sleep.

As unusual as her sleep habits are, it's even more unusual that her sleep irregularities started when she was very young, at the age of three. "As far back as I remember my parents used to be drove nuts by me not sleeping," she said. "I guess I was pretty ornery about my sleeplessness. It wasn't a good thing."

Brandie thinks her sleeplessness in childhood could have been due in part to feeling unsafe at times. Her parents fought often. She remembers shoes—and sometimes hands—flying her way. But mostly she didn't sleep because she wasn't sleepy.

Being awake at night had serious consequences. "If [my parents] found me not sleeping there's times when they would spank me and figure I'd just cry myself to sleep. That didn't work, so they'd try getting me to sit in a corner and hold still. That usually didn't work either. I'd be playing on the walls."

Brandie eventually learned to pretend. "I did end up learning that I should fake sleep when they came around," she said. "I listened to other people snore and caught on to how to do that. Anytime they'd come around, I'd just fake it because I was in trouble if I got caught being awake so it became kind of like a game."

Brandie's brother also had trouble sleeping. The two of them joined forces and tried to find nighttime activities that did not attract notice.

At night, she said, "We talked, me and my brother. We hung out together because both of us had a lot of the sleeplessness. We'd just sneak back and forth between bedrooms because you could hear my parents coming from anyplace in the house. So you had warning, and we could sneak back to our beds.

"If we were both having really bad sleepless nights we would entertain ourselves, play games, whatever, and if we got caught in each others' room that was OK because we both were known to sleepwalk. So sometimes if we happened to get too engrossed in whatever we were doing and didn't go to sleep like we were supposed to, we'd just pretend we were sleeping in the other person's room, and that was OK."

Growing up, Brandie never discussed her sleep problem with anyone. "The sleeplessness thing is just something I wasn't ever taught to talk about. It's like the parents fighting or the aunt and uncle fighting. There were things that happened that you just didn't talk about."

Brandie has never sought help from a doctor for her sleep problems and avoids over-the-counter sleep aids, as they tend to "hype [her] up no end." She manages her insomnia on her own, using the time at night to paint, read, and write; do jigsaw puzzles and macramé; and play with her cats.

"It's just one of those things I had to learn to cope with, " Brandie said, "just like my learning disability [dyslexia] as a kid."

But her sleep problem has had a big impact on her life. "It's made me hate other people to some degree because they can sleep. It makes me real frustrated because I really feel like I could use the sleep. But I just don't know how to make my body relax."

Brandie's life sounded difficult and full of challenges, with insomnia high on the list. My heart went out to her as I listened to her story. I was also struck by her resourcefulness. The severity of her sleep problem would place her toward the far end of the spectrum compared to other insomniacs I would later meet. Yet she'd accepted her unusual sleep pattern and built what she felt was an acceptable life around it. And she was managing it on her own without relying on doctors or medication.

This, I discovered later, is a fairly common response to insomnia. For each person who consults a doctor, there are two more who opt not to.[10] Insomniacs are likewise divided in their views on medication. Poll the sleepless about sleeping pills, and you come up with a map of the sort you see on election night: a red-state, blue-state affair. In one camp are the pill abstainers, like Brandie, and in the other, insomniacs who'd sooner dump their iPhones than part with their pills. Exploring these attitudinal differences would become a part of my research.

Brandie's story of insomnia led me back to my own. The first time my wakefulness really interfered with my life was at college. But moving further back in time, I reviewed the wakeful nights of my adolescence. At slumber parties I stayed up long after my friends' whispered confessionals had trailed into gibberish, only to awaken before the others at the crack of dawn. Then there were the many nighttime vigils at summer camp, when the measured breathing of my tent mates left me alone to rehash the events of the day from start to finish. Back further into early childhood, there was naptime in kindergarten, when I feigned sleep and entertained myself by calling to mind the contents of every nook and cranny of the room. In memory after memory, everyone else was sleeping and I was wide awake. Following this track, I asked my mother about my sleep as an infant. She reports I had wakeful tendencies even then. Ringing telephones and the neighbor's barking dog woke me up and made me cry, she says, in an era when other babies were sleeping through roaring Hoovers and Dick Clark's "American Bandstand."

Other insomniacs I spoke with recalled trouble sleeping in their youth. Dan said his was linked to worry and anxiety from the get-go. "I used to have a lot of trouble sleeping when I was a grade-school kid," he said. "I was so nervous and worried about school and getting beaten up by the other kids that I missed entire nights of sleep. I was scrawny and anemic: the kid that was intellectual in a county elementary school where all the other kids' parents were coal miners; the kid that liked books and stayed to myself and read all the time."

But the situation changed in adolescence. "When I got taller in sixth and seventh grade, I could talk mean enough that I didn't have to worry about getting beaten up any more." It was then that Dan's sleep improved.

This has been the pattern throughout Dan's life: periods of poor sleep coincide with stress, and sleep improves when the stress has passed. Returning to college to get a degree in English, he went through years of smooth sailing. "I had my own work schedule and could go in and out when I pleased. I could take long, leisurely walks with my stepdaughter in the open field and enjoy the weather and have a really nice time. That was a relaxed period. I was able to set my own hours and not feel manipulated or controlled by anybody or anything."

But his sleep problems returned when, following twelve years as an English instructor, he took an eight-hour-a-day job as a college administrator and, at about the same time, his father suffered a serious stroke. "It seemed to really destroy the rhythm and sense of well-being I'd developed through the years. I started having that nervousness again, feeling anxious—a lot like I did when I was a child in the first five years of grade school."

Tired at the end of the day, Dan is usually asleep by 11:30 p.m. But he's awake again at 2:30 or 3 a.m., thinking anxious, depressing thoughts. Once this happens, he may never get back to sleep. "I have a bad tendency to fixate on things," he said. "It could be something minor, like having to come in and send a fax about insurance, but I will blow it completely out of proportion. I'll tell myself I've got to quit thinking about it, but I don't have control of my thoughts. Or it could be about those life goals or big issues. For instance, I have a brother who's very successful. He's the vice president of a corporation. I might think in terms of how much success he's had and how I'm still working and struggling and trying to earn enough to make ends meet. They're always negative thoughts, deep and gloomy, much more so than what you feel if you've been awake for two or three hours."

Dan attributes his sleep problem mainly to generalized anxiety; his doctor has treated him on and off for anxiety neurosis and depression, prescribing antianxiety meds and antidepressants. Occasionally Dan has taken hypnotics (sleeping pills) for help with sleep. Some pills have eased his anxiety and helped his sleep, but often he's unhappy with the side effects. He's still waiting, he said, for "that perfect pill."

Meanwhile the insomnia continues to drag his spirits down. "It creates more nervous anxiety and less joy than you could have if you felt refreshed," he said. "You just don't have the happy edge you'd like to have."

Like Dan, a majority of insomnia sufferers have more than one chronic health problem. Mood and other psychiatric disorders top the list, with physical disorders co-occurring to a lesser extent.[11] It used to be that when insomnia occurred with another disorder—depression, for example—the poor sleep was regarded as merely a symptom of the depression. Treat the depression, so the thinking went, and the insomnia would disappear. But this strategy has not always worked. Taking an antidepressant may get rid of the depression, but the insomnia remains.[12] When insomnia occurs in conjunction with another disorder, say the experts today, it's important to attend to the insomnia, too. The material in this book will be relevant to insomniacs of all stripes.

The majority of insomniacs I interviewed did not report other diagnoses. But mention of depression, anxiety, heart problems, and colitis occurred from time to time, pointing to an unsettling truth: People with persistent insomnia are more likely than normal sleepers to have other health problems. Not only are our odds of experiencing depression and anxiety greatly increased, but insomnia also correlates with a host of medical conditions. Compared to good sleepers, insomniacs report higher rates of heart disease, high blood pressure, neurologic disease, breathing problems, urinary and gastrointestinal problems, and chronic pain. As a group, insomnia sufferers are sicker than normal sleepers. We are absent from work more often and require more health care.[13] The more I learn about chronic insomnia, the clearer it is that we ignore it at our peril.

Dan's and Brandie's sleep problems began in childhood, but the sleep Amy recalled in her youth was sound and untroubled except for occasional sleep-walking incidents. Things changed when the pressures of adulthood began piling up.

The first challenge came with the birth of her daughters. "I was forced to get up to feed them every two hours," Amy said. "So I started sleeping just four to six hours. They conditioned me to be alert and awake through the night." Amy went from being a sound sleeper to a light sleeper, and she's stayed that way ever since. Another challenge was contending with her husband's mother and his son from a former marriage, who came to live in the family's new home. A third source of stress came when Amy took a full-time job as a kindergarten teacher. "Every day I started with frustration: me getting ready, being nice and getting the girls up on a happy note, and then facing my kindergarteners. There was a lot of dysfunctional behavior there. It was a charter school, and there was no support. I had ADHD kids, and everybody every day crying."

The pressures coming from all sides took a toll on her sleep. "I would have stress dreams," Amy said, "very stressful dreams where I couldn't get out of a situation. I was just constantly rolling around, and that's what finally woke me up.

"At the time, nobody said, 'This is too much for you.' It was like, 'Get her on something so she can manage!'" So Amy's doctor prescribed an antidepressant to help keep her on an even keel emotionally and a sleeping pill to improve her sleep. But the drugs didn't solve her problems.

"I went through that first year. But by the second year, I decided I couldn't do it anymore. June, July, and August was not long enough to recover, so I gave my notice and quit by Thanksgiving. By then I'd decided there just wasn't a big enough pill."

Quitting her job was a mixed blessing. It was a relief to get away from the stress, but it was depressing to realize she wasn't cut out to do what she wanted to do: earn a decent salary, and be a mover and a shaker. "I was really disappointed in myself that I didn't have that personality after going through all the teacher training I went through." So she stayed on the antidepressant.

By then she was off the sleeping pill but her sleep was forever changed, and it has remained in a pattern she describes as "dysfunctional." Her situation at home is easier now that the girls are older, and she's taken a part-time job as coordinator of a nursery school that she enjoys, but her insomnia persists. Sometimes she can't get to sleep until late at night, while other times she awakens for long stretches in the middle of the night. Most days she wakes up feeling unrested and less energetic than she'd like to be.

"At times I'll even avoid a morning shower," she said. "I'll wonder if I really need to, and look at my hair and decide instead to spray it a little bit. I always put on my makeup and brush my teeth, but I know I don't have that 'all-together' look."

Amy will sometimes mention trouble sleeping to her husband, or commiserate with the director of the nursery school, who also has a sleep problem. Otherwise she keeps it to herself. "I really don't want people to know I'm sleep deprived," she said. "I don't want for them to think that I'm not able to make a good decision or that I'm mentally unstable. I want to be reliable, and I know I am. But here I am on an antidepressant, I have sleep problems, and then when I'm PMS-ing . . ." She worries about how it all looks.

Insomnia doesn't always clip wings, but it can. Like Amy, some insomniacs bow out of chosen careers when the pressures start interfering too much with sleep. Others admit to thinking twice about accepting new challenges and to eyeing promotions with ambivalence. Always at the back of their minds is this question: how will it affect my sleep?

Attitudes about insomnia have an impact, too. Some insomniacs talk freely about their sleep problems to family and friends, but others are leery of speaking out. "It's what people do with their imperfections," a long-time insomnia sufferer remarked. "They try to keep other people from knowing, and I certainly did."

Yes and no, I was thinking as I replayed this particular conversation in my head. It depends on the sort of "imperfection." I find it a lot easier to talk about my bad back than about my insomnia. There's something suspect about insomnia, something that engenders doubt—as do many disorders lacking objective and definitive criteria for identification. Aren't insomniacs really making a mountain out of a molehill? We may not actually hear the question posed out loud, but we suspect others of wondering about it. And sometimes we wonder ourselves. We may suspect, too, that we're culpable to some extent, and worry that insomnia reflects negatively on our character. Like mental illness, insomnia can suggest emotional instability and weakness of will. It carries a stigma.

The stories of Brandie, Dan, and Amy point to topics explored in this book. Insomnia occurs for many reasons and affects people in different ways, but there's a fair amount of shared experience, and this will serve as a starting point for a look at the night- and daytime symptoms of insomnia in early chapters. One aim of this examination is to give shape and heft to the affliction and underscore the attention it deserves. Another is to present new research relating not just to the nighttime symptoms of insomnia but to the daytime symptoms as well.

Despite advances in understanding, help for insomnia can be hard to find. Many insomniacs choose to manage on their own, turning for relief to alcohol, antihistamines, melatonin, herbal supplements, and teas. It's worthwhile knowing what the literature says about the benefits and risks of these remedies close at hand. But even insomniacs who look to the doctor for assistance may not find it. Knowing the limitations on encounters in the consulting room can be helpful to insomniacs in search of better options.

How people think and feel about insomnia is another part of the experience, covered in chapter 5. Sleep therapists talk about the advisability of rejecting "dysfunctional beliefs about sleep" and developing healthier attitudes, but there's little talk of the messy attitudinal issues that spur some insomniacs to seek treatment and keep others suffering in silence. An examination of history and culture sheds light on the stigmas attached to insomnia and our ambivalence about medicalizing the problem.

The biology of sleep and waking is not completely worked out, but the basics are known. One force that controls the sleep–wake cycle is the circadian system. The other is the homeostatic mechanism that keeps track of how long we're awake and propels us into slumber. These systems work in coordinated opposition, and understanding them is crucial for insomniacs in search of better sleep. Other information in this book is more hypothetical. The

association of insomnia with hyperarousal is a topic still under investigation, as are the neurobiologic mechanisms suspected to play a
role in poor sleep.

At last comes the million-dollar question: what can be done
about insomnia? Cognitive-behavioral therapy (CBT) is considered
by many to be the gold standard in treatment for those who want to
steer clear of drugs. This book follows five insomniacs undergoing
treatment and surveys the efficacy of CBT. Also reviewed are various approaches to tamping down arousal, such as yoga, meditation,
and exercise. Medications deserve close scrutiny as well. With drug
companies hyping their products, scare stories looming large in the
media, information on the web not always reliable, and physicians
not always well informed, insomniacs need a comparative overview
of prescription sleep meds on the market today and in the pipeline.
Finally, a look at novel treatments not widely available and those
under development will acquaint readers with therapies coming in
the future.

Anecdotes, science, history, and medicine are interwoven
throughout this book, and the material in some chapters does not fit
neatly into a single category. But for the benefit of readers inclined to
be selective, personal narratives figure strongly in the early chapters;
history and science, in the middle chapters; and insomnia treatments, toward the end.

So whether you're an occasional insomniac or a chronic sufferer;
whether it's your only complaint or one of many; whether you're a
newcomer to the insomnia club, a lifetime member or merely close
to someone who is, read on. This book is intended to inform and
benefit insomnia sufferers and friends.

2

A Night at the Races

They are always inclined to sleep, yet they can scarce sleep at all, but seem, like Tantalus, to stand always up to the Lips in the River Lethe, for sipping of which, whenever they sink themselves deeper, the yielding Waters always subside lower.

Thomas Willis, *The London Practice of Physick*, 1692

Insomniacs don't have a lot of warm, fuzzy feelings about the night. I've met a few who say they sometimes think of wakefulness as an opportunity: a sculptor who gets ideas for art projects when she wakes up in the middle of the night; a writer who during periods of high insomnia gets a lot of writing done. An art aficionado spoke of beautiful skies he has seen on nights of insomnia—the aurora borealis in northern Michigan, the moon setting over the Gulf of Mexico—after recounting, blow by painful blow, a torturous night when he hadn't slept a wink. For most of the chronically sleepless, nighttime ranks low on the happiness scale.

"You just dread going to bed because you don't know if you're going to sleep or not."

"Your bed becomes an enemy. It's just that a bed is a haven for most people at the end of a day and, for me, it has not been."

"I ended up being—and still am—'narcophobic.' It isn't darkness that scares me; it's actually nighttime."

A few insomniacs spoke disparagingly of sleep itself: "I think it's a total waste of time," an insurance executive confided to me. "Other than the fact that you've got to renew your body everyday, I would prefer not to have to sleep. I just feel that a little bit of you is dying every time you go to sleep. I feel that way about eating sometimes: can't we just skip lunch?"

With such colossally negative attitudes, how can insomniacs expect to sleep?

Bad attitudes can be changed, say the sleep cognoscenti. We'll take a close look at this proposition in later chapters, and at biological and behavioral factors known to interfere with sleep. But we're going to start by charting the subjective experiences of people on shaky terms with the night, now and in times past.

Ordinarily this aspect of insomnia barely gets a nod, assumed to be tedious and stale. But the accounts I heard of people's experiences were anything but boring or similar from one to the next, and much was too personal for ordinary conversation. "These feelings at this time of the night, they're not discussed," said one thoughtful insomniac. "There's this shade about it. It's almost like crossing into another world."

Chronic insomnia involves more than being unable to sleep. We can't take its measure without acknowledging the many ways it blights our lives, starting with its effects on the night.

❨

I don't remember when I began to call my wakefulness "insomnia." I can't recall the moment I felt compelled to name the thing I had, turned the word over in my head, and decided it described my situation as well as any I knew. It certainly did not occur during childhood. Then, I had no quarrel with lying awake for long stretches at the beginning of the night. I accepted it as part of my nature, like my taste for ketchup and patent leather shoes.

For several years my bedtime was 10:30, not so early for a girl in upper elementary school. As my parents watched Johnny Carson and my sister fell asleep in the bed next to mine, I lay in the darkness searching for undigested nuggets of experience whose examination might enlarge my understanding of the world.

Item: a scene I'd witnessed in the school parking lot. I was waiting with my friend and her mother for the friend's father to give us a ride home. He finally came and rushed out of the car. Without a word, he grabbed my friend's mom and kissed her. Not only was the kiss full on the lips, but he tilted her backward so that she was almost perpendicular to the blacktop. It was a kiss like you saw in the movies; nothing like the chaste pecks my father and other fathers in central Illinois were wont to plant on the cheeks of their wives. What kind of a father did that? And in public? What would it be like to have parents that carried on that way? Thinking about incidents like this could sustain me long into the night. Another thing I liked to do in bed at night was read.

Lying awake only bothered me when I experienced what my parents called "growing pains." When these occurred, I waited to see if they would pass and, if they didn't, I went out to the living room to complain. Then my father would follow me back into the bedroom and rub my arms and legs. The rubbing and the attention helped, and eventually I'd fall asleep.

The most disagreeable thing that happened at night occurred not as I lay awake reading or thinking but rather once I fell asleep. It was a recurring dream in which I found myself adding long columns of figures with two or three digits apiece. In my mind's eye, I added up the ones, made a mental mark below the sum line, carried my tens back up to the top of the list, dumped them in single stroke, and began the whole process again. Adding the figures took enormous effort. Yet once the process started, I felt compelled to continue, my brain cranking and cranking away. Eventually I woke up feeling sweaty and anxious and exhausted.

Like my musical parents, I was sensitive to sound. A starling built a nest in the eaves outside my bedroom window when I was twelve. For several days the rasping, plinking sounds of the bird pecking and scrambling around woke me at the crack of dawn, and I could not get back to sleep. Several days of these early awakenings left me feeling dull and headachy in the morning, and they eventually roused me to fury. "*Do* something!" I shouted at my father. I stormed around the house until he took care of the problem by sealing up the eaves.

The first hint I had that my sensitivities were unusual came when I moved into that chamber of horrors euphemistically called the college dorm. Nothing at home had prepared me for the conditions in that place. At my house, sleepers ruled. Anybody who was up after hours had better show consideration—speak in a hushed voice, creep up the stairs at a zigzag to keep the floorboards from creaking, turn the knob before closing the bathroom door to keep it from clicking shut—or they would face a reprimand the next day.

These rules did not apply in the dormitory. There the night gave rise to behaviors that in my house would have merited grounding for a week—people clomping down tiled hallways, slamming doors, playing Pink Floyd at full volume, shouting out windows, and knocking on walls—and nobody else seemed to care. At hall meetings, not a single complaint about noise ever crossed my dorm mates' Max Factored lips. Once I walked in on the third-floor drama queen entertaining her friends with a story about a boy's clumsy attempts to undress her in the backseat of a Volkswagen, to derisive hoots from her friends. Through it all, her roommate was quietly snoring in her bed. It dawned on me then that this was normal behavior and that I, bothered at night by the tapping and dinging of a Smith Corona in the room next door, was the strange one. And strange in a way that did not set me up for easy living with others close at hand. The awareness made me lonely.

Reading the diaries of Franz Kafka in a literature course acquainted me with the figure of the insomniac. The picture Kafka conjured up was of a gaunt, middle-aged man with a haggard face and haunted eyes. I knew I wasn't that. But neither was my sleep robust like that of my night-owl friends. They partied late and slept in late in the morning. No matter how late I stayed up or what I was doing—socializing, consuming platters of pizza, or lying in the darkness doing mental calisthenics before tests—I was awake by 7 a.m.

My nights became seriously disagreeable in the weeks leading up to my master's exams. If I have to point to a time when insomniac nights became the rule rather than the exception, when the early part of the night slid from being a time of quiet reflection to a time of struggle, this was it. The minute I went to bed, a relentless stream of psychobabble mixed with rhyming and word play let loose inside my head.

"Structural linguistics: learning inductive, the blank slate. Noam Chomsky: language-learning abilities innate. Colorless green ideas sleep furiously. Sleep curiously, spuriously, mirthlessly. The Chomskyan Revolution. A Marxist revolution. Newtonian physics, Jacksonian democracy, Freudian psychology. Brownian motion: but what was that? And who was Brown? A scientist, something to do with the movement of particles. Was that sixth or seventh grade? It couldn't have been Miss Ziegler. Could it have been Mr. Craig?" Like this, my brain could go on for hours, abetted by a racing sensation radiating from my torso to my extremities, and body heat that would drive me to toss off my blankets even in the dead of winter.

At the time, I was renting a room in the home of an elderly couple who allowed me full run of the house. Conveniently for me, they were hard of hearing. I could quiet my brain at night by playing the piano downstairs. A friend had given me some sheet music, and one by one I ran through my stash of golden oldies. Sometimes it worked. No sooner had I rolled the first chord of "Star Dust" than I felt myself on the threshold of a fantasyland as haunting as a midnight train whistle.

"And now the purple dusk of twilight time," I sang as I played, "steals across the meadows of my heart . . . "

Why did this help? I didn't know or care. What mattered was that it anesthetized the verbal part of my brain. The frayed, brown edges of the music and its slightly musty smell were comforting too, hinting at bygone, simpler days. I could play and play and lull myself into torpor. On good nights it followed me up the stairs and put me to sleep.

But the path from piano to bedroom was never safe. Why was the shopping list on the dining room table when it belonged on the refrigerator? Because it contained evidence of something I'd promised my landlady and then forgotten to do. How would I smooth things over? No way could I fit another errand into my schedule the next day. Damn. And there was David's toothbrush lying on the windowsill in the bathroom upstairs. Would he ever come over to reclaim it? Why had Emily become more interesting to him than me? Was I fatter? Dumber? Less sophisticated? Why not do a point-by-point comparison, starting right now?

In the time it took me to cross the first floor, climb the stairs, and walk back into my bedroom, all sorts of unsettling business could present itself for inspection. Matters I'd filed away to examine later or considered too trivial to waste time on took on exaggerated importance at night. Bam! An object or a thought was all it took to send me galloping out of the starting gate.

On these nights I wanted to shriek or throw the radio, the phone book, anything I could get my hands on. Why couldn't I turn my mind off? Why couldn't my brain assert its sovereign need to sleep? I would have tried almost anything if I thought it would put me out of my misery. In fact, I did have something on hand. My piano teacher had given me two jugs of home-brewed plum wine and, in the weeks leading up to my exams, I drank it. A glass and a half could knock Noam Chomsky and any relationship troubles right out of my head. The orange liquid left a bitter aftertaste that made my mouth pucker up like I was chewing on lemon peels. Yet I craved the oblivion it brought me. It was a fairly dependable soporific at a time of need.

"Psychophysiologic insomnia" was the medical diagnosis I received twenty years later when I finally saw a sleep specialist, a type of insomnia marked by "conditioned sleep difficulty and/or heightened arousal at sleep onset."[1] In the beginning, the diagnosis didn't sit well. Who could fail to note that the "psycho" came before the "physiologic," implying that in the eyes of the medical establishment, mine was an affliction driven mainly by psychological factors? This was an assumption I heard repeated time and time again and grew to hate.

That assumption was mistaken, I found out not long ago from Michael Perlis, associate professor of psychology and director of the Behavioral Sleep Medicine Program at University of Pennsylvania. I sat in on Perlis's three-day course in cognitive behavioral therapy and he then spent an afternoon fielding my questions about insomnia. Psychophysiologic insomnia "is primarily a physiologic condition that is modified by behavioral and cognitive factors," Perlis said. "It should actually have read 'physio-psychologic insomnia,' but nobody could pronounce that." "Psychofizz," as Perlis refers to it, is a common diagnosis given to people who have excessive focus on, and anxiety about, sleep; fall asleep at unusual times and places; are prone to intrusive thoughts or involuntary rumination; and feel physically "wound up." My symptoms match up with this profile more or less, at least as far as it goes. Psychofizz, are you me?

Among the other types of insomnia is "idiopathic insomnia," or lifelong insomnia with a presumed organic component, in its pure form said to be rare. Could this be me, too? My wakefulness in childhood wasn't troubling the way it later became, but it was a marked proclivity, my mother says. As an infant I was easily awakened by everyday noise, and emotional distress tended to make me restless at night, beginning with the birth of my sister when I was not quite two years old. Regardless of what my sleep problem eventually became, my mother's observations suggest the seeds began to germinate early on.

"Paradoxical insomnia" is yet another type, occurring when "a profound discrepancy" exists between a person's experience of poor sleep and that person's sleep as measured by polysomnography, a test that records activity in the brain and changes in physiological functioning. (We'll look into polysomnography in chapter 4.) Two other types are "physiologic insomnia," perpetuated mostly by organic factors; and "inadequate sleep hygiene insomnia," the diagnosis given to someone who flaunts the do's and don'ts in the advice columns, who drinks coffee at night, and (sin of sins!) watches TV in bed. Last comes a cryptic diagnostic category called "insomnia NOS," or insomnia "not otherwise specified."[2]

To my inexpert ears, these categories sound kind of muddy, and in this the experts agree. The validity of these types of insomnia is still being debated at conferences and in medical journals. Insomnia is a complicated business, and the experts haven't yet devised a classification system that fully and accurately reflects the differences between one person's insomnia and the next.

Nor do they know exactly how insomnia develops, or why it develops in some people and not others. A small group are seemingly poor sleepers from birth. As for the rest, those who develop insomnia later in life, one ingredient in the recipe appears to be stress. Many insomniacs can single out a stressful event that marked the beginnings of their problem.

The bombing of Pearl Harbor destroyed novelist Ella Leffland's peace of mind and disrupted her sleep. Like the adolescent protagonist in *Rumors of Peace*, the young Leffland was afraid the Japanese were going to attack her town. She kept a vigil every night listening for the air raid siren, afraid that no one else would hear it in time to get the family downstairs to safety.

"I was utterly terrified by the war," Leffland told me as we talked in her San Francisco apartment. "I was sure they were just going to bomb us to pieces. Back then, there was no television, only radio. People were frightened, everyone was sure that the West Coast was going to be bombed. Then months passed and nothing happened, but I continued to be terrified." The fear got her in the habit of staying awake at night, a habit that returns periodically and unpredictably.

"I find often when I turn off the lamp when I'm really sleepy and I've been reading, as soon as I find myself dropping off, I jolt myself awake—not that I wish to," Leffland said. "It's maddening. It's as if there's a demon inside of you that makes the decision."

Once she's jolted awake, Leffland is overwhelmed by negative thoughts and feelings. "My thoughts are so horrendous I can't bear them," she said. "They're usually of things that have happened in the past that I can't change now, things I feel horrible and guilty about." Leffland's anxious thinking may persist for hours.

"I get the feeling of actual despair, of helplessness and anger at myself," Leffland said. "I just hate it. It's the worst thing in the world to lie there wanting to sleep and wanting to sleep and being unable to do it. I get to the point where I want to hit myself!"

Despair, helplessness, anger: hardly emotions conducive to sleep. Yet they're perfectly natural responses to being thwarted from satisfying a basic need. Another insomniac I interviewed described a similar reaction: "When I can't sleep and am just laying awake, I'm very frustrated," she said. "I get really angry because I just wonder, why is this happening to me? Why do I have to go through this? I want to punch a wall, that's how mad I get!"

Frustration and anger drive your heart rate and blood pressure up, making it still more difficult to fall asleep. In fact any emotional response to insomnia will likely worsen it, including fears that insomnia may evoke: of the night, of sleeplessness, and of daytime deficits linked to poor sleep.

Joan spoke frankly about her fears. She first experienced insomnia as an adult, as she was recovering from an eating disorder. The sleep problem quickly spiraled out of control.

"I became aware of my own ability to worry myself out of sleep," Joan said. "I didn't have the power to allow myself to let go into sleep; I only had the power to wreck my sleep. It sounds very deeply disturbed, when I think of it. It started me on this path where I realized that, once the thought entered my head that I might not sleep, that was kind of it as for my sleep."

The fear would kick in on nights before Joan was facing a challenging task the day ahead. "It became like a humiliating prospect to me that somehow I would perform poorly," she said. "The fear of that would also insinuate itself into my fears about not sleeping."

The feeling was overwhelming, she said. "I can almost be on the edge of panic that I'm not going to sleep, and the cycle will begin and go on forever. I'd wind up getting only three or four hours of sleep."

At times Joan berated herself for her inability to control her fears. And sometimes she was convinced the problem had more to do with her genes. "We're torn," she said, "between blaming ourselves and cursing the gods."

Fear of sleepless nights and sluggish days eventually became part of my own struggle with sleep. The fear would fade into the background sometimes, but never for long. It was always ready to pounce at the slightest provocation. A few bad nights could start it up. Or it could come out of nowhere when the house was quiet and distractions were few. No matter how relaxed I might feel, the sight of the day deepening into twilight or the thought of going to bed could make my stomach clench. Would I be able to get to sleep, or would I be up half the night? And what about the next day: Would I have enough stamina to finish my work? Or would the story I filed be clumsy and stale? And what about my health? During bouts of bad sleep I was more susceptible to colds. Infections that might slow others down a few days could keep me coughing and blowing for two or three weeks. There were a lot of reasons to feel anxious about my sleep. And thinking about them inevitably made my insomnia worse.

I believed then (and believe now) that my wakeful tendencies were to some extent inborn: the work of the gods, to borrow Joan's language. I was a light sleeper as an infant, and my father's "fair to middling" sleep, together with my parents' insistence on absolute quiet at night, suggests their sleep was fragile, too. I couldn't blame myself for my genes.

But the anxieties my wakefulness provoked were another matter. In principle, I could see how they might develop. Who *likes* the feeling of craving but being unable to sleep? Who *likes* a yammering brain, tension in the stomach, or a racing sensation in the chest? If these experiences occur night after night, wouldn't it follow that sleep could become wedded to anxiety, the way successive asthma attacks might give rise to anxiety about breathing? I could understand how my fears had come to exist, and I had no doubt but that I'd be better off without them. But try though I did, I could not seem to will them away. After a slew of short nights, if I was facing yet another, I found it hard to look on myself with kindness. No matter how many stones I hurled at the gods, I lobbed quite a few at myself.

My worst fear was not getting *any* sleep, and there were odd nights when I was so wound up that I never bothered going to bed. So when I considered the plight of insomniacs whose problems came later at night, I felt some envy. At least they could count on getting *some* sleep. But I wasn't quite so envious after hearing their stories.

Juan's problem was his frequent awakenings between 2 and 4 a.m. "I always had an extremely light sleep," he said. "I needed everything in silence. Not a lot of light, no interruptions. If somebody woke me up in the middle of the night, it would be almost impossible for me to go back to sleep.

"Once I wake up my mind becomes extremely active, almost like it's running at high speed. It's like a constant review, a 'zzzzzzz,' on and on and on. If I haven't done something, it's reminding me of all the things I have to do. If something unpleasant happened, I will be reviewing that, too. It's even happened that I had a song I didn't like, and it keeps repeating and repeating in my mind."

If Juan does get back to sleep, he said, "I'm in a state of mind where I'm half asleep and half awake, basically resting in bed. I go through a process where I'm awake but I'm dreaming. I don't think I'm asleep, though, because I hear noises and am aware of things going on around me. I hardly ever now feel like I get a full night's relaxation and rest."

Penny, too, is distressed about not being able to get a full night's sleep. In the past, she woke up once or twice in the middle of the night but was always able to fall back asleep within an hour, a pattern she could live with. At menopause, things changed. She still falls asleep between 11 p.m. and midnight, but now by 3 a.m. she's up for good.

"Now when I wake up, my eyes are wide open," Penny said. "I'm just, like, up.

"People say, 'Why don't you get up and do something, or read a book or clean?' But I'm in a fighting-back mode, like, I *will* go back to sleep, I *will* go back to sleep, and I watch the hours pass by on the clock. I try to relax my body and try to stop thinking about things. I try as hard as I can to go back to sleep. But usually, I don't."

Sometimes Penny feels her problem is annoying. Sometimes, "days and days and days go by, and it gets to the point where it gets a little scary. I do want to go to sleep and my body's not letting me. It ranges from annoyance to fear that I'm *never* going to sleep."

Penny's and Juan's nights sound miserable to me, and their stories and those of other middle and late insomniacs have made me doubt nighttime awakeners are any better off than insomniacs like me. The night is a trial for anyone with chronic insomnia, no matter what type of insomnia you have or when it occurs.

For the seasoned insomniac, sleep is flighty even under the best of conditions: a fully functional family, a fab day at work, a dark and soundproof room that sports a comfy bed with eight-hundred-thread-count sheets. But woe to the light sleeper whose sleeping conditions are less than ideal.

Motherhood pushed Abby's shaky sleep over the edge. "It was really physically draining to be pregnant," she said. After she had her first baby, "I let him nurse all night, and it was just exhausting. I put myself in a situation where I couldn't relax anymore. I was so used to forcing myself to be awake because I had to take care of the child whether I'd slept or not. Even after I weaned him, I found I couldn't sleep."

Abby's insomnia can strike anywhere in the night: beginning, middle, or end. "What usually happens is either I can't get to sleep—it takes me a couple hours to relax—or something will wake me up that definitely will set it off." It could be her two-year-old crying or her husband turning in bed. Internal sensations can awaken her, too. Whatever the trigger, Abby awakens with a racing heart and racing thoughts.

"I feel like, oh, here we go again. Sometimes if it's a third or fourth night of not sleeping, I start to feel like, what's the use? Definitely the word is 'despair.' I feel like I'm never going to be able to rest, and that my life is flashing before my eyes. I feel like I'm not a good mother and I start to obsess. I have no control even to rest or relax."

For Heather, being on call for her job at night pushed her sleep from bad to worse. Never one to sleep much anyway (a habit shared by both parents), she'd developed insomnia following the birth of her first child. But when she accepted a job as a programmer analyst, agreeing to be available to troubleshoot three weeks a month should her company's computer system go down at night, her sleep went down the tubes.

"Being on call at night is horrible," Heather said. Her company might page her at 12:30 a.m. to alert her that she might be needed later that night. "If I get paged, it's very hard to get back to sleep. Just knowing that I'm likely to get woken up puts me on edge."

Heather prepares as best she can. "I always have my computer turned on at night and in a mode so it boots up quickly. Because the longer I'm awake, the less likely it is that I'll ever be able to get back to sleep. But even if I'm awake just ten minutes, it's going to be two hours [before I get back to sleep]." Calls for help can come at any time. She might get paged at 2 a.m., and then again at 4 a.m. Figuring out what the problem is, correcting it, and trying to wind down again can keep her awake nearly all night. "And then you're expected to be at work at your regular time the next day and put in a full eight hours."

Heather's work conditions sound practically unsustainable for the best of sleepers, and the more so for a person with insomnia. Yet her situation is far from unique. Many jobs today involve night work or bringing work home. According to the National Sleep Foundation's 2008 *Sleep in America* poll, 20 percent of the American workforce now spends ten or more hours a week doing work-related activities (outside of regular work hours) at home; at least a few nights a week, 23 percent of these people do work within an hour of going to bed. *The New York Times* reported in January 2012 that about 40 percent of working Americans now work some form of nonstandard hours, including evenings, nights, weekends, and early mornings. Night work, which clearly poses challenges for people with insomnia, can create sleep problems anew. About 10 percent of the people who do night and rotating shift work complain of sleep problems and are diagnosed with "shift work sleep disorder."[3]

Nighttime responsibilities can disrupt anyone's sleep. But insomniacs are also challenged at night by sensory stimuli that normal sleepers block out. Light, for example, can halt the synthesis of mela-tonin, a hormone secreted at night that helps to quiet the brain. Insomnia sufferers who spend the evening hours on the computer, awaken to moonlight streaming in an open window, or step into a well-lit bathroom may find themselves too aroused for sleep. (Ways to avoid light exposure include dimming lights, covering windows, and wearing eye masks.) The temperature-sensitive may find it hard to sleep when it's too hot or too cold. (Ideally, bedrooms should be a little cooler at night than a comfortable room temperature during the daytime.) But noise is probably the insomniac's biggest environ-mental bugaboo. At night, our ears become giant satellite dishes, capturing every stray murmur the universe sends our way.

This creates problems for apartment dwellers like Colleen. "I hear people's daily noises," she said. "Footsteps, anything like that keeps me awake: hearing other people's stereos and talking and TV. With everybody else, you can watch TV and they can fall asleep, but I can't. You have to keep it off or I'll lay there all night."

For the insomniac, hell is other people's noise.

My frequent awakenings in babyhood make me think I must have been sound-sensitive from birth. This trait has its advantages. In music I can enjoy everything from Brahms to Celia Cruz, and be as fascinated by the whoosh and clank of a steam engine as by a solo violin. But for people who have a hard time sleeping, sensitivity to noise is a curse.

Almost every apartment I rented in my twenties and thirties calls forth memories of a nocturnal soundtrack. In one apartment, it was the slurping, sloshing sound of the landlord's son mixing something in the basement beneath our living room. (What was he up to at 1 a.m.? He was an oddball loner, and the weirdness of his nocturnal activities made it even harder to sleep.) In a French *pensione*, it was the rhythmic grunts of a man in the next room visited by prostitutes day and night. In Seattle, it was the nighttime shouting matches of the couple downstairs. In every instance I was an involuntary voyeur because darkness affords no protection from sound waves penetrating walls. My Mack's earplugs were never quite up to the task of masking all the noise.

The need for a quiet, dark place to sleep has social consequences, too. It doesn't always square with the habits of others close by. So it becomes a liability.

"Let's say we have a family reunion," Juan said. "If somebody comes and turns on the TV, there goes the night for me. It creates friction. I try to make them aware that I have difficulty sleeping and that they need be quiet or be careful with the lights. Most of them respect that, but I've had problems sometimes with my brother. We were all on vacation so he would come back late. He would turn on the lights and make noise and wake me up. Then he would fall asleep immediately while I was awake the rest of the night."

Andrea can rarely bring herself to ask for the quiet she needs. "I'm not very good at putting people out," she said, "so I'll suffer. I go stay at my Mom's, and they're up really late there. My younger brother will have his friends over, and they might not go to bed all night. So they're up and they're playing video games or music and stuff. I'll just lay in bed awake, because there's too much going on. You don't want to say anything, because it's really their house. It's their normal routine. But for you, you just think, 'Oh, no.'"

Trying to negotiate peace and quiet can also make the situation worse. Even the most innocuous request (as in, "Hey, guys. Would you mind turning that down a bit?") can backfire. I got a taste of that the first week in my college dorm, when on a Thursday night I asked my roommate and her friend if they could turn down the volume on the friend's stereo across the hall. Their response was swift and unambiguous: they set the speaker in the doorway to my room and turned the volume up full blast.

As for night noise associated with urban living—live music, parties, construction projects, HVAC systems, sirens, and the like—most communities have ordinances that prohibit "excessive, unnecessary, and unreasonable noise" at night. Yet what's tolerable to the normal sleeper may be intolerable for the insomniac. In the community where I live, night noise is considered excessive if it exceeds 55 decibels, which is just shy of the noise level of a normal conversation or a sewing machine. Not too many insomnia sufferers could sleep through that.

Peace and quiet can also be hard to find when you're sleeping away from home. High-end hotels are fairly reliable when it comes to providing the particular comforts insomniacs require; others, less so. At night they may explode in a cacophony of revelry, clanking air conditioners, and highway noise. Even so, some insomniacs find that springing for a motel room works better than spending a wakeful night cooped up in a bedroom of friends or relatives. But the arrangement itself can lead to awkwardness.

Marilynn has trouble explaining her need for special sleeping quarters to friends. "It makes visiting people and maintaining friendships difficult, especially when people get scattered," she said. "When people say, 'Come visit,' and I go to get a motel room, they're offended. I do that because I love them, not because I'm shirking them." To do otherwise would probably result in a bad night, she said. "At night I get up and prowl around. That's very uncomfortable in someone else's house."

Insomnia inevitably affects intimate relationships. Your partner or spouse shares in its care and feeding, whether they like it or not. And the insomniac's demands can be exacting. No phones in the bedroom. Shades drawn, curtains closed. Don't touch me when I'm sleeping. Turn over, you're snoring. The list goes on.

Most insomniacs I spoke with said their partners were understanding and tried to accommodate their needs. But once asleep, bed partners can't always abide by the insomniac's rules. They may snore, scratch, toss and turn, grind their teeth, and talk in their sleep. For the chronic insomniac, even minor disturbances in bed can spell doom.

"I'm such a light sleeper that if somebody snores, I can't even be in a relationship with them," Beatrice said. "The person I'm involved with . . . I have certain sleep requirements, like he can't come near me when I'm sleeping. Because if he touches me and I wake up, then that's the end [of sleep] for me. I have to have a special kind of mattress, too. You cannot *imagine* what I go through to try to maintain or create a sleep hygiene environment."

Insomniacs with noisy, thrashing partners may resort to sleeping in a spare bedroom or on the living room couch. Among those I spoke with, the decision to do this was rarely made lightly. In Western cultures, to share a bed with your partner is the norm. It can be off-putting to do otherwise, even for couples whose sleep proclivities are completely mismatched. Sleeping separately deprives you of the feeling of skin against skin, and the warmth and comfort it affords. It lessens opportunities for sexual arousal, intimate conversation, and the sharing of dreams. Yet several insomniacs told me they sleep solo at least some of the time, opting to forego intimacy in favor of a better night's sleep.

Sleeping separately all or some of the time may not be so hard to tolerate for couples in well-established relationships. But for the chronic insomniac who's looking for a partner, being unable to share a bed with the one you're courting is definitely a turn-off—even, perhaps, a deal breaker.

Keith felt his wakefulness was part of the reason he'd never managed to form a long-term relationship. When I caught up with him, he'd consulted with doctors at the Stanford Sleep Center for Sleep Sciences and Medicine and spent years in therapy trying to resolve his sleep issues. No solution had worked, and he was particularly distressed about the toll insomnia was taking on his love life.

"There've been times in relationships with women where I'd have problems with them being upset that I was awake," he said. "I'd have problems going away for a weekend with someone and not sleeping, trying to take care of myself by going in another room, trying to relax, and causing difficulties with that person. I'm starting to choke up a little bit."

We look to the night for rest and restoration, yet insomniacs can't count on these basic comforts. Ultimately the blame may lie with genetic factors that predispose us to sleep problems, and/or life experiences that eventuate changes in the brain, which make sleep less robust than before.[4] But whatever the causes of insomnia and whatever its course, the angst it gives rise to is deeply disturbing to contend with night after night. Add to this the challenges of child-rearing, night work, or an unfriendly environment, and the prospect of rest and restoration can come to feel like a distant mirage. No wonder insomniacs harbor negative feelings about the night.

Troubled Nights in Times Past

It's common to assume the night was more peaceful, and insomnia rarer, before the Industrial Revolution. Like kudzu creeping up from the South, choking every green thing in its path, mechanization and the changes it wrought—crowded cities, faster-paced living, keener competition, and twenty-four-hour light and traffic—have encroached on our nights, blighting what in centuries past would have been a tranquil period of repose. We live in a "sleep-sick society," wrote the pioneering sleep scientist William Dement, and our nights get shorted in favor of extending work and leisure activities.

While on a camping trip, Dement imagined what the night must have been like for our ancestors: "With the stars as our only night-light," he wrote, "we are rocked in the welcoming arms of Mother Nature back to the dreamy sleep of the ancients."[5]

The poet Christopher Dewdney has expressed similar thoughts. "The pace of modern life conspires to eat up more and more of our time, and we juggle increasing responsibilities. There's a price. Work-a-holic-related sleep deprivation and a plethora of sleep disorders are burgeoning into an epidemic of insomnia."[6]

Human sleep patterns have changed as a result of advances in technology. Consider the impact of the electric light bulb. Light prolongs wakefulness, and, before the spread of electrical lighting in the nineteenth century, human sleep patterns were more in sync with the natural alternation of daylight and darkness.

"It was the advent of the light bulb that changed everything," said NBC's chief medical editor Dr. Nancy Snyderman on "The Today Show," reporting on the National Sleep Foundation's 2008 *Sleep in America* poll. "We used to go to sleep when the sun went down. We'd rise when the sun came up, and now just having a computer terminal in your bedroom that you don't make go to black can be enough to disrupt your sleep at night."[7]

Electric lighting allows shift work to occur right around the clock, sleep expert Michael J. Thorpy has noted, and international travel enables the rapid crossing of time zones. These cultural developments have led to the disruption of circadian rhythms and other sleep problems.[8]

Eluned Summers-Bremner, senior lecturer in the English Department at the University of Auckland, points to much earlier cultural developments that altered human sleep patterns. One such development was the clock, which came into use in Europe in the late Middle Ages. Another that occurred at about the same time was the rise of the merchant class. Before that, farmers and trades-men set their own hours, favoring a schedule that was largely task oriented, alternating between bouts of intense labor and rest. But when merchant intermediaries arrived on the scene, producers of goods and commodities found themselves subject to different time constraints. "The gradual emergence of a mercantile economy meant that it was future profits . . . rather than approaching nightfall, that began to dictate the length of the working day," exerting a negative impact on people's sleep, Summers-Bremner claims.[9]

Historian Jean Verdon has cited other cultural factors that troubled the nights of medieval Europeans. Darkness in the Middle Ages provided cover for much political violence and many criminal acts. "Violence seemed to be everywhere," he writes, "particularly at night, fostered by drunkenness or by the explosion of resentful passions." The night watchman was a poor deterrent to the looting, arson, rape, and murder that more commonly took place at twilight and after dark. The prospect of these very real dangers took a toll on people's sleep.

Dread of evil supernatural forces increased in the late Middle Ages and was also detrimental to sleep, Verdon says. Satan's minions—witches, werewolves, ghosts, and demons—were believed to be out and about at night looking to harm the imprudent and the weak. "At twilight, the Devil manifested himself especially in fields and forests. The disquiet prevailing over uninhabited areas gradually penetrated into human habitations. Those who could not sleep, the ill, and the dying found themselves alone, without help, in the dark."[10]

Add to these cultural factors the anxieties that arose in the fourteenth century as members of a nascent middle class jockeyed for position, and, says Summers-Bremner, "we are close to finding ideal conditions for the production of insomnia."[11]

All this may be true. But writings from every era suggest that irrespective of cultural trends, wakefulness has troubled the nights of human beings, and been treated as a health problem, for thousands of years.

Hippocrates wrote about sleeplessness using the Greek term *agrypnia.* He viewed it as a sign of illness. "Disease exists," he said, "if either sleep or watchfulness be excessive." The best time for sleep was the night, and the next best time, the morning. "But the worst of all is to get no sleep either night or day," he observed. "It follows from this symptom that the insomnolency is connected with sorrow and pains, or that [the patient] is about to become delirious." Among the myriad health problems afflicting the aged was want of sleep.[12]

Aristotle connected wakefulness at night with literary study, noting that mental activity was typically unfavorable to sleep. But not all kinds of reading and thinking were problematic. "The intellectual activities which cause wakefulness," he wrote, "are those in which the mind searches and finds difficulties rather than those in which it pursues continual contemplation." Aristotle cited poppy, mandragora (or mandrake, a plant in the nightshade family), wine, and darnel (a grass whose seeds have narcotic properties) as substances known to induce sleep.[13]

Physicians who practiced medicine in ancient Rome also administered to the sleepless, those plagued by excessive "vigilantia." Aretaeus of Cappadocia recognized it as a harbinger of physical and mental ills: "Watchfulness . . . produces crudities, wastes the body, is laborious and tiresome, deadens the spirits and affects the mind, wherefore the patients are frequently seized with mania and melancholy."

To combat watchfulness, physicians prescribed an array of soporific herbs. Galen's favored remedy was a mixture of mandrake root, the seed of black henbane (another nightshade with narcotic properties), opium, and lettuce juice, to be taken internally or applied to the temples. Aulus Cornelius Celsus advocated gentle but thorough massaging of the insomniac's body. To those for whom massage didn't work, he prescribed draughts of decoction of poppy or hyoscyamus (henbane).[14]

References to nocturnal wakefulness appear in the Bible. Jacob complains of the misfortunes that visit him while laboring for his uncle Laban: "In the day, the drought consumed me, and the frost by night; and my sleep departed from mine eyes." Job, too, suffering myriad troubles by day, is plagued with "wearisome nights," "full of tossings to and fro unto the dawning of the day." "My bones," he says, returning to the topic later on, "are pierced in me in the night season: and my sinews take no rest." And the Book of Psalms contains this moving lamentation to God: "Thou holdest mine eyes waking: I am so troubled that I cannot speak."

Wakefulness at night continued to be treated as a health problem during the Middle Ages. The Islamic physician Avicenna, writing in the tenth and eleventh centuries, said quite a lot about it in his *Canon of Medicine.* "Insomnia (or tossing about in bed) is bad for all the bodily states," and can result in a "weakening and confusion of the reasoning power . . . and acute illnesses." The hygienic measures Avicenna recommended to ensure proper sleep have a familiar ring.

One should not try to sleep on an empty stomach; after eating, one should delay going to bed until "after the flatulences and eructations . . . have subsided." A hot bath with plenty of hot water poured over the head can induce sleep. The wakeful that require "a still more efficient method" of obtaining sleep should take an herbal preparation containing opium, mandrake, and henbane.[15]

Physicians and intellectuals in the fifteenth and sixteenth centuries wrote about sleeplessness, or "watching," in English and other vernaculars. But when it came to explaining its cause, they held fast to the belief system established in ancient Greece. Wakefulness at night, like all other health complaints, was caused by imbalances in the four bodily humors—blood, phlegm, yellow bile, and black bile. The Italian philosopher Marsilio Ficino, who wrote about sleeplessness in a treatise on the health of intellectuals, saw it as an affliction of learned men with melancholia: a dysfunctional state characterized by too much black bile and a cold, dry brain.

Long bouts of sleeplessness were very harmful to health, Ficino explained. Thus "every effort must be made against this great evil." His list of remedies included compounds taken orally, oils applied to the body, scents held under the nose, and leaves strewn in the bed. Not least, the wakeful melancholic's ears should be soothed "with low songs and sounds."[16]

André du Laurens, a sixteenth-century French professor of medicine, attributed the sleeplessness of the melancholic to fears and negative thoughts. Such men were subject to "continuall watchings," he noted. "I have seene some that have abode three whole moneths without sleepe. The feare that is in them doth continually set before them tedious and grievous things, which so gnaw and pinch them, as that they hinder them from sleeping."[17]

The sixteenth-century Dutch physician Levinus Lemnius observed his patients as they slept and made notes. These light sleepers awakened at the least stirring and appeared to process goings-on around them even during sleep. "I have known many," he wrote, " . . . who in their sleepe, plainly and perfectly understoode every word spoken by the standers by . . . beinge awaked [with] the least noyse . . . they could . . . rehearse [the] most part of those things which had bin there spoken and uttered." Among the results of immoderate watching were the impairment of memory and the consuming of grace, beauty, and comeliness.[18]

Persistent wakefulness at night should not be treated lightly, warned the French surgeon Ambroise Paré. The patient prone to excessive watching could come completely undone. "It hurts the temperature of the braine, weakens the senses, wastes the spirits, breeds crudities, heavinesse of the head, falling away of the flesh, and leanenesse over all the body, and to conclude, it makes ulcers more dry, and so consequently rebellious, difficult to heale, and maligne."[19]

These physicians offered elaborate recipes for soporifics in the form of oral compounds, ointments, plasters, pomanders, and nodules to insert in the nostrils. There were also sleep-inducing clysters, or enemas. Paré set down a recipe for one such clyster, specifying precise amounts of barley water, violet and water-lily oils, plantain and purslane juices, camphor, and egg whites.

Other insomnia remedies proposed by these learned men would have given even the stout-hearted pause: "Sheepes lungs taken warme out of the bodies, may be applied to the head, as long as they are warme," wrote Paré. "There are some which with good successe doe applie Horseleaches behind the eares," wrote du Laurens, "and having taken away the Horseleaches, they put by little and little a graine of Opium upon the hole." In his *Anatomy of Melancholy*, the clergyman and scholar Robert Burton mentioned this old soporific: anointing the soles of the feet with the fat of a dormouse and the teeth with earwax of a dog.[20]

Some remedies were based in folklore and superstition and, if they succeeded in putting people to sleep, they probably worked through power of suggestion alone. Yet the ancient soporific mainstays— opium and its derivatives, and plants containing hyoscine, atropine, and scopolamine (mandrake, henbane, and darnel, for example), which remained in use through the early twentieth century—were no mere placebos. "The most widely used ancient herbs and potions have all turned out to contain chemicals which do indeed produce sedation and sleep," says Ernest Hartmann, a physician and director of the Sleep Center at Newton-Wellesley Hospital.[21] Some were deadly in too large a dose. "In the use of all these stupefactive medicines taken inwardly," du Laurens wrote, "wee must take heed to deale with very good advise, for feare that instead of desiring to procure rest unto the sillie melancholike wretch, wee cast him into an endlesse sleepe."[22]

Treatises written by Renaissance and early modern physicians make no mention of how frequently these powerful plant-based soporifics were prescribed. But the fact that they *were* used suggests that sleeplessness was not regarded as a trifling affliction. The great seventeenth-century physician and scientist Thomas Willis, who called insomnia "the Watching Evil," observed that "Immoderate Watchings arising alone, without any other known cause, seems to be a Disease as it were of it self." And as a disease, sleeplessness called for strong medicine. Want of sleep was first among the proper uses of the opiates, in Willis's opinion.[23]

The sleepless in seventeenth-century Britain could also turn for advice to the popular press. *The Skilful Physician*, a medical book targeted to the general public, stressed the importance of sufficient sleep. To relieve "immoderate Watching," it listed seven recipes containing mixtures of food, herbs, and breast milk. English almanacs promoted fresh dill as a sleep aid. They also contained advertisements for patent medicines with opium derivatives sold to improve sleep. Almanac writer William Salmon promoted his cordial pill as the "greatest and most excellent Preparation of all the Opiates yet invented."[24]

Nights in the seventeenth and eighteenth centuries, although plagued by fewer uncertainties than nights of more lawless times, were not free of anxiety or wakefulness. People then often described their sleep as "restless," "troubled," and "frighted," says historian A. Roger Ekirch. Not only did the lower classes sleep in inhospitable conditions; not only did the nighttime bring with it increased risks of assaults, burglaries, and arsons; but people also continued to fear the machinations of the devil at night, as well as the harmful effects of "noxious air." Our forebears took these and a host of other anxieties to bed with them, Ekirch claims, and he documents numerous instances of wakefulness among them: A Scottish parson complained in his diary that anxiety had robbed him of more than half his ordinary sleep for nine or ten days; a British lady wrote that when she went to bed free of bodily pain, mental anguish kept her awake. The eighteenth-century physicist Georg Christoph Lichtenberg wrote of his insomnia: "I have gone to bed at night quite untroubled about certain things and then started to worry fearfully about them at about four in the morning, so that I often lay tossing and turning for several hours."[25]

To combat wakefulness at night, wealthy insomnia sufferers typically used laudanum, a mixture of opium, alcohol, water, and spices. Commoners turned to cheaper solutions like alcohol. Sleeping drinks were one of many measures the early moderns took to ensure a safe and worry-free passage through the night.[26]

We'll pick up on the historical aspects of insomnia in chapter 5, starting late in the eighteenth century, when explanations for and attitudes toward the affliction began shifting, leading to the attitudes we hold today. But by now it should be clear that insomnia is not just a phenomenon of the past 150 years. Contributing cultural factors may have changed over time, but nocturnal wakefulness by its many names—agrypnia, vigilance, watching—is at least as old as recorded history. Ancient physicians regarded it as a serious health problem, as did physicians in the centuries that followed, and proffered remedies at least as powerful as those in current use. Wakefulness at night was troubling to our ancestors just as it troubles us today.

Some sleep experts have suggested insomnia may be as old as humankind. The claim makes sense if we consider the environment where humans evolved, and the purposes sleep in early humans may have served.

First, human beings are not well equipped for survival in a world full of predators, Michael Perlis, director of the Behavioral Sleep Medicine Program at University of Pennsylvania, observed as we chatted about the functions of sleep. "We're slow, we have no big fangs, we have no big claws, we're not prepared to fight, we can't run fast, we don't see well, we don't hear particularly well. There is just nothing about the human being besides our brains that is very useful for surviving in a hostile environment." The dangers multiply exponentially after dark, as noted by the eighteenth-century philosopher Edmund Burke: "It is impossible to know in what degree of safety we stand; we are ignorant of the objects that surround us; we may every moment strike against some dangerous obstruction; we may fall down a precipice the first step we take; and if an enemy approach, we know not in what quarter to defend ourselves."[27] So the most fundamental purpose sleep would have served in early humans would be to enforce immobility during darkness, the time of maximum vulnerability.

But even immobility would not have assured safe passage through the night, nor would sleeping in protected spots like trees and caves. A degree of wakefulness would have been adaptive in a hostile environment. The ability to maintain vigil or awaken frequently, to snap to attention at the first low growl, crackling leaf, or rattler's hiss, would have afforded extra protection against the perils of the night. In fact, human beings are well prepared to detect danger during sleep. Our brains awaken several times each night (although most people are not aware of these awakenings).[28] This is much better life insurance than we'd have sleeping deeply through the night.

But for insomniacs the insurance policy comes at a price. Being well endowed in the threat-detection department is indispensable when you're up against mortal perils like tigers and roving bands of marauders. But it does little for people who sleep behind locked doors protected by electronic security systems . . . unless you're fond of lying awake and obsessing over lesser threats like home foreclosures and losing your job. Or maybe you're one of the lucky ones able to put your wakefulness to use. "What is insomnia but the gift of more time," says Perlis, who uses early awakenings to get work done. Well, OK. I admit my insomnia can work to my advantage in a few situations, especially when it comes at the end rather than the beginning of the night. But if we're talking chronic insomnia, it's the rare sufferer—the Ciorans of the world perhaps, whose sleepless nights bring them closer to the ecstasy of the saints—who would not trade the extra time spent in consciousness for more regular sleep.

And there's a reason. Insomnia makes it less likely you'll reap the full benefit of the *other* functions sleep performs. Exactly what these functions are is still being sorted out, but research suggests sleep in humans probably affords many benefits, including conserving energy, restoring body tissue, and consolidating memory. Impair sleep, and you infringe upon its blessings. The impact of chronic insomnia extends far beyond the night, as we will shortly see.

A. Roger Ekirch has suggested that far from experiencing an epidemic of insomnia, Americans today are probably sleeping more soundly than our ancestors. Overall, we're safer from violence and inclement weather and less vulnerable to deadly disease. Our sleeping conditions are more hospitable, our beds cushioned and free of bedbugs and lice. We no longer believe in the harmful supernatural forces that frightened generations in the past.[29]

These creature comforts are undeniable boons for human sleep. But the night for the sleepless is still a time for devil's play. And the long night's journey is just a prelude to the insomniac's day.

Running on Empty

*Sleepless nights end not of themselves. In time
the mind loses . . . its self-control during the day.
The nervous system seems to be made of threads
of glass, and while the man is exempted from
none of the labors of life, he is unfitted both in
body and in mind for performing them.*

"Wakefulness and Sleep," *Christian Register*,
December 1850

Haven't slept a wink? No problem. Circadian forces come to the
rescue and set about preparing us for the day. Well before dawn,
the body clock sounds a wake-up call, triggering a flurry of internal
activity. Production of cortisol rises sharply in the second half of the
night. Our core body temperature, at its nadir in the hours before
wake-up time, begins to rise. The ascending arousal system then
comes online, innervating and awakening the higher centers of the
brain. Billions of neurons are soon firing away, discharging neurochemicals that help prime us for the day ahead, increasing alertness

and dexterity and elevating mood. Daylight assists in the process, helping rid us of any leftover impulse to sleep.[1]

So fortified, insomniacs strike out into the world. We go to work, school, the store, the bank. We interact with colleagues and acquaintances, we become part of the pack. Gone is the night and the lonely affair with insomnia.

But not by many measures does it feel like we march in step with our peers.

Take, for example, our overall sense of wellbeing. The December 3, 2004 issue of *Science* published the results of a study on how people use their time and how they feel about their daily activities. The authors were surprised by some of their findings. Income and level of education have little impact on people's enjoyment of their days, they concluded. Rather, aspects of temperament and character affect our sense of wellbeing much more strongly. Right up there with depression in its negative impact on our day-to-day lives was poor-quality sleep.[2] Who knew?

Insomniacs did, and do. We connect the dots between poor sleep and feeling "off" during the day. And the picture isn't pretty. If our nights are wakeful and fraught with tension, our days are effortful and short on pleasure.

"I feel I'm running close to empty."

"It's like pushing a boulder."

"It's like I'm 50 percent all the time."

Exhaustion was just one of the daytime complaints voiced by insomniacs I interviewed. Poor sleep also put them in a bad mood, strained relationships, interfered with thinking and memory, reduced their productivity at work, and sapped their motivation to do anything more than get by. Yet until recently there wasn't much scientific evidence that during the daytime insomniacs had anything to complain about. Experiments involving naps showed that we weren't sleepy during daylight hours. We didn't perform worse than normal on simple psychomotor and memory tests.[3] Perhaps the impairments insomniacs complained of weren't so bad after all?

That story has begun to change. Newer studies suggest that chronic insomnia *is* associated with demonstrable daytime impairments, and that it also has serious effects on long-term health. So let's look closely at what ails insomniacs in our waking hours and what science is saying about us now.

An Empty Tank

"Mentally, I'm always fine," said Juan, who manages building space on a university campus. "I'm very organized, able to accomplish what I need to accomplish during the day, but I feel extremely run down. I don't feel the stamina I'd like to have." Coffee is a poor substitute for the sleep Juan feels he lacks. "In order to pretend to be energetic at the workplace, sometimes you'll bombard yourself with caffeine, but inside you're just barely holding on."

Juan and some of the other insomniacs I interviewed singled out fatigue as their main complaint. They reported feeling "sleepy," "groggy," and "tired," and struggling to stay alert to the end of the workday. Some mentioned taking "power naps."

Others, though they might feel tired, spoke of an edginess during the daytime that kept them up and on the go despite their fatigue. "Sometimes," said Kay, an architecture student, "I almost get to where I feel a sort of high sensation, like I'm running on some kind of altered energy state. I'll be ultra-creative or ultra-excited. It's almost like I've gotten beyond the exhaustion to another level."

The notion of feeling exhausted and yet incapable of relaxing into a nap might seem like a contradiction, yet this captures the visceral experience of many insomniacs. Sleep can be elusive even at times when fatigue is extreme. As at night, when our wake-up and go-to-sleep signals seem to be working at cross-purposes, so our bodies manufacture mixed signals during the day. A majority of insomniacs given opportunities to sleep during the day are no more likely to do so, say sleep experts, than people who sleep well at night. In fact, some studies show it actually takes insomniacs longer than normal sleepers to fall asleep during the daytime.[4]

Scientists are not sure how to interpret this. Some say it implies insomniacs really *are* getting enough sleep at night to satisfy our biological sleep need; some propose that behind insomnia is a trait-level hyperarousal that interferes with sleep both night and day. Others say it may have to do with a dysregulation of the "sleep homeostat"—that insomniacs may require greater-than-normal sleep loss to increase our sleep drive both night and day.[5] I'll say more about these theories in later chapters.

Whatever proves to be correct, weariness and depleted energy are the daily fare for many chronic insomniacs. "The tank is empty," is the way a friend of mine described how it feels to live with insomnia day to day. "The tank is *so* empty."

Science can't yet explain why insomniacs feel as fatigued as we do. To most of us, the explanation is obvious: we feel tired because we're short on sleep. But for all this seems like a no-brainer, sleep experts are not so sure.

"In patients with insomnia," Michael Perlis said, "it is fundamentally unclear whether they're sleep deprived at all. Is it possible insomniacs need eight [hours] and are only getting six, that they're low in the tank for a very long time? It is possible. But since we have no way of measuring sleep need, we don't know."

Some investigators are skeptical that lack of sleep is the real problem for insomniacs, and not because they think we have nothing to complain about. Rather, it may be that both insomnia and fatigue are attributable to a lack or an excess of something else. And whatever that "something else" is, our fatigue may be compounded by the efforts we make, consciously or unconsciously, to compensate.[6] Lacking stamina, we push ourselves harder to meet obligations and do what needs to be done. "Pushing a boulder" and "running close to empty" speak to the sense of exertion and depletion that in insomniacs go hand in hand.

Fatigue has a huge impact on work, a topic we'll get to later in the chapter. It also affects how we use free time, and can turn what should be pleasurable activities into grinding chores.

"I work out at the Y," said Dan, a college administrator. "I burn four hundred or five hundred calories on the elliptical trainer or the stationary bicycle. But instead of feeling rejuvenated, I feel really tired. I'm just not with it."

Liz's fatigue compromises her enjoyment of social occasions. "I sometimes meet friends after work to go to movies," she said. "Quite frankly I would much rather be home here trying to have a nap, but you can't do that. You've got to just fight your way through."

Some insomniacs *do* succumb to fatigue and pull away from activities they enjoy. Keith's lifelong struggle with insomnia led to his eventually leaving a cycling team.

"I was involved with it for five years," he said. "We did hundred-mile rides, and I'd never know if I was going to get a good night's sleep and be able to ride the next day. Usually I'd just struggle through it—but sometimes the struggle was enormous."

Fatigue compels other insomniacs to scale down social commitments. "I still go about my day," Kay said, "but I'm really low energy. I don't want to do anything I don't have to do, and I don't want to make plans to do anything" such as go on outings or take on extra responsibilities.

Internal pressure to follow through with plans may trump concerns about fatigue. But negotiating these activities in the context of unpredictable sleep and energy levels can be tricky, especially when other people are involved.

"If I'm on a trip," said Colleen, an administrative assistant for the United Way, "and I have an itinerary that I'd like to stick to, I can't always do it. I can't keep up when I'm just exhausted because I wasn't able to sleep the night before. It impacts other people's lives and schedules too, which makes me feel anxious."

Studies of the public health burden of insomnia exist, as do studies of insomnia's effects on workplace productivity. This is unsurprising given the societal costs involved. But, while research suggests insomniacs' overall health and quality of life is diminished compared to that of good sleepers, and that insomnia has an impact on mortality, few researchers have looked at insomnia's impact on free time, on pursuits that fall not in the "have to do" column, but in the "want to do" column because they enrich our lives.[7] This chunk of time, small though it may be compared to time spent earning a living and taking care of chores, is probably one of the areas hardest hit by insomnia. Even if we can't slow down at work or skip fixing dinner, we can certainly forego a workout at the gym or an evening at the theater. But the only ones to suffer here are us.

Threads of Glass

Insomnia is unkind to the emotions.

"I feel," Dan said, "like it wears your sensitivities down, like it sands them down sandpaper thin, to where you're almost at the edge of tears. If somebody said something to you, you'd feel like breaking down."

Bouts of insomnia bring Ella down, physically and emotionally. "Very often I feel extremely tired and worn out and also depressed," she said. "It's as if all the light and color goes out of life."

I experienced similar feelings at college, where rock music and dormitory chatter at night turned me from a skittish sleeper into an insomniac. The fading of color from my surroundings was one of the first changes I noticed. The campus looked grayer, flatter, less attractive. This continued into my years in graduate school. My insomniac nights cast an inky film over everything I saw. The washed-out look of the houses and streets matched my washed-out mood. I felt less social, more cut off from people and things I usually enjoyed. I kept up life as a student, attending classes, consulting with teachers, going out for coffee with friends. But some part of me was unable fully to engage. And sometimes I felt weepy for no apparent reason, like Dan.

Many insomniacs report symptoms of depression, and there is solid evidence that insomnia and depression are closely linked. Insomnia correlates strongly with anxiety, too. In fact, a recent epidemiological study concluded that insomniacs are nearly ten times as likely as good sleepers to have clinically significant depression and about seventeen times as likely to have clinically significant anxiety.[8]

Research looking at the biomarkers of insomnia and depression shows these disorders to be both distinct and similar. While insomniacs tend to experience increased high-frequency brain activity during periods of quiet sleep, depression is associated with abnormalities in rapid eye movement (REM) sleep, when the brain is more active and when most dreams occur. But people with both disorders tend to have deficiencies in deep sleep, a type of sleep associated with feelings of restoration. Elevated levels of cortisol, a stress hormone, and interleukin-6, a protein that stimulates the immune response, are also common to both groups, as is a decrease in natural killer cell activity.[9] The significance of these elevations and declines, and the relationship between the two disorders, remains unclear.

But the latest evidence suggests that insomnia is actually a causal factor in depression. Recent surveys of medical literature over the past thirty years show that people with persistent insomnia are two to six times as likely as normal sleepers to develop depression down the line. And even insomniacs who do not develop clinically significant mood disorders are more prone to symptoms of depression and anxiety.[10] It looks like insomnia and psychological morbidity go hand in hand.

Also high on the list of emotional complaints linked to insomnia is irritability. "Crabby," "cranky," "grumpy," "moody," and "irritable" are words I heard a lot during my interviews, accompanied by concerns about their effects on relationships.

Terry's irritability put a strain on relationships at his job. "If I'm tired enough, I can be grumpy," he said. "I can get pushy with corporate clients and tour operators. But when you work in a corporate setting, you can't survive any other way. You push, they push, and everybody gets castrated. Sometimes you eat it, you internalize it. You're angry, but there's nowhere for that anger to go." It's a vicious circle, he added, with the stress at work exacerbating the sleep problem and insufficient sleep making him more volatile at work.

Karen, who manages investment properties, has found that her temper has a corrosive effect at home. "We've had a lot of screaming fights that honestly were nothing but the product of my being really, really tired," she said. "I have profound regret over outbursts I've had toward my brother, my husband, even my dad or step-mom. It's that inappropriate anger toward people because I didn't have the self-control I should have had."

Are the irritability and volatility some insomniacs experience directly attributable to insufficient sleep? The experts are not sure. But lack of sleep has emotional consequences, and to the extent that insomniacs *do* fail to get the sleep we need, our emotional stability is likely compromised.

Sleep Loss and Mood

Here I have to make an important distinction: While most people assume insomnia is equivalent to sleep deprivation, in the world of scientific research, the two have different meanings. Investigators of insomnia study people who can't get the amount or quality of sleep we'd like even when we have the opportunity. Those who study sleep deprivation are generally studying normal sleepers whose sleep is arbitrarily restricted—either completely, as in subjects being kept awake all night, or partially, as when subjects' sleep is restricted to four hours a night for several nights in a row. The two populations are not the same. Whether and how much insomniacs are sleep deprived, and how relevant sleep deprivation studies are to insomniacs, are unanswered questions. That said, many experts acknowledge that insomnia may involve a degree of sleep deprivation, so I'm going to talk about sleep deprivation now and its effects on emotional stability.

Scientists are still uncertain about the functions sleep serves. On a subjective level, everyone knows from experience what good sleep brings: physical refreshment, mental alertness, good humor, and the ability to sustain these feelings through the day. But when it comes to understanding the biological functions that take place during sleep, there are many convincing hypotheses but none are proven.

The work of Rosalind Cartwright, author of *The Twenty-Four Hour Mind*, suggests that one function of sleep is the downregulation of negative emotion. Cartwright's study of dreams, REM sleep, and REM sleep deprivation have led her to conclude that normal dreaming has a calming effect on mood.[11]

Twice as many of our dreams with emotional content are disturbing as are pleasurable, Cartwright notes. For this, the mood regulatory function of dreams theory would suggest, there is a reason. Disturbing dreams enable humans to process negative experiences we have during the daytime. These waking experiences get reactivated during sleep, carried forward into REM sleep, and matched to memories of earlier experiences of a similar emotional tone. What results during dreaming is not the forgetting of recent disturbing events but rather the defusing of their emotional charge. The sleeper then awakens in a more positive frame of mind.[12]

What happens when you deprive people of REM sleep, the sleep stage characterized by rapid eye movement and dreaming? Experiments show that normal sleepers deprived of REM sleep in the laboratory awaken in a bad mood.[13] Electroencephalogram (EEG) studies, involving the recording and analysis of electrical activity in the brain, have not shown that insomnia is a disorder characterized overall by a deficiency of REM sleep. But anyone who doesn't get the full *amount* of sleep they need is liable to pay for it emotionally. Here's why.

Sleep during the first part of the night is heavy on quiet, or non-REM, sleep, including, importantly, deep sleep; it's during the second half of the night when the bulk of REM sleep and dreaming occurs. "It is clear," Cartwright has written, "that short sleep inevitably results in a reduction of the amount of REM, since most REM comes at the end of the night." No matter whether you get to sleep too late or awaken too early, REM sleep is typically the thing that gets short-changed. And "loss of REM," Cartwright says, "may equal direct expression of negative mood."[14]

Matthew Walker is another sleep scientist who studies the effects of sleep and sleep deprivation on emotion. Sleep is protective of emotional stability, Walker has found, and sleep deprivation results in emotional reactivity. "A night of sleep," he says, "may 'reset' the correct affective brain reactivity to next-day emotional challenges."[15]

One study that demonstrates the emotionally destabilizing effects of sleep deprivation was conducted on medical residents in Israel.[16] Medical residency typically involves long hours of work and disrupted sleep, and the authors of this study looked at how sleep loss affected residents' emotional responses to events that occurred during the day. It turned out that sleep-deprived medical residents were significantly more disturbed by disruptive daytime events than their colleagues who slept well. Also, the sleep-deprived residents derived less satisfaction from events that were stimulating and positive. The study suggests that sleep loss not only increases our emotional reactivity to negative events, but it also blunts our ability to take pleasure in events that should make us feel good.

Seung-Schik Yoo, a sleep researcher at Harvard Medical School, and colleagues expanded this inquiry into the effects of sleep loss on the emotions by using functional magnetic resonance imaging (fMRI) to ascertain what was going on in subjects' brains during the viewing of an emotionally provocative slideshow.[17] (An fMRI scan detects changes in cerebral blood flow that occur in response to neural activity in the brain.) Before the experiment, half of the subjects were allowed a normal night's sleep, and the others were kept awake all night. Then, while positioned in a scanner, each subject watched a slideshow whose images progressed from neutral to negative.

As the images grew more disturbing, the brains of subjects in both groups showed increasing neural activity in the amygdala, a part of the brain associated with fear. But the amygdala activity in the sleep-deprived subjects was 60 percent greater in magnitude than in the control group, and more of the amygdala was involved. What's more, images of the non-sleepers' brains revealed less neural connectivity between the amygdala and the medial prefrontal cortex—a region of the brain known to inhibit and modulate activity in the amygdala. In other words, in the sleep-deprived subjects, there was a disconnect between the emotionally reactive amygdala and the moderating influence of the prefrontal cortex. While the well-rested subjects had a mildly negative reaction to the aversive images, the non-sleepers found them deeply disturbing.

Studies that demonstrate the emotional consequences of sleep loss, and others that zero in on which emotion-related brain functions are compromised, add to our general knowledge of the purposes sleep serves. What they reveal about insomnia is an open question. But in cases where insomnia involves even mild sleep loss, emotional stability may be one of the first things to go. Speaking at a conference, Walker said, "Sleep resets the magnetic north of your emotional compass. With sleep deprivation, you're all gas pedal and no brake."[18]

Dial-Up Mode

Christie worries most about the way insomnia affects her mind. "It's really hard to go into work when I haven't slept for days, because I can't think clearly," she said. "I just can't concentrate, and I make a lot of careless errors. A customer will walk up and say they want to cash a check. I enter their account number, and then I can't remember whether they said 'deposit' or 'cash' a check. I'm embarrassed because I have to ask them again what they said. Or I'll be in the middle of a conversation and I'll forget what I was talking about."

Liz, in contrast, doesn't feel her insomnia gets in the way of doing her work at the library. But her lack of energy, both physical and mental, *does* affect her motivation to learn new things.

"When it comes to learning new things I'm not as sharp as I used to be, and a little bit less willing," she said. "I'm a bit more resistant to anything that might be difficult. There was a time when I was very willing to take night school courses and just learn for the sake of it. I took an economics course just because I wanted to know. I wouldn't even attempt something like that now because I know I would quit halfway through because I'm just too tired and my concentration levels just suck."

After a few bad nights, the insomniac brain can feel like it's operating in dial-up mode. But objective evidence that insomnia impairs cognitive processing is not overwhelming. Research teams comparing the reaction time and accuracy of insomniacs and good sleepers on various psychomotor tasks have come up with conflicting results: some have found evidence of mild impairment and others have not. It could be, say the experts, that in some test situations, insomniacs can exert sufficient compensatory effort to enable us to perform as well as our normal-sleeping peers.[19] But one point of agreement seems to be this: When a task is simple, such as pressing a key when a figure appears on a computer screen, or memorizing word pairs, insomniacs typically perform as well as normal sleepers.[20] But insomniacs' performance falls down as the tasks get harder and more complex.

For example, in a recent study by Jack Edinger, a sleep researcher at Duke University Medical Center, and colleagues, insomniacs' speed on a simple reaction time test—pressing a computer key every time a square appeared on the screen—was about equal to that of normal sleepers.[21] Not so on the more complex "switching attention test." In this task, subjects were presented with conflicting cues on a screen and, to successfully complete the task, they had to take note of the cues and then respond based on a command that followed. The task had several steps and required, in the authors' words, "intact concentration, attention, response inhibition, and rapid decision making." Here, insomniacs were significantly slower to respond, and more variable in their responses. All else equal, it seems that in terms of processing speed, the insomniac brain can hold its own when a task is simple. But as the tasks get complicated, we lag.

As a writer, I trade on my ability to think and compose, and the sluggish brain that comes with insomnia is one of my biggest complaints. I have smart days and dumb days (and, yes, the dumb days tend to coincide with bouts of insomnia). On dumb days I spend a lot of time staring at words already on the computer screen. It's a strain to come up with the right analogy or a deft turn of phrase. I'm impatient with the thought that hovers just outside my grasp. Smooth transitions fail to materialize, and the paragraphs I *do* manage to eke out sound labored. Composing on bad days is like trying to chip away at a slab of marble with a kitchen knife.

And I wonder all the time: what exactly is going on in my brain to make me feel this way?

Recent neuroimaging studies offer clues. Research conducted by a team of Dutch investigators suggests some of the cognitive impairments insomniacs perceive may have to do with reduced activity in the prefrontal cortex, near the front of the brain. In this study, good sleepers and insomniacs underwent fMRI as they were performing a series of simple verbal fluency tasks.[22] The insomniacs performed the exercises just as well as the good sleepers—their performance was slightly better, in fact! But, in the brains of the insomniacs, the scanner recorded *reduced* neural activity in regions of the prefrontal cortex associated with verbal fluency. Performance of the task was not affected, but activity in the prefrontal cortex was clearly compromised. After the insomnia subjects underwent six weeks of cognitive-behavioral therapy, though (we'll examine CBT in chapter 8), the activation of the prefrontal cortex returned to normal—a bit of good news.

A group of researchers in California used fMRI to compare neural activity in the brains of two groups, "mild" and "moderate" insomniacs, as they performed a pair of working memory tasks. The two groups performed both tasks equally well. But, as subjects were performing the harder task, the brain scans revealed patterns of neural activity that were strikingly different between groups. Those with mild insomnia registered greater activity in memory-associated areas mostly on the right side of the brain. In contrast, those with more severe insomnia registered increased activity in several brain areas, and more of the activity was on the left side.[23]

The authors offer several explanations as to why these differences may have occurred. One interpretation of the findings, lead investigator Dane Anderson explained to me at the 2011 meeting of the Associated Professional Sleep Societies, is that when insomnia is moderately severe, areas of the brain that would normally be employed to perform a challenging memory task are "tapped out." So to perform the task, he said, "people have to recruit more areas of the brain. They're going from areas in the right side of the brain to activating areas on the left side as the task becomes harder. This could be part of their sense of struggling and not having the same ability as others."

This is merely a hypothesis, yet it sounds plausible. The insomniac brain may process information less efficiently than the normal brain. While insomniacs may get to the finish line as quickly, greater mental effort may be required. This could explain the feeling we have of pushing boulders all the time!

Insomnia and Memory

Insomnia may also interfere with the consolidation of memories that normally occurs overnight, which will likely come as no surprise to veteran poor sleepers.

Jonathan is convinced of the connection between his poor sleep and his diminishing ability to memorize music. "I've been playing classical guitar for over forty years," he said. "When I was younger I could commit music to memory without great trouble. But it's almost impossible for me to memorize a piece anymore. When I play I have to read off the music. To have to have it there as a reminder, it's very frustrating."

The type of memory Jonathan is talking about is called "procedural memory." It's associated with learning how to do things: tie a bow, ride a bicycle, drive a car, play a song without the musical score (musicians call this "finger memory"). To learn skills like these requires conscious attention in the beginning, but then they become second nature and thinking is no longer required.

The other kind of memory is "declarative memory." It is associated with the conscious recall of facts and personal experiences. This kind of memory has always been a stumbling block for me.

Not that in ordinary situations the handicap would show. I can still call up my Spanish when someone lets loose with a "*Como?*" At school my memory was dependable enough to see me through on tests. But most of what I "learned" seemed to vanish once I handed in my paper and left the classroom. As for reminiscing sessions at family get-togethers, usually I'm the one sitting on the sidelines. "Do you remember the time when . . . " my sister and brothers will begin, and nine times out of ten, I draw a blank. It's not just the small stuff I forget; it's major occasions like attending my brother's college graduation or my parents hosting a family reunion at our house. Other family members are quick to recall these events and fashion them into credible slices of life. Yes, I think, it could have happened exactly this way. It probably did. Yet nothing they say—no reminder of a gaffe someone made or a gift I received—is enough to jog my memory. And so I wonder: is there a connection between my poor memory and my poor sleep?

Research suggests it's possible. A body of literature now shows that sleep is important to learning and memory.[24] Sleep first of all aids in memory formation, the "encoding" phase that occurs during waking hours. A good night's sleep prepares your brain to receive new information and know-how and commit it to memory. If you're tested immediately after learning, you're better able to recall factual material and perform procedural tasks than people attempting to learn the same material under conditions of sleep deprivation.

Sleep is also important in "memory consolidation," the process whereby memories become stabilized and enhanced. The stabilization part occurs mainly during waking hours, but the enhancement occurs during sleep. So sleep *after* learning is a crucial part of the process. Overnight, new memories are replayed in the brain and further processed so they become more resistant to loss and deterioration. One result is that sleep actually improves our mental hold on learning that took place the day before.[25]

The Roman rhetorician Quintilian was the first to note this particular benefit of sleep: "[It] is a curious fact," he observed two thousand years ago, "of which the reason is not obvious, that the interval of a single night will greatly increase the strength of the memory. Whatever the cause, things which could not be recalled on the spot are easily coordinated the next day, and time itself, which is generally accounted one of the causes of forgetfulness, actually serves to strengthen the memory."[26]

Scientific research conducted in recent years is generally supportive of Quintilian's observation. Practice your piano scales in the evening, and you'll play them better after a good night's sleep than you did the night before. Likewise, study for a vocabulary test in the evening, and you'll recall more words after a good night's sleep than you would at the end of your study session the night before.[27]

Sleep deprivation has a negative effect on both the encoding and consolidation phases of memory. Subjects who are deprived of sleep *before* learning a new skill or new facts retain less than subjects who have slept a full night. Likewise, subjects who are deprived of sleep on the night *after* learning a new skill or new factual material have less success in remembering it the following day. The consolidation of procedural memories takes place during both REM and non-REM sleep, while declarative memories are consolidated primarily during deep, or slow-wave, sleep.[28] But sleep deprivation interferes with the consolidation of both types of memory.

Insomnia's impact on memory (as contrasted with the impact of sleep deprivation) is not so clear-cut. On tests of new learning and memory, results from a majority of studies show that insomniacs generally perform as well as normal sleepers.[29] The task may involve acquiring a skill, such as learning to trace a star while looking at its image in a mirror (a surprisingly difficult thing to do!). Or it may involve the recall of factual material, such as remembering a set of words after a 30-minute delay. Either way, we insomniacs are usually able to hold our own.

It's during the consolidation phase where the problem seems to occur. After learning the mirror-tracing task I just described, a night of sleep should make you even faster at it in the morning than you were the night before. This is exactly what happened to a group of subjects who were tested on the night of learning and then retested in the morning by Christoph Nissen, a sleep researcher at University Medical Center Freiburg, and colleagues.[30] Both the insomniacs and the normal sleepers were able to trace the star more quickly in the morning. But while the draw time of the normal sleepers improved by nearly 43 percent, the insomniacs' speed improved by only 20 percent. The sleep-dependent consolidation of procedural memories in insomniacs was impaired.

Likewise, getting a good night's sleep after studying word pairs should enhance your performance on a test the following day. But this did not occur in insomniacs who participated in a study led by Jutta Backhaus, a sleep researcher at the University of Lübeck.[31] In this experiment, insomniacs and normal sleepers were asked to learn forty word pairs. Cued with one word, the subjects had to recall the other. The performance of the two groups was identical during the learning phase. The number of learning trials they needed in order to remember at least twenty-four words was the same, and the number of words they recalled in the last trial of the evening was the same. But what a difference the night made! In the morning, as expected, the normal sleepers remembered more words than they had on the final trial the night before. But alas for the insomniacs, they recalled *fewer* words than they had the night before. The sleep-dependent consolidation of declarative memories in insomniacs was impaired.

These studies on the memory effects of insomnia are preliminary. Yet added to research on insomnia's effect on other mental functions, they suggest that in the realm of cognitive processing, insomniacs have grounds for complaint. Insomnia interferes with our ability to concentrate, learn, and think, and it likely compromises memory. Combined with other daytime symptoms, these impairments put us at a disadvantage in a marketplace that values cognitive abilities and skills.

Tote That Barge, Lift That Bale

For many insomniacs of working age (most insomniacs I interviewed fall into this category), work is a proving ground of sorts, a place where we have to accomplish things while contending with our daytime symptoms. This can create performance anxiety.

Rebecca is constantly concerned about passing muster at the publishing house where she works. "I supervise people, and I think about my relationships with them and my relationship with my boss. Does he think I'm doing a good enough job? Am I functioning at a high enough level?"

Rebecca's performance concerns are internal. Other insomniacs report their fatigue and irritability have attracted unwelcome attention from bosses, colleagues, and clients.

"It makes you a liability if you're not performing well because you have insomnia," said Laura of a period when she worked as a personal trainer. "There were times I wasn't functioning—that definitely makes it harder to attend to things when you're in a fog. But if I got called out on something that was directly or indirectly due to my lack of sleep, I would never share it with them. I did a lot of covering up." The effort involved in covering up was a further drain on her stamina. "It takes more effort to interact with others," Laura said. "You have to smile, you have to be pleasant. You don't want to have to explain to people, 'Well, I don't sleep well at night and that's why I'm grumpy now.' You do what you have to do."

Angie, a business consultant, feels a need to hide the evidence of her poor sleep when she's working. "I can put on a pretty good act to other people," she said. "But when you're trying to look awake, it takes more effort. It actually makes you *more* tired."

How many insomniacs find themselves "covering up" at work, or "putting on a pretty good act?" It wouldn't surprise me if more insomniacs were in the closet on the job than gays. Of course, whether the discretion is actually necessary is a separate question, and the answer doubtless varies from place to place. But let's face it:

having to struggle with the daytime symptoms of insomnia is never going to enhance a person's value in the eyes of an employer. That message came through loud and clear the one time I was careless enough to admit to fatigue on the job. I was a newspaper reporter working a midday shift. My boss Ray would charge in to work at 3 p.m., often in heated discussion with the publisher and the business manager, barreling down the narrow hallway at his side.

"How you doing?" Ray would bark at whoever was in the way.

I was on deadline that day, working on a sensitive story about race relations. Two of my prime sources were backing down and refusing to talk. I'd had a bad night before and was totally stressed out. Midway through the afternoon, wondering what lengths I was going to have to go to now to find other sources in the next few hours, I happened to step out of my office into the path of Ray and his entourage.

To Ray's usual question, I blurted out unthinkingly, "I'm exhausted!"

"Exhausted?" he repeated, frowning. "I don't want reporters who are exhausted. I want you ready to kick butt."

The rebuke came as no surprise, but it stung. Well, I thought, in Ray's shoes, I wouldn't want a stable of exhausted reporters either; I wouldn't want a single one. So although I might feel completely wiped out, admitting to it at work was a mistake I never made again.

Ted was vigilant in his efforts to keep his poor sleep and fatigue from affecting his work as a college professor, and he felt his efforts paid off. "I was considered very patient, " he said. "I would be there whether I was tired or not. I think I was able to hide it. I would work harder not to let the tiredness show because I would feel it's unprofessional, and that I shouldn't let that interfere."

But he acknowledged there may have been hidden costs. "No doubt I experienced more stress as a result of that," he said, adding that he could only speculate about how that stress may have affected his health overall.

Working harder, consciously or unconsciously making an effort to compensate for the impairments we feel, is one way insomniacs negotiate passage through the workday. It's survival through brute force, it's powering through exhaustion despite feeling we'd rather slow down.

But most of us have our little assists as well. One is caffeinated beverages. (And after decades of finger-wagging at insomniacs for drinking too much coffee, some sleep experts now acknowledge that the judicious use of caffeine—meaning not too much, and not after mid-afternoon—can be therapeutic after bad nights, helping to combat brain and bodily fatigue.)[33] Another is frequent trips to the water fountain, as much to stretch and move around as for the sake of hydration. But any insomniac's survival guide would be incomplete if it didn't include tips like these:

Schedule work when you're most likely to be alert. "Every job I've had," said Moss, a psychopharmacologist, "I've been able to make arrangements to make sure there's never going to be a strict requirement that I'm ever at work before nine. I usually get to work by eight, but I like to be able to get that extra hour of sleep in the morning if I need it."

Dive into the challenging work on the good days, and do easier work on the bad. As a small business owner, Keith can do that. After a string of bad nights, he said, the kind of critical thinking required for some of his tasks is beyond him, so he doesn't push himself. "My business is very computerized and I do a lot of the programming on a database myself," he said. "If I haven't slept well for a couple of days, I find that I can't think clearly enough to understand my own programming from even a week before. I've learned I have smart days and not-so-smart days, and if I'm not having a smart day, I just won't let myself do that particular function."

Catch up on work at home. Kathleen also runs a small business and can set her own hours. "There's days that I opt to stay at home and work and not go into the office," she said, "because I had a terrible sleep the night before! I can't tell my staff that's the reason I'm not coming in, but I actually do some work, even though it's in my housecoat!"

Accommodations like these can make the workday more tolerable for insomnia sufferers whose jobs permit flexibility. But by far the most common workday survival tactic I encountered among those I interviewed was just to power through: "Every day is a battleground for me," Liz said, "and you just have to fight it because otherwise you'd be doing nothing if you succumbed."

So, does fighting our way through the workday turn us into worker bees whose productivity is equal to our colleagues'? For some people, it may. But sadly, large-scale studies tell a different story.

The data show insomniacs are twice as likely as good sleepers to be absent from work. We're more expensive, too. Khaled Sarsour and his team of research scientists at Eli Lilly recently used health claims data from over 1,300 workers in an effort to calculate how big an impact insomnia had on costs associated with both absenteeism and presenteeism (reduced productivity on the job). The results of the analysis showed that altogether, the lost productivity costs for the moderate and severe insomniacs were 72 percent higher than for the normal sleepers.[33]

The higher rate of absenteeism may be due in part to the fact that insomnia sufferers as a group are sicker than normal sleepers. Not only is insomnia predictive of depression, but it also correlates with a host of chronic medical problems. Compared to normal sleepers, people with chronic insomnia are more than twice as likely to report suffering heart disease, high blood pressure, urinary problems, and chronic pain. They are more than three times as likely to report suffering neurologic disease, breathing problems, and gastrointestinal problems.[34] Other studies have demonstrated a link between insomnia with short sleep duration (as confirmed by polysomnography) and obesity and type 2 diabetes.[35] Not surprisingly, insomniacs visit the doctor more often than normal sleepers and incur higher healthcare costs. In the Sarsour study cited above, the healthcare costs of workers with moderate to severe insomnia were 75 percent higher than for workers without insomnia. Statistics like these are not encouraging, either for employers or for us.

A handful of insomniacs I interviewed experienced daytime symptoms onerous enough for them to call in sick. For Betsy, a medical biller, the "wiped out," headachy feeling that comes following a poor night's sleep can make the prospect of going to work seem dismal, leaving her in a quandary about what to do. "I think to myself, can I really call in and say, 'Hey, I didn't sleep last night?' I mean, is that enough of a reason? I could say I'm sick, but that's a fib. It doesn't quite feel like a valid reason to call in sick, though there are days when I do call in."

None of the insomniacs I spoke to missed work without misgivings. "It's really embarrassing to have to call in because I can't sleep," said one. And another: " I look like a total flake."

Whether or not health problems and symptoms associated with insomnia actually keep us away from work, they can certainly drag us down, and it's at work where many insomniacs have to contend with this. Some react by making adjustments that are adaptive. We arrange to work when we're most alert, get up to move around a lot, and make sparing but strategic use of caffeinated beverages. And some react in ways that may inadvertently make the situation worse: we worry about job performance, strive to "cover up" and pretend to feel energetic, bombard ourselves with caffeine, and drive ourselves to the point of exhaustion. Either way, the daytime symptoms of insomnia limit what we can do and be.

The psychic burden that accompanies this sense of reduced capacity can be substantial, leading some insomnia sufferers to revise career goals. Not only did some insomniacs report that poor sleep was a drag on day-to-day functioning, but they also felt it kept them from pursuing meaningful work or advancing their careers. Two lost jobs because of insomnia-related tardiness. Others lost or quit jobs they felt exacerbated their sleep problems, and found work that was less stressful. One was fired from her job as a tax lawyer and went into property management. Another left a job on Wall Street for one in publishing. Yet another left a job in teaching to become a stay-at-home mom.

A few made their career adjustments without much distress. More insomniacs I spoke with did so reluctantly.

Joan declined to go on promotional book tours, citing concerns about insomnia's effects on her performance. "There was period of time when we were first making decisions about who was going to go on book tours for our cookbooks," she said. "I was one of the people that was being considered, but I just knew I couldn't go. I knew I couldn't count on sleeping. I knew I wasn't going to be bright and beautiful for TV spots. I knew I'd really have to be sharp, and I knew I couldn't do that," she said, adding that it was disappointing to feel she had to withdraw from consideration, and "it was just sad that this [insomnia] would have an impact on it."

A much bleaker account of the impact of insomnia on professional development came from Bill, whose serious trouble sleeping had driven him to a host of medical specialists and much independent research on insomnia in an effort to improve his sleep. Bill viewed his career in home maintenance and landscaping as a comedown from the one he feels he might have had if he hadn't had to contend with disabling symptoms related to insomnia.

"It's caused me to lead a fraction of a life," he said. "I had to drop out of school. I'd like to think I'd have my PhD in one of the ecological, biological, or zoological sciences if I hadn't had to drop out. My take is that I had to drop out because of lack of sleep."

Would many insomniacs consider their sleep problems severe enough to have played a role in shaping life decisions? I don't know. But whether we experience insomnia as profoundly debilitating or profoundly annoying, it compromises our health and chips away at every aspect of daytime functioning, eroding pleasure in leisure activities, destabilizing mood, coloring social interactions, and undermining efforts at work. Surely our daytime symptoms are as deserving of attention as our poor sleep at night.

It's encouraging that scientists are turning up evidence relating to these daytime complaints. Impairments that can be measured are more likely to become targets for therapy. But insomnia sufferers are looking for remedies right now and, for the inquiring insomniac, the promise of help lies just a mouse click or a phone call away. So next we'll take a look at over-the-counter remedies—alcohol, sedating antihistamines, and herbals—and the help insomniacs may get from family doctors.

4

Looking for Help

Because day and night alike I am always
concerned about our common affairs and
because I am not easily able to fall asleep, I
drink wine when I am preparing to go to sleep.

Roman general Lucius Papirius, fourth century BCE

"Twenty-seven-year-old woman seeks help with insomnia"—or so my personal ad to the universe would have run the summer of 1982. By then the bouts of sleeplessness I'd known in college had become a semipermanent fixture in my life. I was having trouble sleeping several nights a week and had no idea what to do unless it was to seek a chemical fix. So, newly married and newly insured, I made an appointment at Group Health Cooperative down the street.

I was not looking forward to the appointment. Insomnia was such a nebulous, intangible problem. All the doctor would have to go on was my story. And how convincing would that be? I rode a bicycle to work and went hiking on the weekends and, except for a bum knee, looked perfectly healthy. There were no dark circles underneath my eyes. My problem was internal, undetectable with any instrument or medical procedure I knew of. With no proof that something was wrong, how easy was it going to be to make the

doctor understand how awful it was to feel exhausted but unable
to sleep? How discouraging it was to watch the hands of my alarm
clock pass into the twos and threes before I finally drifted off, only
to awaken early the next morning and feel wiped out by the afternoon?

Even less was I looking forward to talking about sleeping pills.
The idea of using them spooked me a bit. Every article I'd ever read
about sleep ended by urging readers to avoid them like the plague.
Sleeping pills were *habit forming,* a phrase that conjured up unspeak-
ably grim images: wastrels in foggy opium dens, and prostitutes
leaning against the grimy bathroom walls of speakeasies, removing
syringes from their bags. I wasn't sure that sleeping pills wouldn't
land me in a similar predicament. Yet I couldn't believe the sort of
flattened-out existence I led was the life I was meant to live. My
willingness to consider sleeping pills at all was a measure of just how
bad my insomnia was making me feel.

So I limped into Group Health with my knee injury and my
insomnia. I had an appointment with a female resident, which
pleased me. Discussing my sleep problem with a woman near my
age was a much friendlier prospect than talking about it with an
older man.

The doctor announced herself by throwing open the door and
pausing at the threshold. "Dr. Lee," she said, striding into the room
and pumping my arm.

My knee she dealt with quickly. The cartilage was likely worn
down, she said. The knee would repair itself if I stayed off my bicycle
for a while.

The doctor's manner was a little brusque. But as we talked she
loosened up. I mentioned I had just gotten married, to which the
doctor replied that she was a lesbian. No doctor had ever shared this
sort of personal information with me before, and I took her candor
as an extremely hopeful sign. It put us on a more equal footing and
was just the sort of opening I needed to broach the subject of my
insomnia. Which I promptly did: I told her I was spending many
hours awake at night, and I'd like to try some medication.

Dr. Lee's eyebrows came together in an unmistakable frown.
"Sleeping pills are habit forming," she said. "Once you take them,
you're hooked. No way am I going to write you a prescription for
those things."

I did some furious mental backpedaling as I tried to adjust to what she said. How could the tenor of our exchange change so quickly? In word and tone, Dr. Lee had just conveyed to me that in her view, the matter was closed. Yet how could this be the end of the discussion? I had waited several years to bring my insomnia to the attention of anyone who might be able to help. I scrambled to find a way to get the doctor to reconsider.

I wouldn't use the pills often, I said, maybe once or twice a week. And I didn't have addictions. I didn't smoke or use illegal drugs. As for alcohol, three or four beers a week was my absolute max. The plum wine I'd used to knock myself out during my comprehensive exams at graduate school was long gone.

But sleeping pills were not on the table for discussion with Dr. Lee. Nor did she suggest any alternative ways of managing my insomnia, though by the early 1980s other treatments were in use. This resident's bag of tricks contained nothing for the sleepless.

I left Group Health that day with dashed hopes and no clue about how to solve my problem with sleep. Insomnia, I saw clearly, was something I was going to have to handle on my own.

Help for insomnia can be hard to find. Even now, some thirty years later, I discovered while conducting interviews, there's no predicting what we'll come away with if we take our problem into the consulting room. We might get a prescription for sleeping pills, or the doctor may refuse to prescribe them. We might be told insomnia is a problem for psychotherapy, or to come back when we've *really* got a problem. We might be given an antidepressant, and we might be sent home with a fact sheet on sleep hygiene. If the solution or advice proffered strikes us as on the mark, well and good. If not, it's hard not to feel discouraged and decide we've got to fall back on our own resources. There are several reasons for these difficulties, and they're important to be aware of as we search for better options.

To start, though, at least two-thirds of insomnia sufferers never seek the help of doctors at all. Research suggests that even severe insomnia does not necessarily prompt a visit to the doctor. "Investigations of practice habits among physicians reveal that even severe insomnia problems are undetected in over 60 percent of affected patients," Michael Sateia, director of sleep medicine at Dartmouth–Hitchcock Psychiatric Associates, has written.[1] Even some of the worst afflicted tough it out on their own, availing themselves of remedies close at hand.

Forty percent of insomniacs who self-treat turn for assistance at some time to alcohol and over-the-counter sleep medications. About 5 percent try herbal and other alternative remedies.[2] These numbers are not negligible, so before we look at professional help available for insomniacs, these self-prescribed sleep aids deserve a look.

The Nightcap

Wine has long been a celebrated soporific. "Whoever drinks to his fill," says Hesiod, "the wine becomes maddening for him, it binds together his feet and his hands and his tongue and his mind with invisible bonds, and soft sleep loves him." The poet and playwright Eubulus cautions against over-imbibing, but counts sleep among the healthful effects of drinking in moderation: "Three bowls do I mix for the temperate," says Dionysus, "one to health, which they empty first, the second to love and pleasure, the third to sleep."[3]

Physicians in the Renaissance and Early Modern era prescribed wine for the sleepless, and some used it as a sleep aid themselves. Dr. Nathaniel Hodges, caring for the sick during the London plague epidemic of 1665, found that sherry served both to put him to sleep and to preserve his health. In fact wine was promoted as a harmless soporific through the nineteenth century and beyond. London physician Dr. Francis Anstie, writing in the 1870s, recommended strong wine to improve the fragmented sleep of the elderly.[4]

Though frowned on by medical professionals today, alcohol as an aid to sleep has two points in its favor: it's readily obtainable, and it works. "Initially," wrote Timothy Roehrs, director of research at the Sleep Disorders and Research Center of Henry Ford Health System, in an e-mail exchange, "it puts the person to sleep and the sleep is deep sleep." At least one study has shown that the tension-reducing effects of alcohol are even greater on insomniacs than normal sleepers. But its appeal to insomniacs may also be due to the fact that while alcohol typically interferes with sleep in the second half of the night, moderate doses may not affect insomniacs this way, at least at first.[5]

Let's look at what goes on in the brain at night to understand how this could be. Falling asleep, we move first into non-REM sleep, when the brain is mostly quiet. There, we descend from the lighter stages of sleep—1 and 2—into deep sleep—stage 3—and subsequently move up through the lighter stages again. Then a transition occurs. The brain becomes more active as it moves into REM sleep, when the majority of dreaming occurs. Non-REM and REM sleep combine to form a single sleep cycle, and we typically pass through four or five cycles a night. Cycles at the beginning of the night are heavy on non-REM sleep, including slow-wave sleep. Cycles at the end of the night are heavier on REM sleep. An image of a normal night's sleep as recorded by EEG—called a hypnogram—looks like an inverted cityscape, with the tall buildings, representing deep sleep, clumped together in the first half of the night.

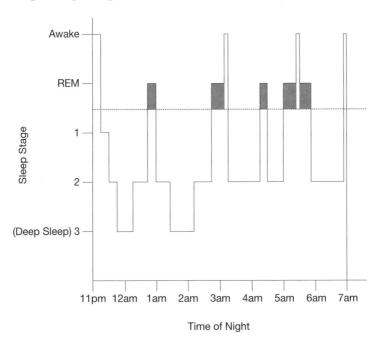

Time of Night

Here's what happens to the sleeping brain on alcohol in experiments involving normal sleepers. During the first half of the night, the alcohol tends to suppress REM sleep and may slightly increase slow-wave sleep. No red flag so far. But the body eliminates the alcohol in four to five hours, and the second half of the night is when the real mischief occurs. To compensate for the altered sleep in the first half of the night, the brain then engages in a riot of REM sleep, light sleep, and wakefulness. So while alcohol conks people out in the beginning, it typically wakes us up later on.

In contrast, research suggests that drinking the equivalent of a couple glasses of wine at bedtime initially appears to improve the sleep of insomniacs. In a study conducted by Roehrs and colleagues at Henry Ford, investigators administered low doses of alcohol or a placebo beverage to twenty good sleepers and insomniacs and then, on subsequent nights, allowed them to choose their beverage in order to compare the effects of the drug on sleep and mood. All subjects who chose alcohol experienced an overall decrease in REM sleep. But in the first half of the night, the insomniacs taking alcohol spent almost as much time in deep sleep as did the placebo-drinking good sleepers. So with alcohol, the sleep of the insomniacs was deeper than usual and looked more "normal" than it did au naturel. But of perhaps greater significance was this: The sleep disruptions that normally occur in the second half of the night following alcohol consumption did not occur in the insomniacs. Insomniacs who drank the equivalent of a couple glasses of wine experienced no increase in light sleep or wakefulness toward the end of the night. The alcohol, investigators concluded, "appears to have improved the insomniacs' sleep without disturbing their sleep in the second half of the night."[6]

So far it sounds like an ideal hypnotic (if you disregard for a moment its negative effects on other biological mechanisms and bodily organs). But of course it isn't. Tolerance and dependency develop quickly, posing a risk to those who use it every night.

Are insomniacs more prone than normal sleepers to alcohol dependency? It seems we are. Research suggests insomnia sufferers are more than twice as likely as normal sleepers to become problem drinkers. A recent cross-sectional survey found that while hazardous drinking was not correlated with any particular measure of insomnia, it is strongly correlated with using alcohol to get to sleep.[7]

This is hardly surprising in view of the ready way the body develops tolerance to alcohol. Experiments on healthy subjects have shown that whatever benefit alcohol affords—getting to sleep more quickly, for example—is lost within three days.[8] The only way to keep getting the benefit is to increase the dose. Insomniacs who use alcohol to get to sleep typically report having one to three drinks at bedtime, a lower dose than that which has usually been studied in normal sleepers. Yet insomniacs, too, habituate quickly. A pair of experiments conducted by Roehrs and colleagues show that tolerance to lower doses of alcohol taken at bedtime develops in insomniacs in less than a week.[9]

So the help alcohol affords the sleepless is short lived. With continuing use it vanishes quickly, leaving sleep even worse than before. Unless of course you increase the dose, in which case you set yourself on the path to dependency. "I would never even advise occasional use," Roehrs said. If drinking is part of the evening routine, do it early in the evening. Avoid alcohol in the three hours prior to bedtime.

Land of OTC

Over-the-counter sleep medications are newcomers by comparison. Developed in early twentieth-century laboratories, first-generation antihistamines came to market in the late 1940s and 1950s as drugs to combat allergies and relieve cold symptoms. But none were free of the side effect of drowsiness. So manufacturers like Rexall and J.B. Williams decided to cash in on that property and market them as drugs to help people sleep.

My first exposure to OTC sleep meds began with the TV commercials of the 1960s, when products were often touted in song. The Sominex jingle, like the jingles for Aunt Jemima's pancakes and Milky Way bars, entered our home via sitcoms like "The Andy Griffith Show" and "The Beverly Hillbillies." These catchy tunes, repeated at every commercial break, gave my sister and me a terrific case of earworm. So when our father wasn't home to object, we entertained ourselves by raucously mocking the jingles that played on the TV and inside our heads.

"Take Sominex tonight and sleep," we'd bellow at the top of our lungs with throaty vibrato, "safe and restful, sleep, sleep, sleep!"

We parodied indiscriminately, regardless of whether the product being advertised actually appealed to us or not. But Sominex in particular struck us as deserving of scorn. A drug you could buy without a doctor's prescription that promised 100 percent safe, "natural-like" sleep? It seemed like a throwback to an era of snake oil and patent medicines, no better than Geritol, advertised in those days for "iron-poor, tired blood." Who was going to fall for things like that?

I never thought to try an OTC sleep aid before my brush with Dr. Lee, assuming by the 1980s that products like Sominex were long gone from the market, exposed as frauds. But no, I found out shortly. A friend recommended the antihistamine Percogesic, so I bought a small bottle and took it home. At first glance the tablets were disappointing. They were dime sized and yellow, and chalky in texture, like Tums. Their appearance did not inspire in me the least confidence that I would sleep. I took two at midnight and settled in for another wakeful night. And as usual, it was 2 a.m. by the time I finally turned out the light.

But my Rip-Van-Winkle awakening in the morning was proof that Percogesic was not snake oil. I opened my eyes to a sunlit bedroom, a languorous body, and a deliciously empty head. How long had I slept? The clock on the nightstand said 8:40, but it felt like I'd hibernated 20 years. The day leading up to my big sleep was now the barest slip in memory. My eyes fell on the plastic bottle by the clock. "O Percogesic," I hymned to myself, "where have you been all my life?" I lay in bed for several minutes before I could rouse myself. It didn't matter that I was going to be late for work; my body felt inert as a cabbage and for once I was going to give in and let it be.

At work, I drifted along like the spaceship in *2001*, floating through the sky to the Blue Danube waltz. I knew my destination: an income statement I needed to produce for a meeting in the afternoon. But I was in no hurry to get there. My head that morning was full of cotton gauze. Lucky for me, the task was routine. Anything requiring real thinking would probably have fallen by the wayside.

I was still under the influence of the drug and I knew it, and the feeling wasn't entirely unpleasant. Gone was the mulish impulse to drive myself forward that I usually experienced after a string of bad nights. That, I was happy to be rid of. Yet drifting through the morning with mush for brains was a poor substitute for the alertness that was mine after the increasingly rare nights when I slept well.

The same thing happened the next time I took Percogesic, and the time after that. While the drug did nothing to hasten sleep, it kept me sleeping longer and left me logy the following day. So I wasn't tempted to use it often. But if it couldn't be a boon companion, at least it could be an occasional friend.

Sales of OTC sleep meds suggest that for some insomnia sufferers, newer sedating antihistamines like ZzzQuil and Unisom work well enough. Americans now spend over $750 million annually on OTC sleep meds.[10] They may confer other benefits as well. Said one enthusiast, "If you make a decision to take a sleep med long term, I think Benadryl's a great one. It's OTC, doesn't cost you hardly anything and, if it works for you, it'll even keep your nasal passages clear." Such a deal!

Some users I interviewed saw sedating antihistamines as a safe alternative to riskier prescription drugs. Others voiced reservations. Might they stop working when taken every night?

This concern may be valid. The active ingredient in most OTC antihistamines is diphenhydramine (some formulations of Unisom contain doxylamine, a similar drug). In a study conducted to assess how quickly tolerance develops to diphenhydramine, fifteen male subjects were given either 50 mg of the drug or a placebo twice a day. By the fourth day, the subjects taking the drug were no sleepier than those taking placebo. With daily use their bodies had quickly developed tolerance to diphenhydramine and it was no longer producing soporific effects. Of course, people using antihistamines for sleep take them at bedtime only, and whether and how quickly tolerance develops under these circumstances is a question this study does not answer. But, the authors conclude, "While other antihistamines and dosing regimens may differ, these results suggest that tolerance to the sedation produced by these drugs develops with remarkable rapidity."[11]

As for the efficacy of OTC antihistamines taken at night for sleep, two recent studies suggest it is modest at best. In a two-week study, diphenhydramine moderately increased subjects' sleep efficiency (i.e., more of their time in bed was spent sleeping rather than awake). In another two-week study, older insomniacs taking the drug experienced a small reduction in the number of times they woke up at night.[12] These are meager gains.

"There's absolutely no systematic evidence for the efficacy of the antihistamines" as sleep aids, said Sonia Ancoli-Israel, professor of psychiatry at the University of California San Diego and director of the Gillin Sleep and Chronobiology Research Center, "and there are significant concerns about the risks." Antihistamines have a lot of side effects: daytime sedation, diminished cognitive function, dry mouth, blurred vision, urinary retention, and constipation. "All of these are not particularly things we want to see in older adults," Ancoli-Israel said.

The main complaint I hear about antihistamines—apart from the fact that for many insomniacs they don't work—is the one about daytime sedation. "I was doing Sominex for a while," said Dale, a marketing executive. "I found *that* one left me just too raggy in the morning. It was really hard to get up and it kept me in a fog for too long."

The hangover effect is probably attributable to these drugs' relatively long elimination half-lives, Ancoli-Israel said. (Half-life refers to the time it takes for a dose of a drug in the blood plasma to decrease by half.) Diphenhydramine has an elimination half-life of 2.4 to 9.3 hours. In some users, a significant amount of the drug remains in the bloodstream well past normal wake-up time, causing morning drowsiness. The half-life of diphenhydramine tends to increase with users' age. The half-life of doxylamine, the active ingredient in some formulations of Unisom, is about ten hours and typically longer in older adults. It, too, may cause morning grogginess.

One antihistamine user I spoke with got around this problem by taking half the recommended dosage at night. Others experienced no residual sedation and were satisfied that OTC sleep aids were the way to go. Except for the side effects and the possibility of developing tolerance with nightly use, research hasn't turned up other reasons to avoid sedating antihistamines . . . if they work.

Alternative Solutions

Herbal remedies for insomnia today are considered to be alternative and complementary, yet they were pharmacological mainstays for thousands of years. The ancients relied heavily on poppy, mandrake, and henbane to alleviate sleep problems. In fact these plants contain chemical alkaloids that promote sleep (opium alkaloids, scopolamine, hyoscine, hyoscyamine, and atropine). A popular hypnotic in the Middle Ages that utilized some of these ingredients was the "spongia somnifera," a sponge steeped in a mixture of wine, opium, lettuce, hemlock, hyoscyamus, mulberry juice, mandrake, and ivy. Placed under the nose, it was used as an anesthetic and to induce sleep. Many of these substances continued in use as hypnotics through the end of the nineteenth century.[13]

Herbs in use for insomnia today, including valerian and hops, have not been recognized for their soporific properties for quite so long. In ancient Roman times, Pliny and Galen mentioned valerian as friendly to sleep, but it's only beginning in the eighteenth century when valerian comes into common use as a sedative.[14] Interest in using hops to promote sleep was likely rekindled, say the authors of a comprehensive reference guide, at the beginning of the nineteenth century. One night when King George III was sick and highly agitated, court attendants laid his head on a bag of warm hops, a folk remedy for sleeplessness. The king slept more than eight hours that night and woke up tranquil "with the fever abated," thus giving a boost to the idea that hops was an effective soporific.[15] The Shakers, who maintained a lucrative business in medicinal herbs in the eighteenth and nineteenth centuries, described hops as "valuable as a sedative to produce sleep" and valerian as useful in cases of nervous debility and hysteria.[16]

What does contemporary research tell us about the efficacy of these and other herbs in combating insomnia? The authors of a recent review of herbal medicine for insomnia and mood disorders summarize the properties of a handful of sleep-friendly herbs as demonstrated in the laboratory:

- Both chaste tree (also called vitex and chasteberry) and hops act on the melatonin system. (Melatonin is a sleep-friendly hormone the body secretes at night.)

- Sour date, used in traditional Chinese medicine, inhibits some of the brain's arousal pathways, and its active ingredient has increased the total sleep time of rats.

- Valerian enhances the action of GABA, the brain's main inhibitory neurotransmitter, and has lesser sleep-promoting effects on the serotonin system.

- Two other herbs that are potentially beneficial for insomnia are passionflower and American skullcap.[17]

The word to pay attention to here is "potentially." When you look for information about the impact of any of these herbs on the sleep of human beings, the medical literature yields slim pickings. The majority of existing studies lack methodological rigor and cannot be used to determine whether the herbs improve sleep or not. That leaves a very small number of studies upon which to draw conclusions.

Valerian alone has gotten much attention from the research community. But only six studies of valerian—all randomized controlled trials, or RCTs (studies where subjects receiving treatment are compared with a group that does not receive treatment, or that receives a sham treatment, and participants are randomly assigned to the different groups)—were deemed rigorous enough to include in a recent review of alternative treatments for insomnia. One found that valerian was modestly more effective than placebo at helping people sleep. Another found that while valerian alone did not improve sleep, a valerian-hops combination was "significantly superior to placebo" in hastening the onset of sleep. In a third study, 600 mg of a valerian extract was as effective in helping people sleep as 10 mg of oxazepam (a benzodiazepine used to treat anxiety and insomnia) and rated as "very good" by 83 percent of the subjects who used it. The other three studies found that valerian or a valerian-hops combination was little or no better than placebo.[18]

"The evidence concerning valerian is quite varied," the authors of the review conclude, "and currently does not support its use in treating insomnia." Two other reviews of studies on valerian used for sleep found that the majority had negative outcomes. However, in a still more recent study (an RCT involving one hundred postmenopausal women with insomnia), 530 mg of valerian taken twice a day for four weeks improved the sleep quality of 30 percent of the women, as compared to 4 percent whose sleep quality improved on placebo.[19] While the herb's efficacy seems to vary from person to person, research has shown that it has no harmful side effects.

Herbal medicines may work best to complement other, more rigorous therapies for insomnia, said Jerome Sarris, a National Health and Medical Research Council research fellow at the University of Melbourne and lead author of two of the articles cited above. "It really is tough to treat chronic insomnia with herbal medicine," Sarris said. "It may be useful as an adjunctive to sleep hygiene and psychological intervention and lifestyle modification, but it certainly does not have the head-to-head efficacy and the strength of a benzodiazepine or the zed-class benzos [drugs like Ambien and Lunesta]." Herbal medicines, Sarris continued, "generally take longer to work, whereas some people just want that quick fix. I think they may have more of a role in long-term assistance for sleep rather than as an acute measure" for combating insomnia.

Some GABA-modulating herbs may be much better at reducing anxiety than inducing sleep. "Chamomile is a case in point," Sarris said. Studies in the laboratory have suggested that the herb has anti-anxiety properties, and an RCT recently conducted on patients with generalized anxiety disorder showed that chamomile was modestly efficacious in reducing their anxiety.[20] But no human studies exist showing that chamomile works as a hypnotic, Sarris said, and neither is there good anecdotal evidence.

On the other hand, a few studies show that the amino acid L-tryptophan—sold in the United States as a dietary supplement—may be an effective soporific, Sarris and his colleague G.J. Byrne conclude in their review, citing positive outcomes on two out of three RCTs.[21] "The best results seem to occur in cases of mild insomnia with long sleep latency," the authors state. (People with long sleep latency take a long time to fall asleep.) Sarris added that L-tryptophan, converted by the body into serotonin, may also be effective at alleviating insomnia in people who also have depression.

In any event, those looking to science to settle the question of whether herbal medicines work for insomnia will not find many answers yet. "Aside from mixed evidence," Sarris said, "for some herbal medicines, there's good traditional evidence [that they work], but they just haven't been studied yet. It might be a case of, 'We haven't got around to it,' or 'we haven't got the funding or even the interest.' That doesn't mean it's not effective. It just means it hasn't been studied."

❨

My own continuing search for better sleep thirty years ago took me not to the herbalist but instead to the self-help section of the bookstore. The minute I picked up *A Good Night's Sleep*, I thought I might have stumbled on a fix. Dr. Jerrold S. Maxmen's opening gambit could not have resonated with my experience more strongly. In his view, nobody else—not spouses, friends, or physicians—would ever likely show much concern for my sleep problem, or be able to offer emotional support.

"Ultimately," Maxmen wrote, "you have no choice but to 'go it alone.' Only you experience the sleeplessness; only you can provide the necessary emotional support; only you can rectify the problem."

Maxmen's do-it-yourself message of hope made me think I might be able to turn my sleep problem around. But even more than that, it was his empathy I found appealing. Here was a doctor who took insomnia seriously, understood how lonely it made me feel, and wrote about the affliction from the point of view of an *insider*. He might be not be my spouse, friend, or physician, but it was clear that behind his words was a living, breathing human being who understood what it was like to tough it out through many a sleepless night and washed-out day. He wrote as if he himself had known insomnia and wrestled it to the ground.

Maxmen's goal was to promote the eight-step program he'd developed to help people improve their sleep. But his book was not one of the many screeds typically found in the self-help section at the bookstore. This doctor did not preach. Acknowledging there were no foolproof solutions to insomnia, he offered some basic rules to live by and a variety of sleep management techniques, and he encouraged experimentation. Merely reading Maxmen's book at night was a meditative act; once in a while, it was even soothing enough to lull me to sleep.

Eventually, based on a suggestion in the book, I came up with a technique I called "rhythmic breathing." (Later I learned the technique was known in therapeutic circles as "diaphragmatic breathing.") Lying on my back in bed, I took slow, deep breaths and counted up to six or seven and then back again, my abdomen rising and falling with each breath. When I noticed my mind starting to wander—and it often did—I returned to counting. It worked the first few weeks. And on awakening in the morning I felt practically intoxicated with power. If I could put myself to sleep at will, then what else could I do? Run a marathon? Win a writing contest? Get a job with a decent salary and benefits? For a short while the possibilities seemed endless.

But there were times when I counted for an eternity and still remained awake. And that made me cross. Why, when I was so earnestly doing my part, was my body failing to do *its* part? Reluctantly, I conceded that rhythmic breathing was not the panacea I'd hoped for. Like Percogesic, it wound up relegated to the status of occasional friend. (We'll take a longer look at relaxation and mind–body therapies for sleep in chapter 9.)

Adventures in the Consulting Room

Many insomniacs eventually take their sleep problem to the doctor, and some receive the counsel they seek. Others come away discouraged. Christie, a bank teller, was frustrated with two primary care practitioners who responded to her complaints of sleeplessness by prescribing pills.

"All they do is write me the prescription," she complained. "They say, 'If that doesn't work, just let me know and I'll write something else.'" Christie wanted a drug-free approach to managing her insomnia, but her doctors had nothing to suggest.

Cami, a web master, took her complaint of insomnia to the doctor expecting to get sleeping pills only to learn that her doctor didn't prescribe them. "She doesn't want to prescribe anything as serious as Ambien. She'll prescribe for my migraines and asthma, but not for anything else. All she told me is that I should probably work out more." But Cami was already working out at the gym two or three times a week, and disappointed that she came away from the doctor's office empty-handed. Eventually she obtained sleeping pills through a friend.

Colleen, who works for the United Way, said her physicians haven't shown much concern about her insomnia at all. "I have talked to my doctors about it," she said, "and they just don't seem terribly interested in it, to be honest. They're willing to give me advice to go to bed at the same time every night and get up at the same time every day. But, above and beyond that, I think they're really not interested in treating it."

Why is it hard to get help for insomnia? And why do insomniacs sometimes come away with the message that perhaps insomnia doesn't merit attention at all?

Sleep specialists agree that complaints of insomnia deserve attention, and the earlier, the better. As we saw in chapter 3, chronic insomnia has a host of negative health consequences. It decreases quality of life and productivity at work, is a causal factor in depression, and is a risk factor for medical problems such as hypertension and diabetes. Data suggest that persistent insomnia also has a negative impact on mortality.[22] All else equal, people with persistent and severe insomnia are apt to die sooner than everybody else. (Superlong sleepers, who typically sleep more than nine hours a day, also bear the burden of increased mortality.) Even if we discount quality-of-life and productivity issues, to dismiss something with such potentially serious consequences is like ignoring the early signs of diabetes and heart disease: it's bad medicine. Treat insomnia in the acute phase, say sleep therapists, and you help to head off major health problems down the line.

But most insomniacs do not consult sleep specialists. A majority take their complaints to primary care providers.[23] And among some of these general practitioners and internists, the lack of a known etiology, regulations on prescribing practices, and physician education and attitudes can turn the insomniac into a persona non grata in the consulting room.

One reason insomnia is hard to treat is that its physiological underpinnings are mostly uncharted and there is no solution that works across the board. Helping the insomnia patient is more of a challenge than treating the patient with diabetes or pneumonia, and perhaps beyond what the family doctor is comfortable taking on.

"You have this combination of no cure and no known etiology, especially not a physiologic etiology, and that right away says to the average GP that whatever this is, it's not within my purview," Michael Perlis, director of the Behavioral Sleep Medicine Program at University of Pennsylvania, said.

Time constraints associated with managed care may keep the subject of insomnia from even coming up. When a general practitioner has to assess the health of all bodily systems in a ten- or twelve-minute appointment, sleep may get short shrift. There is not enough time in a patient's appointment to discuss sleep problems, said a majority of doctors responding to a survey conducted for the National Sleep Foundation in 2000. And of the 1,500 Americans surveyed by the National Sleep Foundation in 2005, seven in ten had never been asked by their doctors about their sleep.[24]

Also, primary care physicians may have little knowledge about the differential diagnoses of sleep disorders and the range of treatments available for people with insomnia. The average medical student spends little more than two hours learning about sleep disorders, according to a report published by the Institute of Medicine of the National Academy of Sciences in 2006. "There is no evidence to suggest that medical schools are placing increased emphasis on sleep-related content in their curriculums," the authors state. A 2011 survey shows that Australia, Canada, and the United States are the only countries where medical students now receive more than three hours of education in sleep and sleep disorders. Even so, "there appears to be minimal change from 20 years ago."[25]

So where *do* our primary care providers learn about insomnia? They may read about it in medical journals, but most of their information comes from sales representatives who visit their offices bearing gifts and peddling drugs. Information about insomnia and other sleep disorders is also presented in seminars and short courses sponsored by pharmaceutical companies. At events like these, expert speakers talk up medical discoveries to their fellow physicians, who benefit from exposure to developments in the field. But at the end of the day, the solution to the problem posed by the new information is always a drug or a medical device produced by the pharmaceutical sponsor.

I've attended a couple of these events myself. A dinner presentation billed as a talk on disrupted slow-wave sleep was mostly about slow-wave sleep-enhancing medications, one under development by the event's corporate sponsor. Another dinner presentation, billed as a talk on circadian biomarkers, was a prelude to the message the event's corporate sponsor wanted to impart, namely, that actigraphs (wristwatch-type devices used to diagnose sleep disorders by measuring movement) were now reimbursable by Medicare for physicians using the correct diagnostic code. These presentations were chock full of useful information (and the attendees, well fed). But they clearly served the commercial interests of their pharmaceutical sponsors.

Many recommended clinical practices do not involve a commercial product, and the history-taking recommended for patients with sleep problems is an example.[26] To address complaints of insomnia, said Michael Bonnet, clinical director of Kettering Sycamore Sleep Disorders Center in Miamisburg, Ohio and professor at Wright State University School of Medicine, physicians should first ask a series of questions to determine the nature of the problem. Information about the duration and severity of symptoms, and other health problems that may be associated with the insomnia, will result in more accurate diagnoses, which may involve tests and point toward different treatments. But the differential diagnosis of insomnia complaints is something primary care physicians rarely do, Bonnet said.

"People aren't trained that way," Bonnet told me in his office at the sleep disorders center. "The drug companies just haven't done it, and that's where most primary care doctors' education comes from," he said, adding that the more typical response to patients' complaints of insomnia is to prescribe a sleeping pill.

Yet not all primary care providers embrace pharmaceutical solutions for insomnia, as Cami and other interviewees were quick to point out. Some doctors will not prescribe hypnotics at all. Most sleeping pills are designated as controlled substances by the United States Drug Enforcement Agency, and their prescription, dispensation, and use is tracked through prescription drug monitoring programs. The monitoring of sleeping pills, in addition to safety concerns, may deter some primary care providers from prescribing them, Michael Perlis said.

"Not only is there this bad context—insomnia is not a disease, it's something psychological, there is no cure—but they're not trained in what there *is* to know," Perlis said. "Then you add on top of that, the drugs they would like to prescribe, they're afraid of. So this is a recipe for, 'Get out of my office because I can't help you.'"

Some physicians hesitate to medicalize a disorder they regard as stemming largely from bad behavior. Sleep is understood to be at least partly under voluntary control, say Perlis and colleagues in a paper on intermittent and long-term use of hypnotics, and a common belief about insomnia holds that good sleep simply requires better self-regulation. This can be seen from the responses of primary care physicians surveyed by the National Sleep Foundation in 2000. Asked what factors they consider when diagnosing insomnia, doctors mentioned lifestyle factors most frequently, followed by sleep habits, health habits, and psychiatric problems.[27] Physicians who regard insomnia simply as a lifestyle issue requiring changes in habit will not be inclined to prescribe sleeping pills.

Complaints of insomnia may also be brushed off because of a belief that, in the absence of complicating factors, insomnia is harmless. It's a symptom of some other disorder and will clear up once that problem is addressed, goes this line of thinking; or it's a transient problem with a few annoying but minor consequences, which time itself will correct.

"There is no conviction among primary care physicians that insomnia in particular, or sleep in general, is a serious health consideration," was the consensus of the participants in a workshop convened by the World Health Organization in 1997, by way of explaining why the educational materials on insomnia available to primary care doctors were so infrequently used. "Physicians, including even sleep researchers, tend to view insomnia and the associated complaints of poor mental and physical health as obsessions of otherwise healthy individuals," wrote sleep investigator Alexandros Vgontzas, a psychiatrist at the Penn State University College of Medicine at Hershey, in 2001. "The prevailing wisdom for primary care practice continues to be 'insomnia is a symptom that, at worst, contributes to irritability and/or very modest impairments in interpersonal, social, and vocational functioning,'" Michael Perlis and colleagues wrote in 2008.[28]

Physicians who regard insomnia as inconsequential may take a hands-off approach to treatment, Perlis said, and sometimes doing nothing actually works. In the majority of patients, acute insomnia associated with life stressors like the loss of a job or a partner will disappear once the stress fades away. But epidemiological studies show that some 25 to 40 percent of the people who experience mild insomnia symptoms will go on to develop a more persistent form of insomnia later on.[29] "That's a very large number to be playing the odds with," Perlis said. Doctors who routinely dismiss their patients' complaints of insomnia are going to leave quite a lot of people vulnerable to worsening symptoms that reduce the quality of their lives, increase the odds of their developing serious health problems, and shorten their lives.

As for the assumption that insomnia will clear up once a comorbid health problem is addressed, this may sometimes occur. But it does not necessarily work this way in people with insomnia and depression. A study published in 2007 showed that the insomnia of about 22 percent of the patients treated successfully for major depressive disorder in a clinical setting did not go away. Indeed, among people who respond to depression treatment, sleep problems are common residual symptoms, according to Rachel Manber, a sleep researcher at Stanford University. Manber and her colleagues found that undergoing a behavioral treatment for insomnia in addition to taking an antidepressant was more effective in getting rid of depression and insomnia than taking the medication alone. This suggests that people with depression and insomnia are better served when *both* disorders are attended to.[30] But the results of these and other studies apparently have not trickled down into the consulting rooms of primary care physicians.

In January 2007, three physicians lamented the "epidemic of diagnoses" in an essay in the science supplement of *The New York Times*. Except in cases where the problem was severe, they asserted, we were better off when such "everyday experiences" as insomnia, sadness, and twitchy legs, unpleasant though they might be, were simply accepted as part of life rather than diagnosed as diseases requiring treatment.[31] I'll agree that if by "treatment" the authors mean medication, this may not be the best solution for every person complaining of insomnia who walks through the doctor's door. But the treatment of insomnia is not limited to drugs. What is really objectionable here is the implication that certain chronic conditions are too trivial to merit intervention, and that we'd be better off if complaints of insomnia, sadness, and restless legs did not result in diagnoses, and people bore their pain and suffering with a stiff upper lip.

I doubt most primary care providers are quite so lacking in compassion. At the very least, doctors are usually willing to send insomnia sufferers home with a set of instructions on sleep hygiene (which, despite its popularity, has been shown to be ineffective as a stand-alone therapy for insomnia).[32] There are better ways to handle complaints of insomnia: procedures for making more accurate diagnoses and for implementing therapies likely to help. But about these practices many primary care doctors are still in the dark.

From Consulting Room to Clinic

You might think an overnight sleep study would put insomniacs on the fast track to getting help. This was the thought that occurred to Liz, a light sleeper for most of her life. She reasoned that her doctors would know better how to treat her insomnia if she underwent testing at a sleep clinic and they saw what was going on in her brain. But this did not prove to be the case.

"The only thing they saw was that I never go into deep sleep," Liz said. But no one could explain why. Nor did that sleep study or a second one provide any insight into what to do about her insomnia. "I just got fed up with clinics," she said.

Many insomniacs who undergo sleep studies tell similar stories. "I did go to a sleep clinic two or three years ago," Kay said. "They told me I did not have sleep apnea [obstructed breathing], and that was it. It was ridiculous. Insurance paid for it. It was very expensive and they paid for it, and I got nothing out of it."

"I had a sleep study done," Tom said. "They found I don't get much REM sleep. Getting the diagnosis from the sleep clinic but not being told where to go from there—it was a little bit of a disappointment. I wish there had been more of a solution. But at the same time I was glad I didn't have sleep apnea."

So what does an overnight sleep study entail, and why are they frequently disappointing to people with insomnia?

Undergoing polysomnography entails spending the night in a small bedroom at a sleep clinic. In preparation, patients are wired up like marionettes with electrodes glued to their heads, chest, and legs. The wires plug into a box, and via cables they travel to a computer in an adjacent room, which records electrical activity in the brain and changes in physiological functioning. Various functions are recorded, including muscle and eye movements, heart rate, and breathing. All incoming signals register as oscillations that move across a computer screen in real time, and the scoring of data occurs later on. There's also a hidden camera in the bedroom so technicians can observe people directly as they sleep. These are hardly ideal conditions for slumber! But sleep technicians insist that every patient evaluated in a sleep lab eventually nods off.

Polysomnography is good at detecting nocturnal abnormalities such as obstructed breathing, seizures, cardiac arrhythmias, and movements associated with restless legs or the acting out of dreams. If a doctor suspects a patient's sleep problem is caused by any of these, then an overnight stay in a sleep clinic is a good way to verify it. In fact, for people with hypersomnia, or excessive daytime sleepiness, the polysomnogram (PSG) has been a spectacular success, Perlis said.

"We found out that all these hypersomnic people—people who would doze—have any number of unseen things going on. They stop breathing, they're kicking, they're having seizures, they have alpha sleep." In such cases, he said, the PSG could reveal the cause of patients' excessive sleepiness during the daytime, "and it would be unique, and potentially, if not definitely, a target for treatment."

But so far, the PSG has not proven similarly useful in the diagnosis and treatment of insomnia. The electroencephalogram (EEG)—the graphic representation of brain waves that is produced during a PSG—can show that a person takes a long time to fall asleep or has frequent awakenings at night. Yet the same information can often be ascertained in a clinical interview. "In the case of insomnia," Perlis said, "all we did was validate to one extent or another, 'yeah, they have insomnia.' There was nothing more to be seen." So the American Academy of Sleep Medicine recommends polysomnography for complaints of insomnia only in cases where a clinical interview does not yield a clear diagnosis, treatments fail, or violent behavior is suspected during sleep.

There *is* wake-like activity going on in the brains of some insomniacs at night, and it can be picked up when the equipment is adjusted to detect the entire spectrum of wave frequencies. (I'll say more about this abnormal activity in chapter 9.) People who experience a lot of it are often diagnosed with "paradoxical insomnia," and perceive that they are awake when their EEGs show that they are sleeping. But in a PSG conducted and scored in standard fashion, *this wake-like activity will not show up.* Moreover, as things stand now, to what extent the abnormal activity is present doesn't make a lot of difference when it comes to options for treatment.

While the PSG can differentiate paradoxical insomniacs from "objective" insomniacs (whose EEGs show that they get quite a bit less sleep than normal), it is not very good at discriminating insomniacs from normal sleepers. Up to 50 percent of the time, the EEGs of insomniacs look exactly like the EEGs of good sleepers: the same sleep staging, the same percentage of deep sleep, the same total sleep time.[33] No wonder so many insomniacs emerge from their night in the sleep lab scratching their heads.

The PSG may someday become a useful diagnostic tool for people with insomnia. Meanwhile, diagnosis and treatment continue to be based mainly on clinical interviews. The average cost of a sleep study in the United States is $2,625: a hefty price to pay for a test that, as currently performed, adds little to the diagnostic process.[34]

So where *can* insomniacs turn for help with sleep and daytime alertness? Primary care doctors may not be willing or able to address what ails us. Nor have the vaunted sleep studies afforded much guidance to physicians who wish to help. As for traditional remedies, alcohol is effective as a hypnotic but not very safe. The scorecard for OTC meds and herbs is weighted in the opposite direction: relatively safe but of questionable efficacy.

Insomniacs who look for help online will find a dizzying array of choices. Dietary supplements, each with its proprietary combination of herbs, promise users better sleep. There are homeopathic remedies for insomnia with Latinate names. Aromatherapy is available in the form of herb-scented bath products, body patches, and essential oils. Sound therapy features babbling brooks and murmuring rivers, and music purportedly designed to coax your brain into deeper levels of sleep. The myriad gadgets for the sleepless include handheld biofeedback and ion machines, and devices that evaluate your sleep and "coach" you in how to improve it. Perhaps some of these products are worth a bid if you've got disposable income. But none have been rigorously tested on insomniacs and proven to work.

There *are* better forms of assistance, and that's where we're headed in this book. Readers interested mainly in insomnia treatments may want to skip ahead to chapter 8, and those looking for information about the science of sleep and insomnia may want to skip to chapter 6.

But there's a side trip really worth taking before starting down these paths. Chapter 5 deals with attitudes toward sleeplessness and how they've changed in the past two centuries. History helps debunk some of the myths about insomnia and will pave the way for a more fruitful discussion of insomnia in the chapters that follow.

5

All in the Head, and Other Ideas about Insomnia

All any self-made insomniac has to do is make himself comfortable and close his eyes.

Dr. Paul H. Fluck, "So You Can't Sleep?"
Today's Health, 1950

Concerning my insomnia I like to think I've grown a thicker skin: that any suggestion that it's a trivial problem, or a sign of mental instability or unhealthy habits, glances off me like I'm made of polished chrome.

If by now I've reached that place, I certainly hadn't in the early years of work on this book. I joined a reading group then, and one night some group members asked what I did. I said I was writing a book about insomnia, which I suffered from myself. To that revelation no one said a word. Everyone looked nonplussed, as if I'd just admitted to running an escort service or selling junk bonds. Quickly I offered a few details, aware that a flush was creeping up my neck and spreading over my face. The incident embarrassed and confused me, and it bothered me for days. I was certain insomnia was worthy of a book-length project. Why feel embarrassed at the reactions of these new acquaintances, unless for me insomnia carried a stigma?

Not all insomniacs are so encumbered. But several I interviewed felt their trouble sleeping reflected poorly on them and diminished them in the eyes of family members and colleagues.

"I think most people take sleep for granted," said Laura, who left her job as a personal trainer to study physical therapy, "so not being able to do it just strikes them as odd. There seems to be a stigma associated with it. Like if you have a mood disorder, people assume there's something innately wrong with you. Or if someone has emphysema, I hear people blaming them, like they automatically assume that they smoked and must deserve it. I feel like insomnia is almost the same way. Some people think it's your fault. You must have done something to bring it on yourself."

Negative beliefs like these are easy to internalize. They cause anxiety and a desire to cover up, as happened to Joan, a counselor at Planned Parenthood. She worried about what her insomnia would imply about her mental fitness.

"I felt mortified for a very long time that any public awareness that I suffered from insomnia would betray something about my character, or just about my wholeness," she said. "It would show that I was damaged in some way, that I wasn't balanced, that I wasn't completely mentally healthy." So she avoided talking about it, even with her therapist. "There's something like you're not supposed to talk about insomnia, something that's in the shadows about it, or at least there is for me," she said, adding, "It's almost tinged with shame."

Christie spoke of feeling ashamed of the sleeplessness she suffered every night. "Even my best friend and my mother—I'll go without sleeping for days and I won't tell them," she said. Christie described her mother as "a real spiritual woman," "a comforting type of mother" who listened when she had things to confide. "But I still feel embarrassed," she said, thinking insomnia is a problem she should be able to deal with on her own. She doesn't say much about it "because it's a negative thing. And I don't want everybody feeling sorry for me all the time."

Feeling judged by others; judging ourselves. Feeling embarrassed and ashamed of a problem that is not of our choosing and may not be entirely in our power to cure. What's it all about? Go online to read about insomnia, or pick up a pamphlet at the doctor's office, and the disorder today is described in neutral terms. Insomniacs get lots of advice—don't drink too much coffee, don't read in bed—but it's served up in the same spirit as advice on how to avoid the common cold or control hemorrhoids.

Insomnia lends itself to speculation, though, first because its underlying causes are not well understood. Scientists know a lot more now than they did twenty-five years ago, yet insomnia today is still considered the biggest black box of sleep-disorders medicine. Another problem is the subjective nature of the beast. We know we have insomnia because of our symptoms, and not because of anything a doctor has seen or identified based on a lab test or even a sleep study. Moreover, throughout much of history, insomnia was viewed not as a health problem in its own right but rather as a symptom of some other condition. All this leaves plenty of room for conjecture. With no definitive diagnostic measures or scientific certainty about its origins, at times viewed as a sideshow rather than the main event, insomnia has for some sufferers led to feelings of guilt and shame.

But lack of scientific certainty never kept pundits from speculating about the causes of insomnia or making assumptions about people who had it. On the contrary, physicians in every era have proffered explanations for nocturnal wakefulness and drawn moral inferences about the afflicted. Early ideas about sleeplessness appeared in medical texts. Beginning in the nineteenth century, articles about sleeplessness appeared in the popular press as well. These sources suggest a historical basis for negative attitudes that exist today. Looking at how these attitudes developed over time may help to defuse their power and will pave the way for the more contemporary, science-based discussion to come.

What We Do or Neglect to Do

Physicians from Hippocrates until well into the nineteenth century explained all health problems as imbalances in the four bodily humors. The health of our forebears depended on their innate capacity to balance the humors—black bile, yellow bile, phlegm, and blood—and eliminate wastes. So nature was destiny.[1] An overall blend of humors determined a person's bodily constitution, mental status, and susceptibility to disease. At the same time, the state of his or her health at any moment depended on the interaction between these internal forces and forces outside the body. Unwise dietary choices could throw the humors out of whack, as could insufficient rest and exercise, excessive mental activity, climate change, travel, and even the position of the planets and the stars. A body that could not withstand these challenges and bring the humors back into balance suffered lapses in health.

Sleeplessness was among the lapses. Fifteenth- and sixteenth-century authorities such as Marsilio Ficino and André du Laurens regarded it as a symptom of melancholia, an affliction common among intellectuals and characterized by too much black bile. Sleeplessness then was not cause for blame. Rather, wakefulness at night was to the man of philosophy like a bad back to the laborer or cowpox to the dairy farmer: an occupational hazard. But it should not be ignored. Long bouts of sleeplessness could dry out the brain, warned Ficino near the end of the fifteenth century. He recommended that every effort be made to feed the sufferer a sleep-friendly diet, anoint his forehead with sleep-inducing oils, sing him lullabies, and wash his body with sweet baths.[2]

Medical authorities by the end of the eighteenth century agreed that inherited and environmental factors were still the main determinants of health. But it was also possible to forestall and even reverse chronic illness by adopting sensible habits. People might inherit a proclivity to gout or "nervous ills" like hypochondria or hysteria, but they could avoid these disorders by leading a well-regulated life. "Not from the natural defects of our constitutions, therefore, but the abuse of them, proceed all our chronic diseases," wrote the physician William Cadogan in 1772. And by adopting healthy habits, the development of chronic disease could be reversed. Cadogan counseled a return to health through exercise, temperance, and peace of mind. The physician William Buchan in 1785 concurred. When it came to chronic health conditions, he wrote, "the cure must ever depend chiefly upon the patient's own endeavours."[3]

These attitudes remained in place until the middle of the nineteenth century. Physicians advised that sound sleep would come if the wakeful practiced regular and healthful habits. Was your bedroom small and dark? "This is an important error in the conduct of life," counseled a physician in 1823. One ought to "choose for a bed-chamber a spacious room exposed to the sun, that can be opened in the day for the admission of pure air and the dispersion of the vapours collected in the night." Were you prone to taking daytime naps? "Sleeping during the day is . . . a pernicious practice, which should be carefully avoided," opined another physician. He also warned against retiring after a full meal. One should eat a light supper and wait at least two hours before going to bed. The Scottish physician Robert Macnish suggested that to sleep well, a person should "keep himself in as cheerful a mood as possible—should rise early, if his strength permits it, and take such exercise as to fatigue himself moderately." Above all, no studying should be done late at night. Students should rather "engage in severe studies early in the day, and devote two or three hours preceding bed time to light reading, music, or amusing conversation." Only when sleeplessness resisted changes in conduct was opium advised.[4]

The upside to this take-charge attitude toward the alleviation of chronic health problems was its message of hope: the power to overcome the affliction lay within the sufferer's own grasp. The downside, medical historian Charles Rosenberg has observed, was the implication that you were in large part responsible for your plight.[5] For some among the wakeful, this may have induced guilt, implying that sleeplessness was a torment they brought upon themselves. You made your bed, and now you lay in it . . . wide awake! If efforts to regulate your habits did not improve your sleep, you might feel guiltier still for having failed. Then as now, an affliction presumed to be manageable through choices in conduct could be experienced in two different ways.

Nocturnal wakefulness by the nineteenth century was classified in medical handbooks not as a symptom of melancholia but rather as a disorder of the nervous system or a symptom of "nervous disease." This whole category of health complaints—including fatigue, restlessness, hysteria, and depression—was suspect. Laymen especially, Rosenberg writes, "seemed prone to the belief that 'nervous' ills were in fact imaginary—and thus culpable." Some clinicians held this attitude as well. In practice they dismissed complaints like wakefulness at night and dysphoria as "only nervousness."[6]

But the authors of medical handbooks took the complaints of nervous patients seriously and advised that nocturnal wakefulness be attended to. Unlike practitioners of medicine in later generations, these authorities did not make distinctions between illnesses of the body and illnesses of the mind. The understanding among early nineteenth-century physicians was that malfunctions of the body were always in danger of spreading to the mind, and vice versa. "Every part of the body was related inevitably and inextricably with every other," writes Rosenberg. "A distracted mind could curdle the stomach; a dyspeptic stomach could agitate the mind."[7] Sleeplessness was thus worthy of medical attention if for no other reason than it could develop into something worse.

And sometimes it did. Persistent sleeplessness could shade into insanity, warned Scottish physician Robert Macnish in his book *Philosophy of Sleep*. *The American Journal of Insanity* in 1845 concurred: "In our opinion, the most frequent and immediate cause of insanity, and one [of] the most important to guard against, is the want of sleep." This belief gained traction in the middle decades of the nineteenth century. At a time when incarceration of the insane was on the rise, and when insanity was provoking high levels of anxiety among "normals," the purported link between sleeplessness and insanity would have been alarming to people who slept poorly (as physicians of future generations would later comment). The link was tenacious. The notion that wakefulness at night was a precursor to and even a cause of insanity would be repeated time and time again in medical and popular literature for nearly a century.[8]

An Urban Nightmare

Articles on sleeplessness appeared in diverse publications, from the *Medical Intelligencer* to the *New England Farmer*, from *Godey's Lady's Book* to *Christian Observer*, suggesting broad interest in the topic. But in the first two-thirds of the nineteenth century, the articles did not appear often or with regularity.

Their numbers increased with the spread of the printing press following the Civil War, when there was a change in attitude about nocturnal wakefulness. Writers in the last third of the century tended

to attribute trouble sleeping less to bad habits than to new environmental challenges. Sleeplessness was "the great foe of great cities,"
asserted one writer, where life was more stimulating, and at once
faster paced and more sedentary, than life on the farm. "An over
stimulation of all our powers is the besetting evil of our generation,"
disturbing the balance between mind and body and causing sleeplessness, wrote Helen L. Bostwick. Who could sleep in a place like
the New York City Mark Twain described in 1867, where "every man
seems to feel that he has got the duties of two lifetimes to accomplish
in one," and vehicular traffic posed a mortal threat to pedestrians
who ventured to cross the street on foot? The elevated train with its
all-night roar was the worst offender of all, complained a New York
City doctor writing about city noises and their effects on health. "It
seems impossible that anyone should ever be able to sleep in a room
anywhere near it."[9]

Concerns about effects of the urban environment on health
coincided with the birth of neurology as a medical specialty in
the final third of the nineteenth century. Neurology laid claim to a
broad array of health concerns: physical afflictions like paralysis and
chorea, mental afflictions like insanity and hysteria, and common
nervous ailments like dyspepsia and fatigue. Wakefulness at night
was among the common nervous ailments. New York City neurologist William Alexander Hammond singled it out as worthy of special
attention. "At present," he wrote in *On Wakefulness*, published in
1866, "there are, probably, but few physicians engaged in extensive
practice in any of our large cities who do not in the course of the
year meet with several cases of obstinate wakefulness." Insomnia—a
term Hammond helped to popularize—was on the rise.[10]

Hammond saw insomnia as an inevitable consequence of the
cultural changes occurring in America as the country moved from
an agricultural toward an industrial economy. Americans were leaving the farm and moving to the city to take up occupations involving
sustained use of mental faculties. Businessmen, bankers, lawyers,
stockbrokers, accountants, engineers, scientists, and "ambitious
women" who aspired to practice these professions were engaging
in "brainwork" to an unprecedented degree. Hammond applauded
the resulting "advances in civilization and refinement," regarding
them as necessary and beneficial to society overall. But he warned
about the health consequences. Overwork of the brain was plac-

ing increasing strain on the nervous system, destroying tissue and interfering with the body's ability to restore itself through sleep.[11]

By Hammond's time, the concept of disease specificity had entered mainstream medical thought. Rather than every instance of illness being unique, depending on constitutional vulnerabilities and the environmental forces pressing down upon a particular patient at a particular time, it now appeared that people fell ill from specific diseases, each disorder having a unique causal mechanism and a characteristic clinical course. It didn't matter who the afflicted was, what her habits were, or in what climate she got sick. Also gaining ground in the last third of the century was the belief that all disorders— whether physical or mental in origin—involved some type of tissue damage. Scientists might not yet have discovered where the damage lay. But they were confident that lesions of some sort would eventually be located in people suffering from every chronic affliction.[12]

This was the context in which Hammond undertook to explain the causal mechanisms behind insomnia. Based on his observations of a patient with a traumatic brain injury and on experiments that he, and later British researcher A.E. Durham, conducted on animals, Hammond concluded that sleep was associated with decreases in the circulation of blood in the brain. Stimulation of the brain, on the other hand, appeared to increase circulation. Emotion and mental activity stimulated the brain, increased circulation, and kept people awake at night, he observed. And when their wakefulness continued night after night, the cerebral blood vessels, in a state of constant engorgement, lost their normal elasticity. "Like a bladder filled to repletion with urine," Hammond wrote, the blood vessels became "paralyzed and unable to contract upon their contents." Flabby from overuse, the cerebral blood vessels could no longer contract in order to restrict the flow of blood and induce sleep. The result was insomnia, or "cerebral hyperaemia," as Hammond later called it.[13]

Untreated, cerebral hyperaemia could have dire consequences. A physician in a novel Hammond wrote, *Robert Severne,* tells the story of a well-known literary gentleman whose two-week bout with insomnia landed him in an insane asylum. Cerebral hyperaemia could also lead to apoplexy, epilepsy, mania, tumors, and a general softening of the brain. It could even end in death.[14]

But not to worry, Hammond reassured his colleagues and the public. Cerebral hyperaemia could be reversed with treatment from a neurological specialist. Hammond sought to cure his patients with conventional therapies involving exercise and dietary regimens, massage, and warm baths. If these didn't work, he advised cauterizing and icing the nape of the neck, administering low doses of electrical current, and, when all else failed, sedating with the drug potassium bromide. "I have never seen it fail when given in sufficient quantity," wrote Hammond of his preferred hypnotic. The records he kept document a phenomenal success rate in curing cerebral hyperaemia. Over a six-year period, of 507 cases of simple insomnia, Hammond reported curing 478, a whopping 94 percent![15]

Hammond wrote the first important American textbook on neurology, and well-heeled New Yorkers came to him with a variety of neurological complaints. But insomnia was his cause célèbre. He devoted more attention to it than any other physician then or for many decades hence. His explanation for insomnia—that it was caused by cerebral congestion due to flabby blood vessels—was dismissed by succeeding generations of neurologists as undemonstrable in the laboratory.[16] But if Hammond was wrong about the science, his insistence that complaints of poor sleep be taken seriously gave moral legitimacy to an ailment often dismissed as imaginary or "only nervous." Patients accustomed to having their complaints of sleeplessness brushed off found empathy instead. This alone could go a long way toward explaining Hammond's success rate in curing insomnia, which if verifiable would be the envy of any physician working in sleep medicine today.

The sleepless in the nineteenth century found another champion in the neurologist George M. Beard. While for Hammond insomnia was the defining symptom of cerebral hyperaemia, in Beard's scheme of things, sleeplessness was but one of many symptoms of a nervous disorder he called "neurasthenia." Neurasthenia developed in people suffering from "lack of nerve-force." But its pathology remained vague. That some type of tissue damage underlay the disorder was certain, Beard felt, but it would fall upon future scientists to uncover exactly what it was. Meanwhile, neurasthenia would be considered a "functional" disorder rather than a disorder with a known physiologic mechanism.[17]

Insomnia was the first on Beard's list of seventy-nine symptoms of neurasthenia, including fatigue, headache, noises in the ears, inexplicable fears, and "vague pains and flying neuralgias." Poor sleep was a common complaint among the nervous patients who sought Beard's help, "one of the most constant symptoms of neurasthenia." Likewise, improved sleep was often the first sign that a neurasthenic was on the mend. "Sleeplessness . . . one of the most common of all the symptoms, and one of the most distressing to patients, is sometimes relieved in a few days after treatment is begun," Beard said.[18]

Like Hammond, Beard maintained that the incidence of nervous disorders was on the rise, and that the main culprit was "modern civilization." Brain strain, competition, worries about job performance, concern for punctuality, and anxieties relating to business and finance—all elements of the urban lifestyle—were taking a toll on health, Beard said. "Steam power, the periodical press, the telegraph, the sciences, and the mental activity of women" were pushing Americans beyond their natural limits.[19] The result was a dissipation of nervous energy and an increase in insomnia and other nervous complaints.

The belief that heredity was a key determinant of health and susceptibility to illness was strong in the last third of the nineteenth century, and Beard stressed its importance in the development of nervous disease. Each person inherited a fixed amount of nerve-force, he said; in no two people was that amount the same. There were "millionaires of nerve-force," born with enough of the electrical essence to power them through adversity to stunning heights of achievement. Other people inherited smaller amounts of nerve-force; but they, too, could manage if they lived within their means. "The man with a small income is really rich, " Beard wrote, "as long as there is no overdraft on the account; so the nervous man may be really well and in fair working order as long as he does not draw on his limited store of nerve-force." Trouble often arose in people born into the higher social classes. The civilized, the refined, the educated, and those destined for high positions inherited a finer "nervous organization" than the "barbarous" and low-born. The store of nerve-force possessed by the elites was sometimes unequal to the tasks they were called upon to perform. So they were vulnerable to insomnia and other nervous complaints.[20]

Some physicians were skeptical that nervous ailments were worthy of medical attention, and Beard endeavored to correct this error in judgment. "Very many of the symptoms of neurasthenia have been regarded by men of science as imaginations of the patients, proofs of hypochondria," he wrote. Physicians tended to believe in ailments that they could see or feel or measure, and nervous symptoms like insomnia, perceived only by the patient, were suspect. Yet just as people had once mistakenly dismissed the insane as being possessed by the devil, so science would one day prove it was a mistake to regard the "obscure phenomena of the nervous system" as inconsequential. Neurasthenia was not necessarily a portal to more serious illness. But it could be. "When neglected or treated improperly," Beard wrote, "it may, in time, advance to any one of quite a large number of familiar maladies of the nervous system," including insanity, melancholia, hysteria, inebriety, and addiction to narcotics.[21] In line with his belief that neurasthenia was a functional illness, Beard was a firm proponent of physical remedies such as massage and electrical current. Like Hammond, he made liberal use of medical devices in his efforts to treat nervous complaints.

In the end, Beard's crusade to convince his peers of the legitimacy of neurasthenia as a medical diagnosis was successful, helping to remove some of the stigma attached to nervous ailments like insomnia and fatigue. "Within a decade of Beard's death in 1883," medical historian Charles Rosenberg has written, "the diagnosis of nervous exhaustion had become part of the office furniture of most physicians."[22] In fact, neurasthenia—because of its association with status and refinement—came to have cachet.

Concern about insomnia as a health problem in its own right was on the rise in the era of Hammond and Beard, if the number of published articles serves as an indication. Insomnia, the pundits averred, was becoming a national plague. Hardest hit were urban professionals, whose work involved sustained intellectual activity and left little time for physical exercise. But it could also afflict their high-strung wives. Prone to insomnia and nervous exhaustion was the votary of fashionable living, who strove to outshine her rivals in dress and entertainment, "whose existence is one perpetual round of excitement, without adequate time for recuperation." Children, too, were developing extraordinary nervous disorders. Instances of insomnia, "that malady which ought to belong alone to that period of life when the vital powers have been overstrained . . . are also appearing among our little ones," a commentator in *The New York Times* lamented. The cause was too much brainwork and too many hours in school.[23]

Some pundits toward the end of the nineteenth century held that insomnia was a relatively benign and reversible condition, resulting from poor choices in conduct. But more common was the view that insomnia was a serious health problem that, if long sustained, could have dire consequences. Obituary columns of major newspapers reinforced the latter view.

A steamship engineer of Yorktown, NY committed suicide by cutting his throat with a razor. "He was a victim of insomnia," according to the obituary, "and when seen by officials of the [steamship] line several days ago he said that his nerves had been completely unstrung by loss of sleep."[24]

"Richard T. Fussell Driven to Suicide by Insomnia," announced the secondary headline of an obituary of a Washington ice cream manufacturer who checked into a hotel and gassed himself to death.[25]

"Insomnia Cause of Woman's Suicide," ran the headline for the obituary of Eliza Koven, 44, of Jersey City. "She shot herself twice, once in the head and the second time through the heart. Mrs. Koven had been in poor health for six weeks past and complained that she could not sleep."[26]

Wrote a *Washington Post* journalist about insomnia, "Scarcely a week passes during which we do not read of a death—self-inflicted or otherwise—caused by this horrible curse." A steady diet of insomnia-induced suicides served up in the newspaper would have heightened anxieties among the wakeful, as late nineteenth- and early twentieth-century physicians would later attest.[27]

On the other hand, one burden the sleepless did not have to contend with as much as in earlier decades was censure. A few moralistic voices suggested wakefulness at night was the price the insomniac paid for lazy, intemperate habits, and that good sleep was something that had to be earned. But these voices were in the minority. Like William Hammond and George Beard, writers of feature articles and advice columns more often attributed insomnia to environmental and hereditary factors that were not so amenable to change.

Could the insomniac businessman afford to put aside his affairs after dinner if his competitors were burning the lamp at both ends? Could his wife—at pains to manage a household, see to the welfare of her children, and live up to her social obligations—be blamed if she was too overwrought to sleep? Not many writers sat in judgment on sufferers like these. Fewer still advocated turning back the clock to a time when Americans earned their livelihood through healthier pursuits on the farm. If Americans of delicate nervous organization were succumbing to insomnia, it was not their fault. Popular opinion stood firmly with Hammond and Beard in this regard, reflecting, among other things, some of the social anxieties of the Gilded Age. Civilization was evolving faster than the human organism could keep pace with, and good sleep was falling by the wayside.

Overall, insomnia elicited mainly concern and compassion among those whose advice columns appeared in newspapers and magazines. Whether they prescribed old-fashioned remedies or new techniques like deep breathing and thought control, they did so in the main with empathy. Insomnia was a "distressing malady," "one of the greatest of personal afflictions," filled with "prolonged and dreary tortures," and "an unequivocal sign of suffering." For insomniacs who in years past had had their complaints dismissed, the acknowledgment that insomnia could cause significant suffering and was worthy of attention would have been a comfort. In this respect at least, the last third of the nineteenth century was a kinder, gentler era for sufferers of insomnia and other nervous ills.[28]

A Mind Diseased

Many nineteenth-century neurologists prescribed physical remedies such as massage, hydrotherapy, and electrotherapy for insomnia and other nervous ailments, believing these complaints were caused by malfunctions of the body. But by the 1880s and 1890s, some neurologists were beginning to suspect it was primarily the *psychic* value of the treatments, rather than their physical effects, that led to the cure.

During this same period, younger neurologists were seeking to classify the main symptoms of neurasthenia into two categories: physical and mental. There was broad agreement about which symptoms belonged in each category. The main *physical* symptoms of neurasthenia were excessive fatigue, gastric disturbances, and headache. Number one on the list of *mental* symptoms was insomnia, followed by a lack of concentration, depression, unreasonable fears, and irritability. By the 1890s, these mental symptoms were the chief diagnostic indicators of neurasthenia. Associated physical complaints were increasingly regarded as imaginary or psychosomatic. Once seen as an illness caused by malfunctions of the body,

neurasthenia in all its manifestations was now understood to origi-
nate in the mind.[29]

Agnes H. Morton reflects this change in attitude with her
"moral" perspective on insomnia printed in the *Chautauquan* at the
turn of the twentieth century: "The most stubborn cases of insomnia
are not due to physical causes," she wrote, "and therefore do not yield
to physical remedies. The sleepless one rarely confides to a physician the anxieties and the emotional disturbances that are the real
cause of unrest. In vain does the patient follow prescriptions, unless
the physician has the insight and the wisdom to 'minister to a mind
diseased.'" Willpower, asserted Morton and her contemporaries, was
the key to overcoming the worries that most often sabotaged sleep.[30]

This change in attitude did not occur overnight. In 1876, when
George Beard first suggested some nervous diseases might be rooted
in the emotions and that it would be worthwhile to investigate the
efficacy of mental therapeutics, the idea met with scorn. If Beard
were taken seriously, William Hammond averred, "we should go
back to monkery—give up our instruments, give up our medicines
and enter a convent." The notion that mental therapeutics might be
effective in combating nervous ailments at first struck nineteenth-
century American neurologists as thoroughly unscientific.[31]

But lay healers had long embraced it. These healers preached
that bodily ills were psychologically induced, and that talk therapy
could rid people of the negative thinking that was making them
sick. Phineas Parkhurst Quimby, a New England clockmaker,
was the first of these influential nineteenth-century mind curists.
Before his death in 1866, he claimed to have administered his
talking cure to over twelve thousand men, women, and children.
Warren Felt Evans, who consulted with Quimby, gave up his Meth-
odist ministry to campaign for mental healing all over the United
States. Evans went on to establish a Massachusetts sanitarium dedicated to the study of the "word cure" and the practice of mental
healing.[32]

Mary Baker Eddy became the most famous of the nineteenth-
century mind curists. A chronic invalid in her adult years, Eddy
consulted with Quimby, and three weeks later she felt healthy again.
She too became a proponent of the idea that disease was "caused
and cured by mind alone." Marrying her philosophy of illness to
religious doctrine, she founded the Church of Christ, Scientist and

promoted a doctrine of salvation through positive thinking and belief in Jesus Christ. Eddy and other mind curists attracted tens of thousands of followers. Trained physicians, however, viewed them with contempt.[33]

Neurologists by the turn of the century were rethinking their approach to curing nervous ills. Science had failed to uncover lesions or other physiological problems in people with abnormal behavior. Moreover, it was becoming clear in medical circles that the mind curists, uneducated though they might be, were actually curing people using psychotherapeutic methods. This being the case, the neurologist Lewellys F. Barker observed in 1906, then surely psychotherapy would be far superior if administered by trained physicians. Neurologist Sheldon Leavitt was thinking along the same lines. "Why not enter and cultivate a field now running to weeds but capable of developing the richest fruits?"[34]

Psychologists were already on board with the idea that psychic factors lay behind the functional nervous ills. "The mental element undoubtedly plays a very important part, and particularly in maintaining the neurosis after it has been once established," wrote Tufts University professor of medicine Morton Prince. Mental therapeutics could also effect cures. Prince's therapeutic method was similar to that of the mind curists. He explained to his patients that their symptoms were the result of false beliefs and bad habits, which he then endeavored to help his patients correct.[35]

One well-publicized foray into the use of psychotherapy to treat neurasthenics was launched by two prominent clergymen and consulting neurologists in the Boston area. From 1906 to 1910, Episcopalian ministers Elwood Worcester and Samuel McComb conducted clinics in the vestry of the Emmanuel Church. The clinics were for the benefit of patients who were "the despair of the ordinary practitioner," that is, "these nervous sufferers with their insomnias, their shifting hysterical pains, their phobias, their hallucinations, their manias, depressions, and harmful exaltations, their intense irritability, their profound weakness, their moral perversion, their morbid feelings, their bad habits." The message Worcester and McComb communicated to nervous sufferers was filled with hope. The afflicted could overcome their problems by placing themselves in the hands of an authority figure who administered "moral treatment," encouraging the development of new habits and a positive mindset. This message was in perfect harmony with the can-do spirit of the Progressive Era. Interest in the effort spread quickly, and Emmanuel clinics sprang up in several churches in the East and the Midwest.[36]

In fact, the sleepless could cure themselves, McComb preached to the readers of *Good Housekeeping* and *Harper's Bazaar*. Much of his advice was conventional. The sleepless should examine their daytime conduct and "eliminate the physical and mental mischiefs," including heavy meals and intoxicating drinks at night. Deep-breathing exercises could help with relaxation. At night, the sleepless should induce in themselves a state of mental monotony and turn away "from all sad preoccupations such as misfortunes, grief, remorse, apprehension."[37] To those who could silence negative thinking, sleep would come.

McComb placed emphasis on fear of sleeplessness as a causal factor in insomnia, and on the role suggestion played in its genesis and could play in its cure. "Very often insomnia or partial sleeplessness is the result of a bad auto-suggestion," he said, "namely, that one cannot sleep. It is this more or less fixed idea of the impossibility of sleep that makes sleep impossible." But that which the mind created could by the mind be cured. Fear of sleeplessness could be overcome in two ways. One, sufferers could nip it in the bud by mental fiat. "Say to yourself: I don't care a fig whether I sleep or not; if I sleep, well; if I do not sleep, also well. . . . This formula often works like magic." Those for whom the magic failed were advised to employ the power of suggestion: "Let the sufferer from sleeplessness say again and again to himself, I *can* sleep, I *ought* to sleep, therefore I *will* sleep. Let him fill his mind with the enthusiastic hope of sleep, and he will reverse the morbid action of self-suggestion and gain the sleep he needs."[38]

Some early twentieth-century physicians also embraced the idea that insomnia was driven by the fear of sleeplessness, and that it was amenable to cure with suggestion therapy. James J. Walsh, a neurologist and medical historian at Fordham University, explained how this dread of insomnia came to exist and could be overcome. Insomnia started during a moment of crisis. A banker or lawyer suffered a few sleepless nights and then, prey to the newspapers' "sensational cultivation of dreads with regard to insomnia," began to fear for his health and sanity. In turn, he began to obsess about his sleep loss, worsening the insomnia and concluding that he was incapable of sleep at all. Worst among those who dreaded wakefulness at night were the very nerve specialists to whom insomnia sufferers often turned for help, Walsh noted. He likened this phenomenon to "a bald-headed man confidently repeating his visits to a bald-headed specialist in order to be cured of bald-headedness." ("Fortunately for some of us," he quipped, "a man does not wear on his forehead the sign of his insomnia quite as he does in the case of bald-headedness.")[39]

In reality, Walsh claimed, it was hard to find any recorded cases of insomnia sufferers who went on to experience serious consequences as a result. On the contrary, many endured long bouts of insomnia in their working years and lived to a ripe old age. The demon behind insomnia was nothing but a "faulty state of mind."[40]

Moral treatment and suggestion were the keys to the cure. The physician should first establish with the patient "a strong bond of confidence and sympathy." Then, by means of suggestion and persuasion, the doctor should correct the patient's misconceptions about insomnia and instill in him the confidence that he could sleep. Whether during hypnosis or when the patient was fully awake, the suggestion that "to-night you are going to sleep soundly," accompanied by a monotonous noise intended to make the patient drowsy, would put him to sleep. After a series of doctor's visits like this, the patient would be cured.[41]

The notion that insomnia was curable through suggestion must have been a comfort in the early twentieth century, when anxiety about insomnia remained high. Through the early 1930s, obituaries continued to feature alarming headlines like these: "Insomnia Victim Leaps to Death," "Patient Insane from Insomnia Attacked Doctor Called to Attend Him," "Tragic Insomnia: Murderous Rage Caused by Lack of Sleep Proves Fatal to Two People," "Unfortunate Victim of Insomnia Takes Own Life After Doctors Fail to Give Him Relief."[42]

Feature articles about sleep and insomnia contained other distressing information, too. Often cited were the results of a cruel experiment conducted by the Russian scientist Marie de Manaceine in 1894. De Manaceine set out to study the effects of sleep deprivation on ten puppies. She fed the puppies but completely deprived them of sleep by keeping them in constant activity. After four or five days, all the puppies had collapsed from exhaustion and died. This result and her conclusion, "the total absence of sleep is more fatal for the animals than the total absence of food," became the boilerplate in sleep and insomnia articles in the popular press, suggesting that the period human beings could survive without sleep might be very short indeed. The idea that insomnia was a faster-acting killer than starvation was disseminated in medical schools. "Taught to every medical man of older generations and to every medical fledgling of to-day," the physician Frederick Peterson complained, "it finds its way to general public acceptance, begetting in the lay mind terrors of insanity and death which haunt every unfortunate victim of insomnia."[43]

In this alarmist context, the idea that sound sleep could be achieved, either through counseling from a physician or one's own efforts to adopt constructive habits and a positive mindset, was doubtless empowering. Insomniacs confident that they *could* sleep were certainly more likely *to* sleep. It also must have been reassuring to hear that a few nights of insomnia did not set them on the path to madness.

But there was another side to the coin. If moral treatment and suggestion could cure sleeplessness, the implication was that there was nothing organically wrong and that insomnia was conjured up wholly in the mind. And who was responsible for this state of affairs but the insomnia sufferer herself? If early nineteenth-century insomnia sufferers had to answer for intemperate habits, early twentieth-century insomniacs were open to blame of a different kind. Pundits looked behind insomnia and saw a host of mental and moral failings.

A short story that appeared in *The Chicago Defender* in 1913 featured a wakeful protagonist whose insomnia had for some time provoked the solicitous attention of his wife and friends. This he thoroughly enjoyed. But the game was up with the arrival of Mrs. Shandle, "who had known Kellinger at the disillusionizing age of 10."

"Stuff and nonsense, Tommy Kellinger!" she said upon hearing of the chronic complaint. "I think . . . you've grown attached to this sleepless idea and hate to tell it to move on. I'm ashamed of you! And your wife is an easy mark!"

His shameful motive exposed, Kellinger yawned and fell asleep, and never had trouble sleeping again.[44]

The Reverend Samuel McComb had increasingly negative things to say about insomnia sufferers in the years following the collapse of the Emmanuel Movement. The sleepless were prone to worry, unhealthy self-analysis, and brooding introspection, he wrote in 1911. They were "petty," "self-centered," "untrustful," "skeptical," "unbelieving," and possessed of a "pessimistic attitude toward things in general."[45]

Some of the most disparaging comments about insomnia sufferers came from physicians. People "whose insomnia is chiefly 'in their mind,'" Dr. Woods Hutchinson observed in *Good Housekeeping* in 1915, "take a perpetual interest in the disturbances of their own internal mechanisms, because they have not enough to keep them properly amused otherwise."[46]

"It is amusing to see how exacting these insomniacs are, in demanding uninterrupted quiet for their hours of wakefulness," wrote Dr. Josephine A. Jackson in *Woman's Home Companion* in 1923, following publication of her book, *Outwitting Our Nerves*. "No clock must tick, no dog bark, there must be no household noises after they retire, although they never get to sleep until midnight or after!" The real problem for the insomniac, Jackson said, was that he was irresistibly and interminably fascinated with himself. "Little does the insomniac think that he is playing the role of Narcissus, as he stays awake to think over what he has done or to agonize over what is to become of him. Like Narcissus, he is content with contemplation." So content, in fact, that he will resist all forms of treatment. "Alas! To be cured would bring an end to a favorite pastime."[47]

Insomnia was a trivial matter in the eyes of many commentators in the early twentieth century. The sleepless should quit complaining and turn their attention to something else. But insomniacs and their complaints *were* taken seriously by some medical professionals, as we will see later in the chapter.

By 1920, the diagnosis of neurasthenia in the United States was passé, seen as lacking specificity. The moral treatment and suggestion therapy proffered during the Progressive Era had fallen out of favor as well. A more rigorous sorting of health complaints was under way, to be distributed among physicians of ever-increasing specialization. Functional complaints formerly treated by neurologists and general practitioners were now regarded as falling within the domain of the psychologist.

Insomnia was one such complaint. Insomnia was understood to be a symptom of many things, from organic disease such as hyperthyroidism and parkinsonism to bad habits such as working late and drinking coffee after dinner. Physicians often treated it as a medical disorder, with chloral hydrate, sulphonal, paraldehyde, and the increasingly popular barbiturate sleeping pills. But the prevailing view was that in the majority of cases, insomnia was caused by an overanxious and vigilant mind. Like many other nervous disorders, insomnia was regarded as psychosomatic. Insomniacs might think the root of their problem lay in their bodies, but in reality it was the psyche, not some malfunctioning of the central nervous system, that was sabotaging sleep.[48]

Sigmund Freud didn't say much about insomnia. But the little he did say influenced the American psychoanalysts who treated it in subsequent decades. Freud attributed insomnia to a fear of the unwelcome discoveries that sleep might bring. In the waking hours, socially unacceptable desires—murderous impulses toward a parent, for example, or a wish to engage in perverse sexual activity, comprising that part of the psyche he named the id—were successfully blocked from view by an internal censor, the superego. At night this censor went off-duty. Forbidden wishes were then free to reveal themselves in dreams. This prospect could be frightening. "There are some neurotic patients who are unable to sleep and who admit to us that their insomnia was originally intentional," Freud wrote. "They did not dare to sleep because they were afraid of their dreams— afraid, that is, of the results of the weakening of the censorship."[49]

This war between the superego and the id lay at the heart of some insomniacs' inability to sleep, said American psychoanalysts who in the 1940s and 1950s incorporated Freud's ideas into their practice. Unconscious emotional conflicts were keeping insomnia sufferers awake at night. These conflicts and the insomnia they gave rise to would not likely resolve on their own. But they would respond to psychoanalysis. The psychoanalyst's job was to uncover the shameful desires the internal censor was straining to repress. He did this by listening to his patient talk about past experiences and dreams, sifting through this material for the true causes of her wakefulness. Exposure of the emotional conflicts behind the insomnia would enable her to adopt a healthier, more realistic approach to life. The insomnia would then fade away.

What sort of hidden material was keeping insomniacs wakeful at night? Case studies reveal a cast of characters familiar to anyone with passing knowledge of Freud. Some insomniacs were afraid of culturally unacceptable erotic desires, such as homoerotic impulses, incestuous yearnings, or the urge to masturbate. Some had castration fears. There were Oedipal jealousies and death wishes toward parents, and associated feelings of guilt. There were suicidal wishes and fears of death. One psychoanalyst reported a patient who came in for therapy unaware of the anxieties that lay behind his insomnia, the main one being an insatiable and frustrated ambition. Another psychoanalyst reported two patients whose insomnia derived from a fear of cancer, which developed because of hidden guilt over hostility toward a dead rival. Yet another reported a patient whose dream of being forced to slave away on a ship by the captain and first mate led to the uncovering of the real cause of his insomnia: rage toward his dictatorial father and older brother. Whatever the unacceptable feelings, insomnia was the defense the superego used to keep them out of sight.[50]

Psychoanalysts who published case reports were convinced that exposing these internal conflicts could cure insomnia. "States of insomnia due to psychogenic causes are entirely amenable to intensive psychotherapy and are curable when the psychodynamics are ferreted out," wrote psychoanalyst Jacob H. Conn.[51] Some insomnia patients evidently responded to psychoanalysis (and were willing to endure months and years of therapy, and affluent enough to pay for it!). At the very least, the psychoanalyst was a doctor who took the problem seriously, which could only have helped.

Psychoanalysts were never able to show their method was useful for more than a small group of insomnia sufferers, though. "Indeed," wrote psychiatrists I. Karacan and R.L. Williams in 1971, "it has not yet been shown that concurrent, underlying psychopathological conditions are of general occurrence in the development of insomnia symptoms."[52] No large-scale studies were mounted to show that psychoanalysis was an effective treatment for the masses of insomnia sufferers. By the end of the 1950s, mention of it in the medical literature had all but died out.

But it left a legacy in the popular press. Starting in the 1950s, journalists writing about insomnia hopped on the psychodynamic bandwagon. In addition to citing older ideas about the affliction—that it was caused by everyday cares and anxieties and by the fear of sleeplessness—they wrote about repressed internal conflicts interfering with sleep. Insomnia was not just the bane of the worrier or the hypochondriac who frittered away life fearing an imaginary illness. Insomnia by the middle of the century was also a mark of the walking wounded, curable if the sufferer submitted to psychotherapy and got the psychic damage straightened out.

A features writer in *The New York Times Magazine* in 1967 told the story of a young insomniac housewife diagnosed with an anxiety neurosis. "What she feared at bedtime were her night thoughts and the encounter with her inmost emotions," the writer said. "Two months of psychotherapy helped her to sort out the tangle of her emotions; gradually she was able once more to discharge the pent-up pressures of her psyche in dreaming sleep." Like most insomnia sufferers, the writer averred, the housewife had been "upset by emotion rather than biochemistry." Emotion was a function of the mind, and mind and body were separate entities. Thus was insomnia "all in the head."[53]

Some popular writers in the middle of the century looked to environmental factors to explain insomnia. Worry about loved ones in the armed forces kept people awake during World War II, giving rise to articles about "wartime insomnia." And the postwar decade was full of environmental stressors that could sabotage sleep. An Irwin Shaw story titled "The Climate of Insomnia" explores those pressures and their effects on a middling college professor during the McCarthy years, when merely having attended a meeting of the Communist Party and made an impolitic comment about a colleague might cost him his job.[54] Like many men struggling for middle-class stability in the postwar years, Philip Cahill has a stay-at-home wife and a host of expenses associated with a consumerist lifestyle: car payments, tuition for his daughter, insurance, taxes, clothing, the doctor, entertainment. He's barely able to make ends meet. Agonizing over the prospect of losing his job takes a toll on his sleep.

Cahill also worries about the atomic bomb. It is frightening "to contemplate exposing yourself to the atom and the microbe, feeling, too, all the while, that your well-run home, enclosing your wife and children, might at any moment dissolve in radio-active dust or become the harbor for the germs of plague. . . . How," he wonders, "does anyone sleep this year?"

Nothing about Cahill's McCarthy-era world is secure: not his family, not his place in society, not his job. One injudicious slip, or a nuclear holocaust launched upon a madman's whim, could wipe it all out. Hostile environmental forces are pressuring Cahill from all sides and robbing him of life-sustaining sleep.

Millions of Americans were in the same boat. In a period historians have labeled the "Age of Anxiety," housewives and organization men were said to be experiencing unprecedented levels of stress. Whether triggered by an inhospitable environment, everyday worries, or past experience, whether at a conscious or unconscious level, anxiety was interfering with Americans' sleep.[55]

So, did insomniacs in the 1950s and 1960s reach out for help to the psychotherapist? Not for the most part. They sought relief in sleeping pills instead. The consumption of hypnotics grew in the twentieth century by fits and starts, and later by leaps and bounds. Veronal and Luminal were popular among the sleepless after World War I, followed in subsequent decades by shorter-acting barbiturates like Amytal, Seconal, and Nembutal. By the mid-1960s, America was producing barbiturates to the tune of two thousand tons a year. One of the steepest rises in consumption occurred between 1952 and 1963, when retail sales of barbiturates increased by 535 percent (as compared to the average retail sales of all drugs during the same period, which rose by 6.5 percent).[56] Whether or not postwar Americans understood insomnia to be a psychological problem, they insisted on a chemical fix.

Sleep Science Comes of Age

A counter-narrative to the twentieth century's "all-in-the-head" story on insomnia was born in the sleep lab. After the Civil War, neurologist William Hammond had hypothesized that flabby cerebral blood vessels were the physiological mechanism behind insomnia, but his theory was never substantiated by scientific research. Nearly a century later, scientists were studying sleep and wakefulness at night with new tools, and wondering again if physiological factors lay behind insomnia.

Some experiments leading to advances in the knowledge of sleep and waking took place before the middle of the century. Constantin von Economo, a psychiatrist and neurologist working in Vienna during and after World War I, studied the brains of people who died of encephalitis lethargica (a kind of sleeping sickness) and located a center that appeared to regulate sleep. The German psychiatrist Hans

Berger in 1929 was the first to record electrical activity in the human brain with an instrument called the electroencephalograph. Using this machine, the American scientist and inventor A.L. Loomis and his colleagues identified five different stages of sleep, based on brain activity. Dutch neuroanatomist Walle Nauta, carrying von Economo's observations further, studied rats in the 1940s and eventually produced evidence that both sleep and waking centers existed in the hypothalamus. These discoveries, significant though they were, did not challenge the then-dominant belief that sleep was a passive process in which the brain was basically shut down. But the discovery of rapid eye movement sleep (REM sleep) by the pioneering sleep scientists Eugene Aserinsky and Nathaniel Kleitman in 1952, and the demonstration of its association with dreaming, marked a turning point. It was then clear that during sleep the brain was active, making sleep a more attractive subject of research.[57]

By mid-century it was known that sleep brought about a decrease in heart rate, blood pressure, and body temperature. When sleep scientist Lawrence J. Monroe measured these and other bodily functions in good and poor sleepers in the mid-1960s, he found notable differences. The poor sleepers' body temperature dropped significantly less during sleep, and their heart rate was slightly higher. They also moved more during sleep and had more vasoconstrictions, another sign of arousal. The physiological functioning of the poor sleepers was "closer to the waking end of the sleep–wakefulness continuum than for good sleepers," Monroe observed.

Electroencephalograph recordings, too, showed marked differences in the quantity and quality of sleep the groups obtained. The poor sleepers took longer to fall asleep, woke up more frequently, and slept considerably less than the good sleepers. "Phrased simply," Monroe concluded, "self-reported poor sleepers not only sleep less, but the sleep they obtain is more 'awake-like' than that of good sleepers."[58]

Monroe's study and others that followed suggested there were physiological aspects to insomnia. Was it possible this heightened bodily arousal might be a driving force behind the affliction? Early speculation on the topic was confined to academe; studies on the physiology of sleeplessness received scant coverage in the media. But the implications filtered down to the public as advice to the sleepless changed. Increasingly in the 1960s and 1970s, insomniacs were counseled in ways to reduce bodily tension. As sleepless, stressed-out Americans were flocking to their doctors for sleeping pills, advice columnists and physicians leery of drugs were touting the virtues of relaxation, meditation, and biofeedback.[59]

Perhaps the editors of mass publications felt that research on the heart rate and blood pressure of insomnia sufferers was too boring to set before the general public. But the study of brain waves evidently had sex appeal. Starting in the 1960s, journalists began visiting sleep clinics to observe scientists collect data on the sleeping brain. One writer, watching as a subject got hooked up with assorted electrodes to an electroencephalograph, declared he went to bed "looking like the inside of a telephone." Another reported on the scribblings of the machine. "Delta waves have a satisfying appearance," wrote Maggie Scarf. "They look like brain waves of deep slumber *ought* to look— lazy and easy and wide."[60] The images of brain waves that appeared in popular periodicals—resembling tracings from a parkinsonian hand whose tremor grew alternately narrow and wide, fast and slow—were purportedly pregnant with meaning. Dreams had once been called the royal road to the unconscious by a cigar-smoking Jewish atheist who listened as his patients told their stories from the couch. But modern sleep scientists studying the brain wanted none of that. The EEG was the first objective and scientifically valid key to unlocking the mysteries of sleep.

What revelations about insomniacs tumbled out of brain wave studies and into the public domain? Number one, while some sufferers' EEGs clearly set them apart from normal sleepers, other insomniacs' EEGs looked perfectly normal. In fact, the insomniac who complained he couldn't sleep a wink was often sleeping like a log, according to his EEG. He was descending into and out of deep sleep, and in and out of periods of REM sleep, with the same regularity as a normal sleeper. Some insomnia sufferers were sleeping seven or eight hours to boot. "Pseudoinsomnia" was the diagnosis given to this kind of insomniac: pseudo, as in "not actually, but having the appearance of," insomnia.[61] Patients like these—who claimed they hardly slept at all and whose sleep registered as normal on the EEG—were sent home with reassurances that they had nothing to worry about. Their problem was merely one of faulty perception. (The term "pseudoinsomnia" was soon replaced with another: "sleep state misperception." I'll say more about this in chapter 9.)

For decades doctors had contended that insomniacs were exaggerating their plight, and early EEG studies appeared to bolster this claim. "Bad sleepers are much given to self-deception," Hilary Rubinstein said in his book *The Complete Insomniac* in 1974, citing the results of EEG studies and studies of sleep deprivation. "They often claim that they never slept a wink, but this is almost never in fact the case." "Insomniacs cannot provide reliable estimates of their total sleep time," according to a 1980 report in *Working Woman*. "When insomniacs are monitored in a sleep laboratory, their dramatic claims of hours of sleeplessness are seldom borne out."[62] The discrepancy between the amount of sleep insomniacs reported and the amount the EEG recorded cast renewed doubt on the legitimacy of insomniacs' complaints. Rather than calling into question the EEG's capacity to fully evaluate insomniacs' sleep, the discrepancy was often cited in the popular media as evidence that insomnia was less serious than sufferers claimed.

At the same time, EEG studies revealed that the brain waves of insomniacs on sleeping pills were strikingly abnormal. Long-term barbiturate users experienced sleep that was shallow and nearly devoid of REM sleep. When they stopped taking their pills, they experienced "REM rebound": nights full of REM sleep and terrifying dreams. EEG studies also showed that the hypnotics that eventually replaced the barbiturates—benzodiazepines like Dalmane—were also flawed. Long-term use of benzodiazepines tended to decrease the amount of deep sleep users got.[63] The extended use of sleeping pills could degrade insomniacs' sleep and cause "drug-induced insomnia." Thus was the cure by pill said to be worse than the disease, a view long espoused in the popular press and now confirmed by the study of brain waves. (I'll treat this topic at length in chapter 10.)

Psychology Tightens Its Grip

With drugs tarnished as a remedy for insomnia and research on the biology of insomnia in its infancy, it fell to psychologists to continue explaining insomnia and proffering cures. Some offered a story not unlike Freud's. In the mid-1970s and again in the 1980s, Anthony Kales and colleagues evaluated hundreds of insomniacs with the Minnesota Multiphasic Personality Inventory (MMPI), a personality test. Kales found evidence of psychopathology in a large majority of the insomniacs tested. The most common personality trait was that of "internalization of psychological disturbances rather than by acting out or aggression." During the day, Kales said, insomniacs typically denied or repressed their hostile feelings. At night those feelings broke through into consciousness, causing physiological arousal and interfering with sleep. Kales' insomniacs also scored high on scales measuring depression, rumination, and anxiety. All this suggested a causal relationship to Kales. "The homogeneity of the MMPI profiles in our chronic insomniacs should be interpreted as strong evidence of their psychopathology being primary rather than secondary to their sleep disorder."[64]

Kales and his wife, Joyce D. Kales, wrote a book about insomnia, *Evaluation and Treatment of Insomnia*, published in 1984. In it, the authors elaborate at length on the pathologic personality traits of insomniacs (and one gets the distinct impression that they don't much admire the people they're writing about). Patients with insomnia derive "a great deal of secondary gain" from their symptoms, using them to get sympathy from familiars and shirk responsibilities. Emotionally deprived in childhood, they feel inadequate, insecure, and dependent as adults. "They also have difficulty in interpersonal relations," the Kales write. "They need and demand sympathy and support, but are often too self-preoccupied to be attentive to the feelings of others." Insomniacs are also difficult to treat, causing physicians at times to feel "anxious, frustrated, manipulated, and angry." And to top things off, insomniacs typically deny that their sleep problems have a psychological basis (accustomed as they are to denial!). The Kales' MMPI findings give the lie to this denial: psychopathology is really at the heart of sleeplessness, fueling the bodily arousal that keeps insomniacs awake.[65]

The Kales were not the only clinicians talking about insomnia and psychopathology. "The main emotion of insomnia is the insomniac's underlying *anger* at the imperfections in the world," said the psychologist Henry Kellerman, "at not being attended to, and at any impending separation from the person on whom they are dependent." "Many chronic insomniac patients are described as tense, complaining, histrionic individuals, who are oversensitive to minor discomforts and unable to relax easily," stated the sleep researcher Quentin Regestein. The first fifty-four patients seen at

a sleep clinic in Cincinnati had "a disturbed, neurotic profile" sug-
gestive of "depressive aspects to their personality and a heightened
somatic concern of a hypochondriacal nature." Insomniacs seen at
the Sleep Disorders Clinic at Penn State Hershey "appeared to be
a distressed, pessimistic, worried group, who faced the world with
apprehension, anxiety, and self-deprecation." Good sleepers appear
"busier, more active, and more involved in their work and with other
people," wrote sleep investigator E.J. Marchini and her colleagues.
Insomniacs seem "more preoccupied with self."[66] As described by
clinical researchers, insomniacs were not the kind of people you'd
want to spend time talking to at a party, much less go out with on
a date.

The popular press picked up on the link between insomnia and
psychopathology, and ran with it. There, as in medical journals,
the relationship between psychopathology and insomnia was often
alleged to be causal rather than correlational. "Much chronic insomnia is psychogenic, resulting from such very common disorders as
depression and anxiety and from such other emotional conflicts as
neurotic guilt or phobic dread of dreaming or dying while asleep."
"Most insomniacs have underlying psychological problems of
which the sleeping difficulties are only a symptom." "Most victims
of insomnia find it necessary to reject their unacceptable feelings.
. . . The insomniac personality may be described as one that needs to
deny, either consciously or unconsciously, feelings of hostility toward
important people in his or her life." "The majority of insomniacs . . .
seem to have psychological problems, which include a 'history of
chronic anxiety, unhappiness, low self-esteem, and passive dependency.'" "Some insomniacs . . . are given to an excessive degree of
self-pity and dependence upon the emotional support of others."
Insomniacs "take things hard, feel they haven't lived 'the right kind
of life' and are high-strung."[67]

In self-help books, the sleepless were sometimes blamed for
their poor sleep. In *Forty Winks at the Drop of a Hat,* published in
1968, Valerie Moolman says, "You! Are really the major cause of
your own insomnia." The sleepless create their problem themselves
through a neglect of health, excesses of ambition and greed, guilt
complexes, and unfounded fears, in Moolman's view. "The insomniac should quit kidding himself. He has no weird disease or weighty
problem as an excuse for his sleeplessness; he only has himself."[68] I

wonder how many insomniacs took heart after reading statements like that. Other popular writers parroted the Kales' views on secondary gain. "You must arm yourself against the operations of a secret agent known as *secondary gain*," writes A.K. Schwartz in *Somniquest,* a self-help book published in 1979. "The ill wind of insomnia blows some good by way of attention, concern, and displays of love which the insomniac, like all of us, cherishes dearly. . . . Take careful note of each escape from obligation, each release from responsibility, and each expression of devotion which you receive as a result of your insomnia. Your mere awareness, your own acknowledgment of your secondary gain, will, by itself, help to counteract the impact."[69]

The early 1980s were prime time for talk about the psychological underpinnings of insomnia. I don't know how it affected other insomniacs (I didn't know many others then) but it was a big turn-off for me. In denial about my feelings? Full of neurotic guilt? Angry and histrionic? It certainly made me angry that so-called experts were suggesting that the wakeful tendencies I'd had since early childhood could develop from traits I could not possibly have possessed at such an early age. How could a child at two or three have emotional conflicts or repressed feelings? On the other hand, that there might be a correlation between insomnia and personality traits was a proposition I could accept. But how could causality be presumed on the basis of personality tests alone? Wasn't it possible that insomnia and personality both grew out of a combination of constitutional and experiential factors that were yet unexplained?

As for the specific personality traits linked to insomnia, I couldn't deny that some applied to me. I was known in my family as "oversensitive" and to "take things hard." My friends saw me as high-strung; one described me as "finely tuned." Some attributes—being quick to react emotionally and needing time to recover from setbacks—were part of my nature. Other personality traits said to underlie insomnia were not, yet the link between these traits and poor sleep was purportedly solid. Did that make me guilty by association? If psychopathology lay at the heart of insomnia, what assumptions would people who learned of my insomnia make about me?

Even if the association between personality and insomnia actually "explained" something meaningful, it amounted to a big fat zero when it came to helping me figure out what to do about my sleep. To accept that insomnia was predisposed by psychological traits—inherited at birth or developed early in life—would mean I was doomed to suffer sleeplessness in perpetuity unless I could somehow crank my emotional thermostat down a notch and grow a thicker skin. I could accomplish this through psychotherapy? No thanks. Consulting a psychotherapist who might view my insomnia as stemming from guilt or as a ploy to gain sympathy did not appeal in the least.

I eventually found my way to psychotherapy, and it helped to repair some of the psychic damage connected to unhappy periods in my past. But it never did a dime's worth of good for my sleep. Nor, apparently, has it cured insomnia in many other people. "There is not one scientific study demonstrating that psychotherapy is effective in treating chronic insomnia," Harvard sleep scientist Gregg D. Jacobs would write in 1999. "Regarding insomnia as a psychiatric problem just reinforces the stigma associated with insomnia and diminishes self-esteem and confidence."[70]

The idea that insomnia was mainly driven by psychopathology had many supporters, but it wasn't the only game in town. In 1972, a psychologist with a behavioral orientation offered a different analysis of the problem. Richard Bootzin proposed that insomnia could develop in healthy individuals when the bed and bedtime became associated with arousal. This type of insomnia was conditioned, or learned. It developed when people routinely engaged in activities like working, watching TV, reading, or studying in bed or in the bedroom, which over time tended to cue wakefulness at night rather than sleep. Misuse of the bed and the bedroom was the chief problem for insomniacs, Bootzin said, returning the insomnia narrative to a place it had been before: as deriving from errors in conduct. He maintained that conditioned insomnia could be reversed by reserving the bed and bedroom only for sleep (more on this in chapter 8).[71]

Also by the 1970s, sleep researchers had identified several other triggers for insomnia. Drugs and alcohol could worsen sleep, as could sleep apnea, periodic limb movements, and "disorders of the sleep-wake schedule." By the early 1980s, there was mounting evidence of insomnia's association with higher levels of physiological arousal as well.[72] Myriad underlying conditions and behaviors could seemingly set the stage for poor sleep. So once again it became convenient to regard insomnia as a symptom of something else.

In journal articles spanning the 1970s and 1980s the words "insomnia" and "symptom" were joined at the hip.[73] "Insomnia is a symptom, not a disorder" was the mantra sleep investigators adopted as they set about pursuing their various lines of research. Meanwhile, conventional wisdom held that the main drivers of insomnia were psychiatric disorders and conditioned arousal at bedtime.

A Multifactorial Disorder

This bears only faint resemblance to the story I hear at sleep conferences today. In the past quarter century, insomnia has come of age.

For one thing, insomnia is not regarded as a sideshow anymore. Even when it occurs concurrently with another health problem, sleep specialists say that insomnia cannot be assumed to be caused by that problem and should not be treated as secondary to it. In every instance, insomnia merits consideration in and of itself.

As for the explanatory narrative du jour, there are several. Among the older ones is a behavioral model, which suggests that while several factors may predispose insomnia, and that it may be triggered by a stressful life event, it's the response we make to it that turns acute insomnia into a chronic condition. A physiologic model claims that the essence of insomnia lies within the body in the form of a trait-level hyperarousal incompatible with sleep. A cognitive model stresses the centrality of worry and rumination.[74] There's shared territory among these older models, but more disparity. Behind each one lurks the assumption that the main driver of chronic insomnia lies either in behavior, the body, or the mind.

Newer models of insomnia are more inclusive. This is evident merely from the names. There's a "psychobiological" model, a "neurocognitive" model, and now a "neurobiological" model of insomnia. Attempts to create more integrative models are an acknowledgment that the etiology of insomnia is likely more complex than it once was thought to be. Chronic insomnia today is described as a "multifactorial disorder" attributable to an array of factors both inherited and learned. Biology and the environment, behavior and attitudes: all likely play a role in its development.[75]

The moral climate surrounding insomnia has also changed. What I hear at conferences and read in journals is empathic, more like the attitudes that existed during William Hammond's day than in most of the twentieth century. This is surely a step in the right direction.

But older attitudes about insomnia persist. No causal mechanism has been identified, and insomnia and other disorders that share this distinction—chronic fatigue, irritable bowel, and chronic pain, to name a few—tend to be suspect still. "'Functional' ills still bear a burden of moral failure," medical historian Charles Rosenberg reminds us, "or psychic weakness or even conscious malingering."[76]

Insomniacs who feel culpable or who have internalized the message that insomnia is a trivial problem may refrain from reaching out for help. While doctors hear more complaints of poor sleep now than in the past, surveys show that well under half of insomniacs do not raise the issue in the consulting room.[77] In fact, some insomnia sufferers avoid talking about the problem at all. Asked why insomniacs were not organized in the same way as people with other disorders, who join advocacy groups dedicated to pressuring the government for funding and raising public awareness, sleep scientist Peter Hauri said this: "They don't want everybody else to know they have insomnia. Mainly, I think, they don't want to expose themselves."[78] I'll go along with that. Half of the insomniacs I interviewed asked not to be quoted by name. "There's not a lot of good reasons to share this stuff," said one chary insomniac, who "puts a face on" to keep from turning into the butt of gossip at work.

Scientists are now endeavoring to chart the biology of insomnia. Geneticists are homing in on some of the genetic factors that affect sleep ability. Neuroscientists are using new technologies to create revealing portraits of neural activity in the brain. Endocrinologists are studying the neuroendocrine aspects of insomnia, and there's research examining the relationship between insomnia and the immune system as well. Progress toward identifying the biomarkers of insomnia, and the drive to chart the internal pathways by which insomnia develops, is heartening, and it's tempting to think the answer to what ails us lies here. Scientists will identify an insomnia gene or genes, a mechanistic glitch in our sleep–wake systems, a particular set of neurons that are under- or overrepresented in our brains, and the riddle of insomnia will finally be solved.

I doubt this will be the end of the story. But even if for some insomnia sufferers it is, behavioral and psychological factors will not become irrelevant. What we experience, think, and do changes our internal milieu, which in turn can affect the way we sleep. There's solid evidence that habits and modes of thinking can worsen sleep and that changes in behavior and attitude can improve it.

What needs to be relinquished is the guilt and blame attached to psychological and behavioral explanations of insomnia in the past. If insomnia can be shorn of stigma, if we can simply regard it as a health problem that impairs quality of life and long-term health, then we're free to consider it from a truly multifactorial perspective. We're going to take an all-hands-on-deck approach to exploring the science of sleep and insomnia and therapies available now.

6

Battling the Body Clock

One morning I'll rise at five in the morning.
You'll think I'm a go-getter, Ben Franklin's boy;
a healthy, bird-watching, cow-milking Child of
Nature. The next day I'll wake up at seven and
you'll think I'm just like you. The next day I'll
sleep till nine and you'll smile indulgently.

Then I'll get up at eleven and you'll call me
lazy. Then I'll sleep till one in the afternoon, then
three, then five—and you'll call me a sybaritic
clod. . . .

By and by my schedule will roll around till
I'm waking at nine in the evening. I'll be up all
night and you're just a little scared of me now,
aren't you? Aren't you slightly concerned for the
safety of your 9-year-old kid when ghouls like
me are prowling the streets?

George Dawes Green, "The Chains of Circadia"

The narrator of "The Chains of Circadia" has a bone to pick.[1] He lives in a twenty-four-hour world, but his body clock cycles every twenty-six hours. This two-hour discrepancy creates big problems. He can't fall asleep or wake up when he's supposed to (although "Satan's alarm clocks," he says, are always exploding in his ear), and from the start he's an underachiever. By early adulthood he's got a stream of absences, failed interviews, and lost jobs trailing in his wake.

A body clock that's out of sync with solar time is a terrible force to reckon with. But the experience vividly recounted in "The Chains of Circadia" is symptomatic of a rare condition called "Non-24-Hour Sleep–Wake Disorder." It occurs mainly in people who are blind. In sighted people, daylight normally "entrains," or sets, the body clock to a twenty-four-hour period. But in people who are blind, damage to a neural pathway from eye to brain may prevent the sunlight from entraining the internal clock. The clock then runs free, cycling in periods of twenty-five and twenty-six hours. People with "Non-24" have a hard time living ordinary lives without medication.[2]

But you don't have to have a rare disorder for your body clock to become your nemesis. Fly halfway around the world to India, and come nightfall, the last thing you're ready for is sleep. But the next day, as you approach the Taj Mahal, a wonder you've waited all your life to see, tidal waves of sleepiness flood your brain. All you want is to find a sliver of shade so you can lie down and tune it all out. Taj Mahal be damned!

Shift work can wreak similar havoc. The first night on the graveyard shift may not be so bad. Coffee can help you keep up with the production line, monitor your patients, or maintain the night watch (although by 4 a.m. or even earlier it may be a struggle to stay alert). It's when you finally get home in the morning that the chickens come home to roost. Shut your blinds, turn off your phone, make your home a bunker where no trace of light or noise or activity from outside can filter in. Though you're totally wiped out, it may be impossible to sleep.

The body clock will have its way. But it can be reset. With help from the sun, your internal clock will fall into alignment with the light/dark cycle on the opposite side of the earth in little more than a week. After four or five days working the graveyard shift, with the assistance of bright light on the job and dark glasses when you leave, your circadian rhythms will shift far enough to enable you to sleep during the daytime.[3] But the adaptation phase can be brutal. And then you're back in the muck when your shift gets changed again, or when you adopt a nighttime sleep schedule on the weekends and then return to working nights during the week.

The human body clock did not evolve to accommodate transmeridian travel or shift work. It prefers to remain on the same twenty-four-hour schedule day after day.

But we don't all run on the *same* twenty-four-hour cycle. Some people are early risers, and some come alive at dark. The rest fall somewhere in between. Body clock–wise, this last group form the lucky silent majority, whose habits never attract much attention or comment because they mesh so well with normal activity patterns. Good sleepers among them can as easily show up bright-eyed and bushy-tailed for an 8 a.m. meeting as hunker down in the evening to finish a report. They sleep between the hallowed goalposts, 11 p.m. to 7 a.m.

Then there are the outliers, the so-called larks and owls. Larks feel best in the morning; they go to bed and get up early every day. Larks get lots of social approval. "Early to bed, early to rise, makes a man healthy, wealthy, and wise"; "The early bird gets the worm"— that sort of thing. But to find yourself stifling yawns at 9 p.m. makes you a pretty dull date. Owls hit their stride in the evening. The quintessential party animals, and the quintessential party functionaries, they go to bed and get up late.

You might chastise yourself for your party-pooping ways or blame your late-rising habits on a lack of discipline, but in reality we don't have much say in the matter. These predilections— "morningness" and "eveningness"—are encoded in our genes. Scientists have identified a number of "clock" gene variants that determine our preferred hours of sleep. This genetic material gets copied and recopied every time our cells divide, assuring that larks keep nodding off early and owls keep staying up late. (People do tend to want to go to sleep earlier as they grow older, but this has to do with age-related changes in the brain.)[4]

Predilections one way or the other—even predilections that veer to extremes—can be comfortable and even prized. Novelist Anthony Trollope preferred to write early in the morning before leaving for work: "It was my practice to be at my table every morning at 5:30

a.m.," Trollope recounts in his autobiography, attributing his early morning habits to self-discipline. "By beginning at that hour I could complete my literary work before I dressed for breakfast." Trollope wrote with lightning speed. He produced a cool 250 words every quarter hour, timing himself with his watch, and completed ten pages at the end of every three-hour stint (bloggers, drool away!). By the end of his career he'd written forty-seven books.

As impressive as Trollope's output was, it paled next to that of his mother. Between the ages of fifty and seventy-six, Frances Trollope supported herself and her family with money she earned writing 114 books. What was her secret? She picked up the pen at 4 a.m.[5] They were perfect larkish specimens, mother and son, whose matinal inclinations suited them like stripes on a honeybee.

At home on the owlish end of the spectrum is the essayist Anne Fadiman. "I am not fully alive," Fadiman has written, "until the sun sets." Only as others are falling asleep does she find the clarity and focus she needs to write. Then, "three or four hours pass in a moment; I have no idea what time it is, because I never check the clock. . . . I am suspended in a sensory deprivation tank, and the very lack of sensation is delicious." Normally Fadiman tries to live more or less on the same schedule as the rest of her family. But once when she needed to speed up work on a book she was writing, she abandoned that effort. For several months she wrote furiously at night, breakfasted with her family, and slept from 9 a.m. to 4 p.m. "The pages," she wrote, "piled up as speedily as the Tailor of Gloucester's piecework."[6]

If you've got a flexible schedule—if you're an artist or academic, a student or self-employed, if you don't have young kids—then larkish or owlish tendencies may be more of an inconvenience than a problem. They may deprive you of the evening company of a partner, but not necessarily affect the quality of your sleep.

On the other hand, you may be a lark or an owl who can only fantasize about flexibility. You hew to a daily routine set by family members and employers. And that can pose a challenge to your quality of life and health.

I've come across several people struggling with a mismatch between their internal rhythms and the clocks on their bedside tables. The larks' main complaint is their lack of a social life. Here's the way an early bird described her experience in an Opinionator column of *The New York Times*:

Being an extreme lark has great disadvantages. Yes, I can get to work on time, but it's very hard to make friends if ordinary social events are impossible.

No dinner parties for me, no performances except matinees (always full of screaming children). No city council meetings or night classes. No choir rehearsal. No midnight Mass. No New Year's Eve. Everything has to be organized around the fact that I become a zombie at about 7:30. My eyes cross, my head aches, all I can think about is nighty-night.

Owls, on the other hand, face their scheduling conflicts in the morning. Feeling energized till 2, 3, or 4 a.m. is a torture for those who have to get up for early classes and normal jobs. Here's how Larry, a marketing consultant, described his plight:

I was a poor sleeper as a child, with a habit of staying up until very late (3 a.m. to 5 a.m.), then being exhausted during the next school day and napping in the afternoon . . . continuing the vicious cycle. This pattern has pretty much stayed the same throughout my adult life. For six years I worked for an accounting firm where I just had to be there at 8 a.m. and alert all day. There were days when I showed up on zero sleep and just had to fake it for the whole day, working with numbers and details and sitting in meetings with my eyelids pulling shut against my will.

Kathleen, a small business owner, reported a similar experience:

All my life, from a small child (reading under the covers with a flashlight for hours) I've wanted to stay up late. I feel like I'm about three hours behind the rest of the world. No matter how tired I might feel in the evening, I still can't go to sleep until late (or early in the morning!). Sometimes just knowing that I have to get up earlier for a meeting or having to catch an early flight makes me crazy and not able to sleep at all.

Both Larry and Kathleen eventually found their way to careers where their owlish tendencies were not such an impediment. Others I interviewed were not so fortunate. They were struggling to keep jobs with corporate hours. They spoke of tardiness, reprimands from superiors, and, sometimes, quitting their jobs or getting fired. There were emotional repercussions, too. After leaving her job at an investment management firm, Susan confided to me what she was reluctant to admit to others: "I would have been ashamed," she said, "to admit to my husband, and anybody who asked me why I quit this job, that I didn't want to get up in the morning, that this was a factor. I would have been seen as lazy and undisciplined and foolish. Like, 'how could you quit for such a stupid reason?'"

A mismatch between the rhythm of your body clock and terrestrial time is not a stupid or trivial thing. It can result in chronic sleep loss, underperformance, and low self-esteem.

Insomnia is a frequent complaint of people whose body clocks are misaligned with solar time. But medically speaking, their problem is classified not as insomnia but rather as a circadian rhythm disorder, or CRD (from the Latin *circa*, meaning "about," and *dies*, meaning "day"). Larks fall asleep and wake up much earlier than they want to; their sleep phase is advanced. Hence the diagnosis: advanced sleep phase disorder, or ASPD. Owls can't get to sleep until much later than they want to; their sleep phase is delayed. The diagnosis is delayed sleep phase disorder, or DSPD.[7]

The sleep of people with CRDs is fine when they can choose the timing of their sleep, as they would on vacation. Then they can get enough sleep to wake up feeling refreshed, day after day. But the sleep problem returns when they resume their normal lives. The mismatch between their internal circadian rhythms and the light/dark cycle does not go away.

Insomniacs may have the same problem to a lesser degree, say the experts. The timing of our internal sleep–wake cycles may be somewhat out of sync with terrestrial time. Insomniacs may also, in an effort to sleep better, adopt habits that actually interfere with the workings of the body clock and with sleep. We may be trying to sleep when our body's circadian forces are clamoring for us to be awake—similar to what occurs during jet lag. To understand how this could happen, let's take a closer look at the body clock and how it operates.

Hunting for the Master Clock

You might think the "body clock" is just a metaphor. It's pretty hard to visualize a timepiece buried in the brain. Yet the body clock is a physical entity located in the brain's middle region. There, in the front part of the almond-shaped hypothalamus, are two tiny clusters of nerve cells resting side by side. These important clusters—called the suprachiasmatic nuclei (SCN)—constitute the famous body clock. Peripheral clocks are scattered throughout the human body. But the SCN is home to the master clock, the maestro of the circadian symphony that performs the same piece day after day.[8]

The important function of the SCN was established in the early 1970s by scientists experimenting on rats. When the scientists destroyed the SCN in their rodent subjects, the rats' sleep went haywire. The amount of sleep they got did not change, but their sleep became erratic. Gone was the regular sleep–wake rhythm inherited at birth. When scientists went a step further, removing the SCN of a rat and then replacing it with a new SCN transplanted from another rat, its regular sleep–wake pattern reemerged with time. In the rats without an SCN, some bodily functions retained their normal rhythms, attesting to the presence of secondary internal clocks. But the SCN was clearly the master horologe, controlling, among other things, the timing of sleep and wake.[9]

In humans, the SCN is connected via a direct channel through the optic tract to the retina. (Some part of this structure is often damaged in people who are blind, resulting in abnormally long sleep–wake periods.) The purpose of the nerve cells in this channel is to sense and communicate changes in daylight and darkness. Thus the SCN has a dedicated phone line to the outside world. And it's thanks to this phone line that our internal clocks, which may run a little fast or slow, are reset to a twenty-four-hour period day after day.[10]

The SCN is also well connected to a wide range of brain and body tissue. Not only does it have direct access to the important sleep–wake centers in the brain, including those in the hypothalamus, the brain stem, and the basal forebrain. The body clock also has cozy ties to secondary neural relays and hormones, which spread its influence far and wide.[11]

Ascertaining the special function of the SCN was accomplished in laboratories, by scientists in white lab coats whose experimental subjects lived in cages. It involved cutting, destroying, and removing brain tissue, which obviously could not be done to human beings. But when it came to studying how the human body clock behaved, humans had to be the guinea pigs. The first volunteers were scientists willing to experiment on themselves. They knew that studying their internal biological rhythms would necessitate removing themselves completely from all cues relating to time on earth. So to escape from sunlight, noise, people, and clocks, they set themselves up in underground caves.

Tracking Human Biological Rhythms

Kentucky's Mammoth Cave, June 4, 1938: The pioneering sleep scientist Nathaniel Kleitman and his postdoctoral assistant, Bruce Richardson, descend the cave on what will amount to a month-long camping trip 119 feet underground. The purpose of their experiment is to see if human beings can adapt to a twenty-eight-hour day.

Kleitman's dry account of the experience betrays little about how it felt. Yet his descriptions of the living conditions and photos of their underground lair make it plain the trip was no picnic. The air was vapor clogged, the temperature a brisk fifty-four degrees ("conducive," Kleitman wrote, "to frequent strolling"). Among the Spartan furnishings were a pair of chairs and sleeping cots—with legs planted in large cans to keep cave rats from scurrying up into the beds.[12]

The men spent thirty-two days underground, only to end up with a puzzling result. Richardson readily adapted to the 28-hour schedule, but Kleitman could not. What to make of this? Did human beings lack the fixed biological rhythms found in plant and other animal species? Kleitman concluded that in humans (at least, in some humans), biological rhythms were quite flexible, possibly becoming more brittle with age[13]—a conclusion that would be refuted by chronobiologist Charles Czeisler in 1999.

Michel Siffre, a young and intrepid Frenchman, was the next guinea pig. Siffre was a speleologist, and caves were a real passion in his life. But even a gung-ho spelunker would quake in his caving boots imagining the experiments Siffre dreamed up.

The first took place deep in a high-altitude cave in the Alps. On July 16, 1962, Siffre descended a series of "potholes" 375 feet down into a cave, where he took up a two-month residence on a glacier. He planned to study the glacier and the rest of his chilly surrounds, but his main purpose was to see how his stay would affect his bodily functions and sense of time.

Conditions on that subterranean glacier were about as hostile as could be imagined. Think Sir Ernest Shackleton in Antarctica, think Sir Edmund Hillary on Mt. Everest. The pitch-black darkness of the cave, broken only by a feeble light inside his tent, was for Siffre a constant source of gloom. But it was the steady freezing and near-freezing temperatures in that saturated atmosphere, together with the periodic cave-ins of rock and ice (which, had they fallen on Siffre, could have buried him alive), that nearly drove him mad with cold and fear. For two months he lived in a state of semi-hibernation. To leave the relative warmth of his sleeping bag when he woke up became a dreaded ordeal.

But the experiment produced results. While Siffre was in the cave, his perception of time bore no resemblance at all to actual time above ground. A period of waking that he estimated as lasting seven hours was, in reality, twice that long. More significantly, though Siffre had no clue as to the time outside, his pattern of sleeping and waking remained on a fairly steady twenty-four-hour cycle, as recorded by his assistants above ground. His two-month stay in that "time-free" environment is regarded as early evidence that the human circadian clock has an innate period of about twenty-four hours.[14]

It's now known that in healthy adults both young and old, the circadian clock has a period of twenty-four hours and eleven minutes, on average. Using Kleitman's twenty-eight-hour sleep–wake protocol, chronobiologist Charles Czeisler and colleagues determined this in 1999 based on a month-long experiment in which subjects were forced to stay up four hours later every night. Only dim light was permitted during waking hours to avoid entrainment. Subjects' sleep–wake rhythms shifted to a twenty-eight-hour "day," but other circadian functions, such as temperature, alertness, and cortisol secretion, maintained close to a twenty-four-hour rhythm throughout the entire experiment. Czeisler's team concluded that the intrinsic period of the circadian clock is as regular in humans as in other species.[15]

Siffre seems to have been a glutton for punishment. Ten years later he decided to sequester himself in another cave for further study of his biological rhythms, this time for six months. Conditions in Midnight Cave in Texas promised to be more hospitable: where he planned to set up camp, the air temperature was a constant seventy degrees.

But this time the strain of six months in solitary confinement nearly did him in. He'd gone underground knowing he'd need mental sustenance to help while away the lonely hours. But the diversions he brought didn't serve him: his record player broke early on, and mildew made his books too disgusting to handle. As the months dragged on he got depressed and lonely. The experiment came to seem trivial and meaningless; he contemplated suicide. He reached the point where, near the end of six months, the thought of any type of companionship—even that of a mouse he heard burrowing into to his food supplies—thrilled him. He decided to trap the mouse and keep it as a pet. He enticed the tiny creature with jam and slammed down a casserole dish to capture it, killing it instead.

"Desolation overwhelms me," he wrote in his account of this incident in *National Geographic*. A series of accidental electrical shocks Siffre received on his way out of the cave nearly accomplished in fact what he'd contemplated in his darkest hours.[16]

But again the ordeal bore fruit. Records kept by Siffre's assistants above ground showed that during his first five weeks in Midnight Cave, he fell into a twenty-six-hour rhythm similar to that of people who are blind. He "free-cycled," going to bed two hours later day after day, right around the clock. Importantly, his twenty-six-hour sleep–wake pattern moved in tandem with fluctuations in his core body temperature.

A brief diversion on body temperature: Most of us don't think much about it unless we're sick. Then we fetch the thermometer and conclude we're running a fever if the reading is higher than 98.6. In fact, even when we're perfectly healthy, our temperature rises and falls twice a day, varying by about 1.5 degrees Fahrenheit over the twenty-four-hour period. This may not sound like much. But it turns out to be very significant in matters relating to the timing of sleep. When Siffre was free-cycling, completing a circadian period every twenty-six hours, he always fell asleep when his temperature was at its low point.

From day thirty-seven of Siffre's stay underground, this pattern changed. His sleep–wake rhythm broke free of his temperature rhythm, two players in a symphony suddenly following different conductors. His temperature rhythm continued to cycle every twenty-six hours, a steady basso continuo. But his sleep–wake schedule stretched into longer periods of forty and fifty hours. He'd stay up for thirty hours or more sometimes and then sleep for fifteen. This dissociation between his temperature and sleep–wake rhythms did not last long. They would return to moving in tandem, only to become wildly divergent again. Through it all, Siffre himself was completely oblivious to what was going on.[17]

In other studies, scientists have encountered many more instances of this same strange phenomenon. It's called "spontaneous internal desynchronization." When people are living in time-free environments—in underground bunkers or windowless, soundproof rooms—their sleep–wake rhythms can break free of their temperature rhythms. This can occur at any time during the experiment, and for any length of time.[18]

Studies of spontaneous internal desynchronization have led to a trove of knowledge about the human body clock and biological rhythms, knowledge that may have bearing on insomnia. For one thing, the studies have shown a tight relationship between body temperature, mental alertness, and the secretion of the alerting hormone cortisol. In time-free conditions, people's sleep–wake patterns can become erratic. But come hell or high water, these three functions— temperature, alertness, and cortisol secretion—continue to march to the drumbeat of the body clock, cycling in lockstep. In fact, body temperature and mental alertness are virtually joined at the hip. The higher our temperature, the sharper our mental faculties. The lower our temperature, the duller we feel.[19]

Under normal conditions, our temperature dips twice during a twenty-four-hour period. The nadir occurs about one to three hours before wake-up time. So the average sleeper who wakes up at 7 a.m. is typically least alert between 4 and 6 a.m. Graveyard shift workers can attest to the hazards associated with the hours prior to dawn. This is when the greatest number of single-vehicle trucking accidents occur, when the disaster at Three Mile Island occurred, and when Charles Lindbergh on his solo flight across the Atlantic struggled again and again to pull himself back from the "borderland" of sleep.[20] Not for nothing is it called the "zombie zone."

A second, lesser temperature dip normally occurs between 1 and 4 p.m. This time of day, the "circadian slump" (Why can't I remember his name? the title of that book? where I used my credit card last?), is in some cultures a time set aside for the postprandial nap. Yet contrary to popular belief, it's not digestive processes that cause the mental slackness. We crave a mid-afternoon cappuccino because our body temperature is down.

The timing of body temperature lows varies somewhat from person to person. The lows for larks fall earlier in the day. The opposite is true for night owls: their temperature lows occur later in the day—quite a bit later, in some instances.[21] So life can be difficult for owls working corporate hours. When the alarm clock rings at 7, they're still in the zombie zone. (No wonder it's hard to drag yourself out of bed! No wonder you're in a fog. The zombie zone is the time of least alertness in the day.)

But it's not just the timing of natural temperature lows that can make it hard to adapt to a schedule dictated by work and family commitments. Temperature highs can also interfere. Time-free experiments have shown that body temperature influences when people feel inclined to be awake. Specifically, desynchronized subjects tend not to fall asleep when their temperatures (and their alertness levels) are at their peak. The same holds true for people entrained to a twenty-four-hour period.[22]

For the average sleeper, the first temperature high occurs between 8:30 and 11:30 a.m. The second peak occurs between 8 and 10 p.m., in the hours leading up to bedtime. During these hours, circadian forces are doing their utmost to make us feel like staying awake. (I'll say more about this seemingly contradictory phenomenon in the next chapter.) In fact, so marked are people's preferences for avoiding sleep at these times that Peretz Lavie, an Israeli sleep scientist who studied sleep–wake preferences in people under conditions of sleep deprivation, called them "forbidden zones." These forbidden zones, also called "wake-maintenance zones," occur earlier in the day for larks, and later for owls.[23]

In the mid-1970s, sleep scientists Mary Carskadon and William Dement had also found evidence that the period right before bedtime was not conducive to sleep. The subjects in their experiment adhered to an extremely "short day" schedule. They were permitted thirty minutes of sleep followed by sixty minutes of wake time, right around the clock for five days. Subjects on this grueling sleep–wake regimen slept 30 percent less than normal, so they were partially sleep-deprived. Even so, there were some times of day when they just didn't feel sleepy. The very worst time for sleep, Carskadon and Dement discovered, was in the evening right before subjects' normal bedtime: the period chronobiologists later identified as the evening wake-maintenance zone.[24] Not only do people prefer not to sleep in the hours immediately preceding bedtime; this study and others have demonstrated that often, they simply can't.

So let's return to the situation of night owls trying to mobilize at 7 a.m. Maybe this is you. Maybe your body clock (along with the peaks and troughs in your temperature cycle) runs later than normal, by two, three, or even four hours. It's bad enough having to start the day smack dab in the middle of your zombie zone. But notice what happens if you try to behave like a good citizen and go to bed at a reasonable hour. Turn the lights out at midnight and shut your eyes and . . . well, the odds of your falling asleep are about the same as a snowball's chance in hell. Why? You're right in the middle of your evening wake-maintenance zone. No matter that you have to get up at 7 a.m. At midnight your brain is still in party mode. You're damned if you honor your natural inclinations and damned if you don't.

It's not just night owls that face off against the evening wake-maintenance zone. People whose circadian rhythms fall well within the normal range can enter into the same fray. Say you've been having trouble getting to sleep (for whatever reason), and say the situation persists. You decide to take the bull by the horns and make a few changes. Since you've been sleeping poorly, it occurs to you to go to bed earlier to recover some of the sleep you've lost. (In fact, sleep experts say, this is a fairly common practice among insomniacs.) By now it should be clear that this solution is pretty sure to fail. Not only will it fail because in the hours leading up to your ideal bedtime, your body clock is a mule team driver urging you to stay awake. It's psychologically risky as well. Being unable to sleep when you want to sleep can create big-time anxiety. And anxious and sleepless is not a place you want to be.

Joey, a young parole officer I interviewed, had discovered the perils of the evening wake-maintenance zone for himself. "Say, instead of 11 p.m., which is my usual bedtime, if I go to bed at 10 instead, I'll lie awake for several hours if I do not take medication," he wrote. "If I crawl into bed at 11, I can fall asleep more often."

Larks, too, may find themselves battling the body clock. Recall that the dips and crests of larks' core body temperature typically occur a few hours earlier than normal. There are some whose temperatures bottom out soon after midnight. (Perhaps this was the case for Frances Trollope, who began her writing day at 4 a.m.) Getting to sleep is not a problem for these extreme morning types. But they may in some situations find themselves entering "forbidden" territory early in the morning, writes Australian sleep researcher Leon Lack.[25]

Lack's explanation for how this could occur goes something like this: Say you're having to stay up late for work, or play chauffeur for a teenager with an evening summer job. You force yourself to stay up past your normally early bedtime. When you're finally able to crash around midnight, your body temperature is well on the way to its minimum, so you're out cold the second your head touches the pillow. But . . . ring-a-ling! You're awake again at 4 a.m. And you can't fall back to sleep for the life of you! Why? Your body temperature has risen to the point where you're approaching that other wake-maintenance zone, which in normal sleepers occurs considerably later in the morning. A handful of nights like this can push you into the ranks of the sleep-deprived.

Being out of sync with terrestrial time is hard to sustain over the long haul, particularly for extreme owls. Those I came across—whose body clocks ran on Hawaii-Aleutian Time though they had to earn a livelihood in the contiguous forty-eight states—were either permanently on medication or had parlayed themselves into jobs with flexible hours. They became home healthcare workers, consultants, small business owners, and college professors. They found ways to work from home.

But not everyone can find a way to live in harmony with their biological rhythms. And not everyone wants to. "I don't like it," Kathleen said, of her proclivity to stay up until 4 a.m. and sleep until noon. "It's not the way the rest of the world lives."

So another option for larks and owls is to coax the rhythm of the internal clock into phase with the rhythm of the earth. This may sound impossible without medication, especially if battling your body clock has been a lifelong trial. Yet sleep therapists say it can be done, and there's research to back the claim.

Phase-Shifting Effects of Light

Light is the strongest entraining agent for the circadian clock. Exposure to daylight can shift the internal clock by as much as sixty to ninety minutes a day. Appropriately timed exposure to bright light via a light box can effect substantial phase shifts as well. So bright light is the first form of therapy recommended by the American Academy of Sleep Medicine for patients with advanced and delayed sleep phase disorders. (It's recommended as a counter-measure to jet lag and shift work as well.)[26]

Correctly timing your exposure to light is critical. You'll recall that your body temperature is lowest from one to three hours before you normally get up. This temperature minimum (Tmin) is a meridian of sorts when it comes to determining the effect light will have on your sleep. The simple rule to remember is this: Exposure to bright light soon *after* Tmin (in the morning) is going to advance your sleep cycle, or help you fall asleep sooner. Exposure to bright light in the hours *leading up to* Tmin (in the evening) is going to delay your sleep cycle, or help you stay awake longer.[27] Several studies attest to the efficacy of early morning bright light in advancing sleep and circadian rhythms for night owls whose aim is to fall asleep earlier. Research on bright light helping to extend the day is less plentiful, but some gains have been achieved using evening bright light, and there's anecdotal support for the practice.[28] It's worth consideration if you're struggling to keep your eyes open by 9 p.m.

The devil is in the details. To shift your sleep cycle by any appreciable amount—say, by an hour or two—the light has to be intense enough, and the exposure, long enough.

Concerning intensity, you can't do better than daylight. At 10,000 to 20,000 lux on a clear day, daylight is extremely powerful in its phase-shifting potential. People in northern latitudes can take advantage of extended daylight in the summertime, the larks in the evening, and the owls immediately after getting up. But darker seasons necessitate the use of a light box. (Standard room lighting, at 50 to 100 lux, is not nearly bright enough.)

So is one light box as good as the next? I put the question to Charmane Eastman, professor in the Behavioral Sciences Department and director of the Biological Rhythms Research Lab at Rush University Medical Center.

"The bigger the screen size, the better," Eastman said. "The tendency over the years is to make them smaller because they are cheaper, but then they are not as pleasant to sit next to. It is less aversive when the light surrounds you than when it is a little bright spot in a field of dark." Also, to get a phase-shifting effect, the light must be continuously striking the eyes, Eastman said, and this is harder to achieve with compact models such as the goLITE and the Litebook.

It's important to sit close to the light box to ensure sufficient light intensity. Successful phase shifts have occurred in experimental subjects sitting between 40 cm (about sixteen inches) and 70 cm (about twenty-eight inches) from the light box.[29] "The bigger the light box," Eastman said, "then the further the person can sit away from the box."

Duration of light exposure is another important consideration. In experiments where subjects have successfully shifted their sleep–wake rhythms, scheduled light sessions have lasted at least two hours. A two-hour light session in the hours leading up to bedtime may not be such a hassle for larks wishing to extend their day. The box can be used during sedentary activities such as eating, reading, using the computer, and watching TV. It may also be possible to delay sleep by merely brightening up the room. Author and sleep researcher Daniel Kripke reports "solving" advanced sleep phase with very bright room light (about 300 lux) for one to three hours in the evening.[30]

But a two-hour session with a light box can pose a major inconvenience for night owls, whose early morning light sessions will conflict with getting ready for work and getting children off to school. In this case, it may be reassuring to know that exposure to light from the light box does not need to be continuous.

"Intermittent light is OK," Eastman said. Time with the light box can be interspersed with taking showers, getting dressed, making breakfast, and other early morning activities. "But the more time by the light box soon after waking, the better," Eastman said. Delaying light exposure until later in the morning will make it much less effective. "But there is no rule that it has to be two hours. Some people might be able to maintain an earlier phase with less [time spent by the light box]."

For owls wishing to advance their circadian rhythms and keep them from reverting, light sessions must occur on a daily basis. Otherwise, the body clock will quickly shift back to cycling in its default mode. Also, some people are more sensitive to the phase-shifting effects of light than others. "Someone who always wears dark sunglasses and is indoors a lot would be more sensitive than somebody who spends a lot of time outside with no sunglasses," Eastman said. (Bright light can also trigger mania in people with bipolar disorder. If you're bipolar, consult a doctor before starting treatment.)

Human sensitivity to light is keener in the three- to four-hour period after waking up and from late in the afternoon through the evening. For anyone wishing to shift sleep timing, bright light early in the morning or in the evening will yield the biggest bang for the buck.[31] But exposure to light in these critical periods can also shift circadian rhythms in the wrong direction. While a light source must be fairly intense to produce big phase shifts, it's now known that much lower intensities of light can shift circadian rhythms as well if the exposure occurs at a time when the brain expects darkness or dim light. Normal room lighting—possibly even the light emitted by a computer screen—can block the evening secretion of melatonin and delay sleep.[32] If you consistently have trouble falling asleep, light could be part of the problem. Try dimming your lights in the evening, or spending the hour before bedtime with a book rather than on Facebook. Likewise, larks wishing to prolong alertness in the evening might consider wearing dark or amber-colored glasses that filter out bright light on early summer walks.

Exposure to bright light at the wrong time can also worsen jet lag. This can occur after eastward flights crossing several time zones. To get in sync with local time, the body clock will need shift forward several hours. "Unfortunately," Eastman and fellow chronobiologist Victoria Revell have written, "many review papers and websites advise travelers to seek outdoor light in the morning in the new time zone after flying east, which can be the wrong advice, depending on the time of arrival." On a flight arriving at the destination city early in the day, a traveler whose body clock is still in sync with time at the place of departure may not yet have reached his body temperature minimum. Exposure to daylight before Tmin will shift his bedtime *later* rather than to the earlier hour desired.[33] Here's another instance where it would be wise to wear sunglasses or spend the first few hours of a trip indoors.

A Phase-Shifting Supplement

Supplements of the hormone melatonin are another recommended aid for people with delayed sleep phase disorder. (Clinical evidence is lacking regarding the efficacy and safety of melatonin as a therapy for advanced sleep phase disorder). Melatonin is a "chronobiotic"— a substance that alters the timing of internal biological rhythms. It has the opposite effect of light. Taken in the morning (after Tmin), melatonin will delay sleep; it will advance sleep when taken in the late afternoon or early evening (before Tmin).[34]

A recent meta-analysis evaluating the results of five studies of adults found that taking melatonin late in the afternoon or early in the evening advanced the sleep time of people with DSPD by an average of forty minutes. Melatonin used in combination with bright light therapy typically results in larger phase advances.[35] If your goal is to advance the timing of your sleep, supplemental melatonin may be just the thing.

Secreted by the pineal gland, melatonin is a powerful player in the circadian system. It exerts its effects not via the GABA system, like most sleeping pills on the market today, but rather directly on melatonin-sensitive neurons in the SCN, where the body clock resides. There, melatonin works to inhibit alerting forces and thus hastens the onset of sleep.[36]

But following instructions on the bottle to take melatonin shortly before bedtime will not do the trick. By then your body's natural melatonin production is already under way. Melatonin secretion typically starts a few hours before you fall asleep and ends about the time you wake up. Adding to it by taking oral melatonin at bedtime is redundant. You may as well take a sugar pill.[37]

To get a phase-shifting effect, you've got to take melatonin *before* your natural melatonin cycle begins. The idea is to get it into your system early and keep it there until your endogenous melatonin production kicks in. Based on research establishing when to take melatonin to achieve the maximum phase advance, Eastman advises taking 3 mg of melatonin seven hours before you normally fall asleep. So if you usually drop off at 1 a.m., you'd take the melatonin at 6 p.m.[38]

You might worry that taking melatonin before dinner would make you drowsy. If it worked like Ambien, in short order you'd be down for the count. But the hormone of darkness is slow acting. Most subjects who remain upright in the evening have not felt sleepy on the 3 mg dose. By taking it several hours before bedtime, you're creating the expectation that nighttime will arrive sooner, catalyzing an array of bodily processes that eventually lead to sleep. You're tricking your circadian system into behaving as though the day were going to be shorter than it actually is. (People who *do* feel sleepy after taking a 3 mg dose may want to try a 0.5 mg dose, which should be taken five hours prior to normal fall-asleep time.)

As with bright light, melatonin is a maintenance therapy for people with DSPD. When it's discontinued, circadian rhythms quickly revert to their natural cadence.

A combination of late-afternoon melatonin and morning bright light will achieve the best results, Eastman said. When an individual starts therapy, it's a good idea to start out by trying "slightly different timings of the melatonin (for at least a week at a time) to find the optimum for that person." However, "both the morning light and the afternoon melatonin would have to be used every day to trick the body clock into assuming the unnatural (for that person) early phase position."

Melatonin can assist in preventing or lessening jet lag insomnia as well. As a preflight strategy before an eastbound flight, take it as recommended above, either seven or five hours before the previous night's sleep onset, depending on the dose, and advance your sleep schedule and the melatonin by thirty minutes a day. As a postflight strategy following an eastbound flight, research has shown that you may be able to alleviate jet lag by taking melatonin at bedtime, depending on the number of time zones crossed and where the new bedtime falls in relation to your Tmin.[39]

For all melatonin is an effective chronobiotic, it has little to offer as a hypnotic. "Useless," "lousy," "no effect whatsoever" were comments I heard from insomniacs who tried it. The authors of a recent meta-analysis reviewed a dozen studies assessing the effects of melatonin on people with sleep disorders and found that on average insomniacs taking melatonin got to sleep seven minutes sooner than insomniacs who took a placebo.[40] Seven whole minutes! No wonder so many melatonin bottles wind up collecting dust. Melatonin, said sleep investigator Sonia Ancoli-Israel, "has never been shown to be effective for insomnia in any age group."

This may be true because for people with chronic insomnia—not circadian rhythm disorders—the body clock may not factor into the problem. (Or if there is a circadian component, it may be relatively weak.) The main issue is not sleep timing; it's the amount and quality of sleep we get. Even so, an awareness of the workings of the circadian clock can keep us from inadvertently making sleep problems worse.

Sleep may also improve with changes in exposure to light. Take stock of the lighting in your home. If you consistently have trouble falling asleep, try brightening lights in the morning and dimming them in the evening. If you tend to awaken too early, keep lighting low in the morning and brighten it in the evening. Make use of daylight when you can.

But the main thing to keep in mind is the discoveries made in "time-free" and "short-day" experiments. The golden hours for sleep, when body temperature is falling and hovering at its nadir, are bounded on both sides by shorter periods very unfavorable to sleep. These forbidden zones lie in wait for the troubled sleeper, ready to pounce should you stray by habitually going to bed too early or routinely forcing yourself to stay up too late. If you can work with—and not against—the rhythm of your body clock, already you're better off.

Waiting for the Big Wave

What you hope for
Is that at some point of the pointless journey,
Indoors or out, and when you least expect it,
Right in the middle of your stride, like that,
So neatly that you never feel a thing,
The kind assassin Sleep will draw a bead
And blow your brains out.

Richard Wilbur, "Walking to Sleep"

Number one on many insomniacs' wish lists would be a speedy transition to sleep. Laura, a long-time insomnia sufferer, has rarely experienced this at any time of night. Since the age of six or seven her inability to slip easily into slumber has set her apart from almost everyone she knows.

"Seeing things like how people sleep on trains and planes just blew me away," Laura said. "Even under the best of circumstances I couldn't sleep. So how is it that people can just crash sitting up in a room full of strangers with all the lights on and a bunch of noise in the background? My father could fall asleep reading the newspaper with his arms still up—that's talent! I never had that kind of feeling, that I would just be overwhelmed by sleepiness or drowsiness and just pass out."

Insomniacs spend a lot of time watching other people sleep: at home, in public, under the worst of conditions. Who can blame us for feeling resentful when sleep eludes us in even the quietest, darkest bedrooms and the most comfortable beds? We envy and marvel at a quick, neat passage into the Land of Nod.

I witnessed one of these remarkable passages at the birthday party of a three-year-old. A dozen of us were sitting around the table, cracking jokes and keeping up a lively banter between bites of fabulous Sri Lankan food. Someone had given the birthday boy a remote control car, and the annoying "woo woo!" it made as it raced around the floor added to the din. The honoree was standing at the table on his father's lap. To him, the banter was mostly noise, but he was doing his best to join in the fun, laughing with his head thrown back.

Then suddenly Wilbur's kind assassin drew a bead. In an instant the boy's eyes glazed over, his smile went slack, his head rocked forward, and his body collapsed. Just like that, so quickly it was all his father could do to catch him, an excited boy fell sound asleep.

The typical three-year-old is a prodigy when it comes to falling asleep. Animals too have the gift, and can likewise inspire envy. One insomniac commented on the split second it took her cat to fall asleep beside her in bed: "I can't help thinking, 'yeah, but can't I get some of this too?'"

Insomniacs may well be able to get some of it, say the sleep experts. Problems getting to sleep and staying asleep can occur because of insufficient sleep drive, and if this is your problem, you may be able to alleviate it by changing your routine. The aim would be to boost sleep drive and prime yourself to fall asleep (or back to sleep) more easily. There are caveats, and these I'll get to later. First, here's how sleep drive works.

Building Pressure to Sleep

Circadian pressure to stay awake is highest in the hour or two leading up to normal bedtime (the evening "wake-maintenance zone"). Well into the evening, neurons in the brain's wakefulness centers are merrily firing away, making hay and thinking the sun's still shining. The pineal gland begins secreting melatonin, but melatonin onset is gradual, as we've seen. It's not until later in the evening when sleep drive finally makes its bid. At bedtime it triggers a cascade of neural activity that reduces arousal and finally enables sleep.

Sleep drive doesn't march to the regular beat of the body clock, rising and falling at the same time every day. Instead, the strength of sleep drive at any moment depends mostly on how long we've been awake.[1] It's lowest when we wake up in the morning, and with every waking hour it grows. This accumulation of sleep drive is also referred to as "sleep debt." The longer we're awake, the more debt we accrue. In the evening the debt grows large enough to overwhelm the forces of wakefulness.

All sorts of contingencies can interfere with this process, for better and for worse. Worry can hamper the ability of sleep drive to induce sleep, as can pain, which may seem like poor evolutionary engineering. On the other hand, if you were chased by a barbarian with a nose bone, you wouldn't want a drive so powerful that it shut you down. The body's fight-or-flight response overrides sleep drive in life-threatening situations, enabling soldiers to postpone sleep for hours and even days. Sleep drive yields readily to more ordinary challenges as well. You're studying for finals. You're fixing a computer crash. You're caring for a sick child. With enough willpower, light, stimulation, and bodily movement (and, perchance, help from a Starbucks venti), you can put off sleep to accomplish almost any task you really set your mind to.

Nor is sleep drive a match for excitement. All-night cafés in Spain are packed with revelers, and the hardcore among them sip sweetened espressos till sunrise. In another corner of the globe, the Gebusi of Papua New Guinea hold all-night dances and feasts. They make up for their sleep loss by snoozing the next day. The Balinese, too, hold all-night weddings, funerals, and shadow plays. These events typically last for two or three nights, in part so celebrants can experience trance-like states associated with sleep deprivation.[2]

But no matter how successful humans are at postponing slumber, sleep drive eventually prevails. It builds through the day and eventually activates neurons in key sleep-regulatory centers of the brain, notably the ventrolateral preoptic nucleus (the VLPO, a.k.a. the sleep switch) and the median preoptic nucleus (MnPO) of the hypothalamus. In these spots, GABA- and galanin-producing neurons start firing away like mad, tranquilizing the wakefulness centers in the brain and thereby shutting it down.[3] And when after an unusually long vigil we *do* finally sleep, we pay off the debt in a way that alerted scientists to the fact there was something very special about deep sleep.

The Randy Gardner story illustrates this pretty well. At the close of 1963, this 17-year-old high school student decided to ring in the New Year by staying awake for eleven days.

Gardner wasn't the first to attempt this sort of audacious publicity stunt. The end of the 1950s and the 1960s saw a rash of fame-seekers hoping to set records for going the longest time without sleep. One was New York disc jockey Peter Tripp. During parts of his eight-day wake-a-thon in 1959, Tripp was broadcasting live from a glass booth in Times Square to raise money for charity. There was also KPOI radio personality Tom Rounds. That same year, he stayed awake 260 hours—four hours short of eleven days—in the display window of a Honolulu department store.

It was Rounds' record Gardner wanted to beat to gain a place in the *Guinness Book of World Records*. Two fellow high school science buffs agreed to assist him, seeing to it that he stayed awake, testing him, and observing his behavior.

Gardner's experiment did not involve two frigid months in the bowels of an alpine cave. But it was a mission only geeky, glory-seeking teenagers could willingly endure: 264 hours of glaring lights, blaring surfer music, Winchell's donuts, pinball, basketball, cold showers, and death marches up and down halls.

After just one night without sleep, Gardner had trouble focusing his eyes. Things went downhill from there, as recorded by his sidekicks and sleep investigators who later arrived on the scene:[4]

- Day 3: Mood changes, difficulty with muscular coordination, nausea.

- Day 4: Irritability and memory lapses. Gardner mistakes a street sign for a person. He imagines he's Paul Lowe, a famous San Diego Chargers football player.

- Day 5: He hallucinates a path running through a forest.

- Day 7: Speech is slurred, becoming progressively slow and mushy.

- Day 9: Fragmented thinking, fragmented speech. Blurry vision.

- Days 10 and 11: He imagines a radio show host ridiculing him and is indignant.

"It was like someone was taking sandpaper to my brain," Gardner recalled some forty years later. "My body was dragging along okay, but my mind was shot."[5]

Earlier sleep deprivation experiments suggest the impairments Gardner suffered were relatively mild. Others who suffered sustained sleep loss experienced delusions, sustained hallucinations, and paranoia. But the researchers who interviewed Gardner near the end of his eleven-day vigil reported he was "well-oriented as to time, place, and person." And at six weeks, and again at seven months after the experiment, he was pronounced "perfectly normal."[6]

It's the EEG recordings made when Gardner finally crashed that illustrate the importance of deep sleep. During his eleven-day vigil, Gardner lost a total of about eighty hours' sleep. Yet recordings of his recovery sleep show that, when allowed to sleep to his heart's content, he ended up paying back only a fraction of the sleep he'd lost.[7] He slept over fourteen hours at the first opportunity. But he didn't have to pay off his sleep debt hour for hour—not even close.

Instead, the sleep Gardner got on the three nights following the experiment was rich in deep sleep. Percent-wise, he got about twice as much deep sleep as normal. This accords with results of later sleep deprivation studies in the laboratory. "After a waking period of some two hundred hours," sleep scientist Alexander Borbély has written, "the percentage of deep sleep in the first nine hours of the recovery period rises to more than double its level in an ordinary night." In fact, after only a single night's sleep loss, we get more deep sleep the following night. The same holds true in conditions of partial sleep deprivation, say, when experimental subjects are restricted to sleeping four hours a night for several days in a row. Sleep loss great and small leads to increased sleep drive and more deep sleep.[8]

Importance of Deep Sleep

It may be that the depth of sleep—as much as or perhaps more than the number of hours—makes the biggest difference between a good night's sleep and a poor one, between feeling well rested or fatigued in the morning. During periods of deep sleep, sleep is very intense; if ever there's a time when we're oblivious to a partner's snoring or a cat crawling across the bed, this is it.

Characterized by the slow, synchronized firing of neurons in the brain, deep sleep registers in the EEG as delta waves: brain oscillations that look tall and widely spaced. Deep sleep is also called "delta sleep" and "slow-wave sleep," or SWS. Children are prodigies when it comes to their propensity for deep sleep. The average five-year-old spends up to a third of the night in SWS.[9] But the percentage of deep sleep changes radically during adolescence, sleep scientist Irwin Feinberg told me. "The decline in SWS, or delta sleep, which begins at about age eleven and a half in our longitudinal studies, is very steep," said Feinberg, a physician and professor in the Department of Psychiatry and Behavioral Sciences at UC Davis. "In four years of adolescence, there's a 60 percent drop in SWS. Then it declines much more slowly until late middle age. Certainly by age sixty-five it has fallen to its asymptote and does not change further to age ninety." Adults may get as little as 10 to 15 percent SWS.

Slow-wave sleep is now believed to benefit humans in several ways. As we've seen, it facilitates learning and memory, and it enhances daytime performance. It also has a restorative function, promoting healing. SWS is associated with the release of growth hormone, and it has a positive effect on glucose metabolism and on the stress and immune systems.[10]

But back in the 1960s, when Randy Gardner set his record for going without sleep, not much was known about it. Gardner's experiment and others suggested SWS was important in recovery from sleep loss. But it wasn't until the next decade that scientists finally grasped the fundamental role it played in the daily sleep–wake cycle.

Scientists in the early 1970s knew the average adult spent about 15 to 20 percent of the night in SWS. But they hadn't paid particular attention to when the SWS occurred. Nap studies conducted during the daytime had showed that SWS was absent from naps in the morning but increasingly common in naps later on.[11] The demand for SWS seemed to grow as the day progressed.

Then in 1974 Feinberg published a paper in which he analyzed the results of several sleep studies documenting how the amount of subjects' SWS changed over the course of the night. (Recall that humans typically go through four or five sleep cycles a night, in each cycle moving from lighter to deeper to lighter non-REM sleep, and then into REM sleep.) SWS was very prominent in the first sleep cycle, Feinberg found, but it tapered off considerably in successive cycles. SWS apparently was so important that it took precedence over REM sleep, which occurred mainly in cycles later in the night. But the crux of the matter was this: while the nap studies showed the propensity for SWS increasing during waking hours, Feinberg's data showed clearly that it decreased during sleep at night.

Feinberg then postulated the existence of a process now understood to be fundamental to the regulation of sleep and waking: Brain activity during waking hours leads to increasing sleep drive, and SWS reverses that process. In other words, it's deep sleep—not just any kind of sleep—that enables us to pay off the sleep debt we accrue while awake, zeroing out our balance for the day.[12]

This process, "Process S," is also referred to as "sleep homeostasis." Through the build-up of sleep drive during the daytime, it hastens sleep; through the discharge of SWS, it reduces sleep ability. The controlling mechanism is called the "sleep homeostat."

Others have compared the sleep homeostat to the thermostat on a furnace,[13] but I think it's more like the thermostat on an air conditioning unit. On a hot day, you set the thermostat to a particular temperature, say, 77 degrees. Once a certain amount of heat gain occurs, the heated air trips the thermostat. Your A/C unit then comes on and cools the house back down to 77. Likewise, your sleep homeostat has a set point. Wakefulness can only last so long (or sleep drive build so high) before it trips the homeostat. The homeostatic process then endeavors to bring your body back into equilibrium by inducing sleep.

The importance of the homeostatic process would be hard to overstate. While the circadian process controls the timing of sleep, it's the homeostatic process that determines the amount and quality of sleep we get. And is anything more important than how much and how well we sleep? Many experts suspect that homeostatic dysregulation is a major culprit in insomnia. So we're going to examine sleep homeostasis further and look at ways to get the homeostat working to our advantage.

Clocking the Hours

First we'll consider the issue of sleep duration. As I said before, the homeostatic process regulates the amount of sleep we get. So just how much sleep is enough?

Well, most insomniacs would start by saying it's more than we're getting. Here's what some have said:

"I really am an eight-hour-a-night person. I'm OK with six, but I really feel better with eight."

"I probably get between four and six hours. I'd like seven or eight."

"I can fall right to sleep between 11 and 12, but it's usually for two or three hours. I always wish I could sleep through the night: get seven or eight straight hours."

Eight hours' sleep: I grew up understanding that this was the hygienic standard, as advisable as brushing twice a day and wiping from front to back. So where did this time-honored yardstick come from?

The ink spilled on the topic of how much sleep humans need could fill a football stadium. Before the twentieth century, opinions on the subject were quite diverse. In the late Renaissance, many medical authorities were convinced that digestive processes controlled the duration of sleep. People slept as long as necessary to digest their evening meal. Ambroise Paré held that this would vary from one person to the next, but that sleep should not exceed seven or eight hours. A particularly large supper would require a longer night's sleep, said Levinus Lemnius. Other physicians believed that a man's humoral temperament determined how much sleep he needed. A phlegmatic man needed at least nine hours' sleep, wrote Andrew Borde, but sanguine and choleric men could easily get by on seven.[14]

Sleep durations recommended in an eighteenth-century French devotional book varied according to sex and health. Nine to ten hours were appropriate for women and "enfeebled people;" six to seven for men.[15]

The belief that women needed more sleep than men was alive well into the twentieth century. A physician named J.J. Terrell wrote in 1917 that women needed two hours' more sleep than men "to compensate for the handicap of inequality of the sexes." Not only did twentieth-century American women need more sleep than men, Terrell averred; they also needed more sleep than their female forebears. "The social whirl of modern life . . . demands just so much more sleep for replenishment. If seven or eight hours' sleep sufficed to repair our grandmothers' machinery, nine or ten hours is a reasonable allowance for the woman of today." The idea that women needed extra sleep appeared in popular magazines right up to the middle of the twentieth century.[16]

Sleep need was also said to vary according to social class and occupation. In her late nineteenth-century book on sleep, Russian scientist Marie de Manaceine noted that the sleep needs of adults in "civilized" nations were different from those of children and "savages." Observing that "the least developed and least cultured persons" needed more sleep than their cultured counterparts, she recommended eight hours' sleep a night for the latter. In 1932 Episcopalian ministers Elwood Worcester and Samuel McComb expressed similar views. "It is the illiterate, the peasant, the man who hardly thinks at all who sleeps most and who can always sleep, while, as a rule, those whose brains are most active seem to require and to obtain the least amount of sleep."[17]

Children in every era were known to need more sleep than adults, and popular magazines in the early twentieth century were full of charts with sleep times for children based on age. Recommended sleep durations for adults, on the other hand, were all over the map. Health columns in newspapers and magazines advised eight hours a night about as often as six to seven and sometimes nine.

Then in his 1939 book *Sleep and Wakefulness*, sleep scientist Nathaniel Kleitman declared all such prescriptions to be invalid. Kleitman's research suggested that sleep need varied widely from one person to the next. Six hours was sufficient for some people, while others needed nine. "There is no more 'normal' duration of sleep, for either children or adults, than there is a normal heart rate or height or weight," he wrote.[18] Kleitman's claims regarding the variation in sleep need found voice in the popular media as the century progressed.

Yet in the years immediately following publication of Kleitman's seminal book, many pundits lined up behind the advisability of a solid eight hours' sleep. Columnists and feature writers preached this orthodoxy through the war years and beyond, and commentators in later years acknowledged its persistence. "Somewhere along the line we were sold on the idea that everyone needs eight hours," wrote a doctor in *The Washington Post* in 1964, a remark that might just as well have been made yesterday.[19]

There is no objective way to ascertain how much sleep a person really needs. But scientists have looked at how much people *do* sleep, and it turns out that in this, as with sleep timing, there's lots of variation. Sleep investigator Daniel Kripke, who analyzed a 1982 survey of over a million Americans, found that while a majority reported sleeping seven or eight hours a night, about 8 percent reported sleeping nine hours or more, 16 percent reported sleeping about six hours, and 4 percent said they slept five hours or less.[20] Would a similar analysis performed today show that people are sleeping less than they used to, as is often claimed? Not likely, the work of researchers at the University of Chicago suggests. This team recently reviewed data from eight studies conducted between 1975 and 2006, concluding that "the assertion that sleep durations have declined drastically in the U.S. population . . . over the past 30 years may be inaccurate." Only full-time workers appear to be sleeping less than they did thirty years ago.[21]

Do people who sleep less die sooner? Here most data fall into a distribution pattern resembling a U-shaped curve, showing that people in the middle live longer than those at the ends. In the Kripke study cited above, people who reported sleeping 6.5 to 7.4 hours a night had the best survival rate. The increased risk of mortality exceeded 15 percent in subjects reporting more than 8.5 hours, men reporting less than 4.5 hours and women reporting less than 3.5 hours a night. A recent meta-analysis in which investigators pooled data from sixteen studies found that "short sleepers (commonly less than 6 hours a night, and often less than 5 hours a night) have a 12 percent greater risk, and long sleepers (commonly more than 8 or 9 hours a night), a 30 percent greater risk of dying than those sleeping 7 to 8 hours per night."[22]

Of course, if it feels like you're not getting enough sleep, statistics and averages are beside the point. But these figures *do* suggest there's nothing magical about eight hours' sleep.

There are familiar cultural biases associated with the naturally long and short sleepers. And here it's the long sleeper who gets the short end of the stick. Like the night owl who sleeps in late, the long sleeper is purportedly lazy and unambitious. This association dates back to Biblical times: "He that sleepest in harvest is a son that causes shame." "Love not sleep, lest thou come to poverty." It turns up in more recent contexts as well, both religious and secular. The Puritan minister Cotton Mather wrote that sleeping more than a third of each day was sinful because it interfered with the all-important work assigned by God. British theologian John Wesley warned against the dangers of oversleeping: "By soaking . . . so long between warm sheets, the flesh is as it were parboiled, and becomes soft and flabby." Early in the twentieth century, Dr. Fred W. Eastman fulminated against people who slept even eight hours a night: "For the healthy normal human being of sedentary occupation to indulge in siestas or to spend much more than a quarter of his time in sleep, is lazy neglect of his duty to himself and the race, and a reversion toward the stage of the amoeba."[23]

The idea that long sleepers are slackers has currency still, psychologist Stanley Coren claims. So entrenched is it that biographers routinely apologize for the sleep habits of long sleepers who rise to greatness, he asserts, citing biographies of Charlemagne and the mathematician Abraham de Moivre. These men are said to have succeeded *despite* their proclivity for longer-than-average sleep.[24]

On the other hand, short sleepers are—and for centuries have been—held up as models. It goes without saying that God never sleeps. The saints, too, slept little, spending much of the night in prayer. Saint Dominic, founder of the Dominican Order, did not even have a proper bed. Instead he slept briefly wherever the urge overtook him: on a bench, the ground, or the straps at the bottom of a chair.[25]

Secular forces joined sacred in applauding the short sleeper following the Industrial Revolution. The equation was simple: more time awake meant more time for work. Editorialized the *Scientific American*, "The fittest type of man will surely be he who can keep awake the longest, and get through the most work in 24 hours. All the scientific evidence seems to point to the early riser, or, let me say, the short sleeper, as the coming man."[26]

No one was a stronger proponent of this view than Thomas Alva Edison. He famously proclaimed most people could accustom themselves to less sleep than they imagined, and urged everyone to try. He typically slept five hours a night and made a frequent point of saying so.

"It runs in our family to require little sleep," Edison told the *Los Angeles Times*. "My father seldom took more than five hours even when he grew old. My grandfather never went to bed at all. He used to sit in a chair and sleep for four or five hours every night. He lived to be 104 years old."[27]

Current literature on sleep deprivation shows that shorting ourselves on sleep is a risky business. Consistently depriving ourselves of even small amounts of shut-eye results in decreased alertness and performance, cognitive and memory impairments, elevated levels of stress hormones, and a higher risk of accidents.[28] So Edison was doing nobody a favor by suggesting we all sleep less.

But research supports his view of sleep length as a substantially heritable trait. Just as a number of clock gene variants determine whether we're larks or owls, so genetic factors are thought to have a considerable impact on the length and quality of our sleep. And this brings us back to the homeostatic process.

Genes and Sleep Homeostasis

There's strong evidence that homeostatic aspects of sleep are under genetic control (although many specifics remain unknown). Long and short sleep tends to run in families. Studies of identical and fraternal twins suggest the heritability of sleep length and sleep quality is about 40 to 50 percent: similar to the heritability of general intelligence. But scientists who study the genetic underpinnings of the homeostat are not talking about just one or two genes. Rather, sleep ability is likely determined by "a complex underlying genetics with contributions from numerous genes."[29]

A few of these genes have been identified. In 2009, investigators studying early awakeners located a transcriptional repressor—a protein that binds to DNA and prevents transcription of nearby genes—associated with naturally short sleep. They found this genetic mutation in a mother and daughter who normally wake up feeling fine after sleeping an average of six and a quarter hours. Other family members, who average eight hours' sleep, did not have this rare mutation.[30]

A more common genetic factor affecting sleep length came to light in 2011. Scientists studying a large pool of Europeans identified a genetic variant which they claim accounts for about 5 percent of the variation in human sleep duration. Their data show that people who possessed two copies of a common variant of a gene called ABCC9 slept significantly less than people with two copies of another version.[31]

What these two discoveries may have to do with insomnia remains to be seen. But they *do* suggest that sleep duration may be less amenable to change than other aspects of sleep. Situational factors can lengthen or shorten sleep on any given night. Yet overall, it seems that how long we sleep is quite dependent on the blueprint we inherit at birth.

So while an eight-hour night can feel heavenly, to use the eight-hour yardstick as a measure of sleep adequacy on a day-to-day basis does not make sense for everyone. It may also, experts suggest, be counterproductive, leading to habits and worries that have a negative effect on sleep. Besides, how rested we feel may have less to do with sleep duration than with sleep intensity, which is also under homeostatic control.

Insomnia and Homeostatic Compromise

We're going to look into how to enable the homeostatic process to work as best it can, hastening sleep and improving sleep quality. By way of preparation, let's look at how it interacts with the circadian process overall.

Ideally, the two processes work in neat coordination. Right before bedtime, when the homeostatic pressure to sleep is high, the circadian forces promoting wakefulness are diminishing, and vice versa in the morning. This arrangement enables a consolidated episode of sleep at night and a consolidated period of waking during the daytime. It also helps make the transition from one state to the other clean and quick, as it was for the three-year-old birthday boy. Here's a thumbnail sketch of how the two-process model of sleep regulation works.

At the beginning of the night, homeostatic forces direct the show. Once the sleep switch is tripped, enabling GABA- and galanin-producing neurons in the VLPO and the MnPO to calm the brain (as described earlier), sleep drive pushes vigorously for the brain's descent into slow-wave sleep. There's a circadian influence too: rising levels of melatonin. For a while these forces do a nocturnal pas de deux. But sleep drive diminishes during the first half of the night and soon recedes into the background. Melatonin then takes the lead. The hormone of darkness, secreted plentifully in the early morning hours, presses onward in an effort to keep us sleeping through the night, aided by neurons in the VLPO and the MnPO.

About an hour before wake-up time, the circadian alarm clock rings, summoning a whole new cast. With sleep drive spent and melatonin levels falling, body temperature rises and production of the alerting hormone cortisol soars. Suddenly the switching mechanism flips. Myriad forces associated with arousal then come alive. Neurons in the brainstem begin firing away, activating ascending pathways and awakening higher levels of the brain. Orexin-producing neurons in the hypothalamus also become active, helping to maintain alertness throughout the day. These and other circadian forces predominate from dawn to dusk.[32]

In the evening, the brain's wakefulness centers busy themselves with making an end-run effort to stave off sleep. This gives us a second wind after dinner. Then the cycle begins again, with sleep drive gathering forces in the wings. The pineal gland steps up secretion of melatonin. Then come signs that change is close at hand: yawning, drooping eyelids, the mind going slack. With melatonin levels rising and alertness fading, sleep drive makes a dramatic bid to quiet the brain, unleashing a flood of forces that roll through the head like a giant wave. All we need to do now, say the experts, is catch the big wave and ride it to sleep.[33]

Come again?! Falling asleep may be just that easy for the lucky ones. But many insomniacs do not feel anything like rolling waves of sleepiness at bedtime or anytime else. Our journey to sleep feels more like an arduous slog, like the one described in Wilbur's poem.

"I can lie in bed for hours sometimes without sleeping," a frustrated insomniac told me. "A good night will take me about thirty minutes to get to sleep, a typical night is about an hour, and bad nights will have me laying awake many hours, sometimes *all night!*"

Other insomniacs report problems sleeping through the night: "I can fall asleep. But my sleep is broken up. The problem is that I wake up in the middle of the night—usually to go to the bathroom—and I have a hard time getting *back* to sleep."

If your trouble occurs at the beginning of the night, you could be fighting your body clock, as we saw in the last chapter. Courting slumber in the evening "forbidden zone" is for the insomniac almost always a losing proposition. But something different may be going on, or something in addition. Difficulty getting to sleep at the beginning of the night (and failure to sleep through the night) may be attributable to insufficient sleep drive. The drive you've built up may not be strong enough to carry you quickly and smoothly beyond the shoals of wakefulness and keep you there. You're stuck in the shallows of a placid sea, waiting and waiting for the big wave to arrive.

Dysregulation of the sleep homeostat may be the problem here, some sleep experts say, citing research showing that insomniacs' homeostatic response to sleep debt differs from that of good sleepers. Slow-wave sleep enables us to pay off the sleep debt we accrue while awake. Some studies have shown that insomniacs do not get as much (or the same percentage of) SWS as good sleepers. Investigators have speculated that in some cases, insomnia may reflect a deficiency of SWS, suggesting compromise of the homeostatic process.[34]

Other studies have not found insomniacs to be deficient in SWS. But they have pointed to a difference in the way SWS gets discharged. Sleep investigators Wilfred Pigeon and Michael Perlis found it took insomniacs about twice as long as good sleepers to descend into the deeper stages of sleep. This too may signal a weakened homeostatic response to normal sleep deficit.[35]

Nor are insomniacs as sleepy during the daytime as might be expected, as we saw in chapter 3. Since insomniacs typically *feel* sleep deprived, researchers reasoned, we should fall asleep more easily during daytime naps. But we do not, if the standard assessment tool, the Multiple Sleep Latency Test (MSLT), is a valid measure of daytime sleepiness. The MSLT is a test administered in a sleep lab during the daytime. Subjects are hooked up to a machine that records brain waves and then given five brief opportunities to sleep over the course of several hours. The results of MSLTs consistently show it takes insomniacs as long or longer to fall asleep during naps than it does normal sleepers. This lack of daytime sleepiness could be attributable to a trait-level hyperarousal, as some sleep experts have suggested, but it could also signify that the homeostat is functioning in a suboptimal way.[36]

Does the possibility of a dysregulated homeostat mean that our transport to slumber is defective, and that insomniacs are doomed to difficulties falling and staying asleep for the rest of our lives?

No, the experts say. It may be that for insomniacs' homeostats to function well, they require a larger-than-normal sleep deficit, something like a richer grade of gas.

This is hardly music to insomniac ears! Already we feel like we're short on sleep, "functioning" on less than we need, to borrow language from insomniacs I interviewed, "surviving" on a few measly hours, "running close to empty." Talk of needing a larger-than-normal sleep deficit is the last thing we want to hear! Yet researchers have tested this concept and claim that it basically holds.

For example, Edward Stepanski, then a sleep researcher at Rush-Presbyterian-St. Luke's Medical Center, and colleagues conducted an experiment in which insomniacs and good sleepers stayed awake all night. The next day they underwent MSLTs. The insomniacs fell asleep in brief naps just as quickly as the good sleepers. This would suggest our sleep homeostats are functioning, but they need a bigger charge—a full night without sleep!—to work as nature intended. Later that night, during recovery sleep, although insomniacs experienced larger increases in sleep time than good sleepers, they had a smaller percentage increase in SWS. In a similar study where sleep time was restricted to just three hours, insomniacs showed increases in total sleep time and SWS the following night, but their gains were not as great as those of good sleepers. Altogether, the data suggest insomniacs' homeostats are functioning, but they may require more of a sleep debt to work well.[37]

So our cup is half empty . . . or half full. For while the results of these studies are not exactly cause for jubilation, they do offer grounds for hope. Just as insomniacs can work against the body clock, so we can inadvertently interfere with the optimal functioning of the sleep homeostat, and changing our behavior can help.

Let's say you have a couple late nights and allow yourself to sleep late the next morning. You wake up at 10 a.m. feeling wonderful. But when your normal bedtime rolls around in the evening, you're stuck. At midnight you've been awake just fourteen hours, not long enough to build up a sleep debt that will readily put you to sleep. You have a major case of Sunday-night insomnia, no matter which night of the week it is.

Or maybe in that same situation you *are* able to fall asleep at midnight as usual. But without the build-up of sufficient sleep pressure during the day, your sleep debt is quickly paid off. You wind up wakeful in the middle of the night, or awakening early. You may as well be on a stretch of the Alaskan highway for all the likelihood any transport to slumber will pass your way again.

The solution offered by sleep therapists is simple (and doubtless one you've heard before): Avoid sleeping late in the morning. Get up at the same time on weekends as you do during the week. This may raise your hackles (it did mine): If you're already short on sleep, why should you knowingly short yourself further by forgoing the opportunity to catch up in the morning? Normal sleepers routinely catch up on lost sleep by sleeping late on weekends, at no cost to themselves. Why shouldn't insomniacs do the same?

As we've seen, insomniacs' homeostats seem to require more of a sleep deficit to function well. Sleeping late in the morning makes you feel good temporarily, but it creates problems at the end of the day. Not only will it reduce your sleep drive at night. It can also push your body clock out of sync with the cycle of daylight and darkness. Handicapping both the homeostat and the body clock creates the perfect conditions for insomnia.

Napping can likewise reduce sleep drive. If during a nap you descend into deep sleep, then you pay off some of your sleep debt early, just as eating an hors d'oeuvre takes a slice out of your appetite. Reduced sleep drive can result in trouble falling and staying asleep at night.

Now it's true whole cultures have organized their lives around the afternoon siesta and not been known to suffer sleep problems as a result. (And I'd bet that people in more leisure- and less work-oriented cultures suffer fewer sleep problems, but it's just a guess.) Naps can even serve as an insomnia management strategy, I learned from Toby, a puddle-jumper of a sleeper all her life. At night Toby typically descends into sleep for a brief sixty minutes' refueling, and rises into wakefulness again. Then she gets up, drinks decaffeinated tea, reads a romance novel, and then returns to bed for another brief sleep. The cycle repeats itself a few times every night. If she's sleepy during the daytime, she takes naps.

But napping is not a viable management strategy for most insomniacs I know. We don't have time for naps and, even if we did, many of us lack the ability!

For those inclined to take naps, though, it's best to keep them short: no more than twenty to thirty minutes, according to Deirdre

Conroy, clinical director of the Behavioral Sleep Medicine Program at the University of Michigan. That way you'll avoid descending into deep sleep and reducing sleep drive.

Doing one or both of these things—getting up at the same time every morning and cutting out or shortening naps—may help to "prime" a sluggish homeostat. It may enable you to catch the big wave and ride it to sleep, or have a better chance of staying asleep once you're there. And if these tactics are insufficient, there are more aggressive measures, and we'll consider them in the next chapter.

A Closer Look at the Homeostat

We're not quite finished with the homeostat yet. As described so far, the homeostat is just an abstraction. Yes, it works sort of the like the thermostat on an air conditioning unit, tripped when something called "sleep drive" builds up high enough. But what are the biological mechanisms controlling the homeostatic process? While most of the details are beyond the scope of this book, a few deserve brief mention.

For decades, the assumption has been that sleep drive is associated with the build-up of a substance or substances during waking hours and a reversal of that build-up during slow-wave sleep. Many substances are probably involved. One sleep-promoting neurochemical in particular—adenosine—has been the focus of several studies that suggest it's a key player in the homeostatic process.

Adenosine doesn't have name recognition like adrenalin or cortisol, yet there's no bodily substance whose actions people the world over more routinely seek to counteract. We accomplish this jujitsu by drinking caffeinated beverages like coffee and tea. Caffeine blocks the action of adenosine and stimulates the central nervous system. Neural activity in the brain intensifies after a latte or a pot of Earl Grey. We feel more alert, and the alertness enables us to work or drive through the night.

Adenosine is a byproduct of metabolic processes that occur during waking hours. It builds up in the brain during periods of wakefulness and decreases during sleep, as shown, for example, in an experiment involving freely behaving cats. When the cats in this experiment had their wakefulness prolonged six hours by gentle handling, their adenosine levels increased further, building with every additional hour of sleep deprivation. More specifically, keeping the cats awake led to more adenosine in the basal forebrain and the cerebral cortex. Adenosine calms wake-promoting neurons in these regions and is associated with increases in SWS.[38]

Gene studies also suggest that adenosine is an important homeostatic sleep factor. Julia Rétey and colleagues at the University of Zurich reported locating the human gene for adenosine deaminase—an enzyme that converts adenosine to iosine—in 2005. Eight to 12 percent of the Caucasian population they studied possess a genetic variant of the enzyme that slows this conversion down, resulting in increased levels of adenosine in the brain. And these 8 to 12 percent are gold-medal sleepers. Their sleep is more intense, and they have more SWS and fewer awakenings than the rest of us. The researchers also found, in contrast, that a variant of the adenosine A2 receptor gene, associated with sensitivity to caffeine, correlated with more sleep problems and less SWS.[39] Rétey's findings are direct evidence that the adenosine system modulates the quality of human sleep.

But adenosine is not the only substance known to play a role in the homeostatic process. Other substances produced as the result of neuronal activity during the daytime include nitric oxide, tumor necrosis factor, and interleukin-1. These substances have also been found to promote sleep.[40]

Exactly how these sleep-regulating substances induce sleep is not yet known. The traditional theory holds that sleep is imposed upon the brain by sleep-regulatory circuits that direct the process from on high. Whatever substances sleep drive consists of, sleep drive builds up steadily throughout the day until—wham!—it trips the sleep switch, activating global circuits that shut the brain down rapidly. This paradigm views both sleep and waking as whole-brain states in which transitions between states are quick and clean.[41]

A New Model of Sleep Regulation

But new research suggests the dynamics of falling asleep may be more nuanced. James Krueger, a sleep researcher in the WWAMI program, a medical education program in the Northwest, proposes that the homeostatic process is different from that described above. He notes first that the traditional model of homeostatic sleep regulation doesn't account very well for states where people appear to be simultaneously awake and asleep.

"The most obvious example of this is sleepwalking, quite common in adolescence," Krueger said in an interview. "Clearly they're asleep, because you can shake them and wake them up. But parts of the brain are clearly awake, because they [sleepwalkers] can navigate through very complex situations." Another phenomenon that seems to fall outside the traditional paradigm is "sleep inertia," the zombie-like feeling some people have when they first get out of bed in the morning. Tests have shown that upon waking, people need about thirty minutes to reach their full cognitive performance ability. Krueger suggests this too is a situation in which parts of the brain are awake while other parts are still sleeping. The traditional model of the homeostatic process leaves these conditions and other halfway states unexplained.

Based on a series of animal experiments in the laboratory, Krueger and his colleagues have concluded that sleep, rather than being imposed upon the brain all at once, is initiated at a local level, as first one assembly of neurons, and then another, tires out from use. These neuronal assemblies (Krueger also calls them "cortical columns") are very small, yet they're considered a fundamental processing unit in the cerebral cortex. Studies have shown that the longer each cortical column is "awake," and the more stimulated it is during waking hours, the more it's inclined to reverse course and down-shift into delta mode.[42] (Delta waves, you'll recall, are the critical component in slow-wave sleep.)

For example, Krueger said, the more you twitch a rat's whisker, the more the corresponding cortical column is inclined to fall into a sleep-like state. "You can localize and overactivate particular parts of the brain," Krueger said, and thereby induce a sleep-like state in a very specific brain region (while other parts of the brain remain awake). Krueger and his team maintain that sleep is not imposed upon the brain from on high but rather may occur in any brain region in response to its use.[43]

So, according to this model, the brain does not fall asleep all at once at night. Falling asleep occurs as individual neuronal assemblies and then their neighbors, and then the neighbors of neighbors, tire out from use and succumb to a sleep-like state. This can happen rapidly, Krueger said, likening the process to the synchronizing of fireflies in June. It doesn't take long before the hundreds of fireflies in your backyard are flashing on and off at the same time. Likewise, the neural and chemical connections in the brain are inclined to speedy synchronization. "Sleep goes global very rapidly," Krueger said. "If you have a certain fraction of your neuronal assemblies in a sleep-like state, somehow you end up transitioning into sleep."

So what about the involvement of the central sleep regulating mechanisms, that is, the VLPO and the MnPO?

"I think they're playing a very important role," Krueger said. "What the global circuits are probably doing is somehow coordinating the sleep that's initiated at the local level to suit the environment." Exactly how this occurs remains unknown. But according to Krueger, quite a bit of research now suggests that sleep is initiated at a local level by neuronal assemblies. They then trigger the involvement of the central sleep regulatory circuits, and together these forces promote the global shut-down of the brain that occurs in normal sleep.

Krueger's model of the homeostatic process accounts for situations in which some parts of the brain are in a wake-like state while others are in a sleep-like state. Two examples noted before are sleepwalking and sleep inertia. Insomnia is a third. As we'll see in chapter 9, the insomniac brain is prone to wake-like neural activity even as we sleep, as demonstrated in EEG and neuroimaging studies. What can feel to insomniacs like wakefulness at night may actually be more akin to a hybrid state.

It remains to be seen how dysregulation of the homeostatic process might occur in insomnia, and to what extent it's even a culprit in the various flavors of the affliction. Meanwhile, for some insomniacs, medication is the surest path to a swift descent into slumber and fewer nighttime awakenings. (We'll take a close look at hypnotics in chapters 10 and 11.)

But medication is not our only recourse. Another approach that looks as good or better than medication is cognitive-behavioral therapy for insomnia (CBT-I). Even small misalignments in the homeostatic and circadian systems can sabotage sleep; CBT-I aims to turn these two systems from tormentors into friends. So now we'll move beyond theory and consider how to put this information to use.

8

Aligning the Powers That Be

We ought to make the utmost persevering efforts to break the enchantment of bad customs; and though it cost us some uneasy sensations at first, we must bear them patiently; they will not kill; and a very little time will reconcile us to better modes of life.

William Cadogan, *A Dissertation on the Gout, and All Chronic Diseases*, 1772

Many sleep experts say cognitive-behavioral therapy for insomnia (CBT-I) is the answer to our problems. It's drug free—a plus for insomniacs who don't respond to sleeping pills, don't like the side effects, or are just plain opposed to taking prescription drugs. Insomniacs young and old have reported improved sleep following CBT-I, and some report improvements in daytime functioning. CBT-I was recommended as a front-line treatment for chronic insomnia following a National Institutes of Health–sponsored State of the Science Conference in 2005, based on studies showing it to be as least as effective as drugs. And follow-up studies indicate that insomniacs successful with CBT-I continue to reap benefits long after therapy ends.[1]

But for all its virtues, CBT-I is not the silver bullet insomniacs dream of. It's not fast, and for several days you may feel worse. It requires the sort of effort and commitment that swallowing a sleeping pill does not.

When I asked an insomnia sufferer I met in a CBT-I course to recall his experience, he replied, "I think, going into it, if I'd have known *that* was what I was going to have to do, I don't know if I would have agreed to it," he said.

"That" was "sleep restriction," a therapy based on the notion that insomnia sufferers, to get more and better sleep, must start by spending *less* time in bed. If you're new to this concept, it will probably have as much appeal as sleeping on a bed of nails. But sleep restriction has a track record, and we'll look into it later on.

CBT-I isn't just about curtailing your hours in bed. You're also asked to observe the rules you're so familiar with from advice columns and the web: cut out naps, and reserve the bed and the bedroom for sleep and sex. No matter if your brain turns to mush when you miss your twenty-minute power nap, no matter if the TV in your bedroom sometimes *helps* you fall asleep. Eventually you may be able to return to some of these activities (and maybe not). But in the beginning you're asked to cut them out completely to increase your chances of success.

Some of these suggestions are common-sense rules for healthy living. Others—the proscriptions on reading and watching TV in bed, for instance—are part of an approach to improving sleep called "stimulus control." The idea is that refraining from wakeful activities in the bedroom will reduce the associational triggers for wakefulness in bed. Ever since the 1970s when it was first proposed, research has shown it to be effective.[2]

There's also a cognitive component to CBT-I called "cognitive restructuring." Once your habits are in order, the therapist sets to work on your attitudes. All sorts of mental detritus can keep you wakeful at night, including, the experts say, misconceptions about sleep and catastrophic thinking about insomnia. The therapist's job is to convince you that some of your thinking is distorted, and persuade you to adopt a more realistic and productive mindset. The cognitive component involves written homework as well.

If the whole package sounds more like boot camp than talk therapy, I'll agree that it is. CBT-I is highly structured, focused narrowly on boosting sleep drive and removing any psychological and emotional barriers you may have to sleep. But the bottom line is this: 70 to 80 percent of insomnia patients benefit from it.[3] The nature of the benefits, I'll save for later. For now, the numbers suggest that anyone who suffers chronic insomnia should take a careful look.

Diving In

Consider the experience of Andrea, a regulatory specialist at a medical company who entered the University of Michigan's Behavioral Sleep Medicine Program with bona fides that make the complaints of many seasoned insomniacs look puny. Trouble falling asleep and staying asleep had plagued her since childhood, and nights of just an hour or two of sleep were the norm rather than the exception. At thirty-three, she decided the problem was out of hand.

"I don't ever remember not having it," Andrea said. "Even being really young, I remember laying in bed at night, just laying there, and not being able to fall asleep, or waking up. The wind blows, the house creaks, the furnace kicks in, a window rattles—I hear all that. It wakes me up. Then once I'm up, it's very difficult to go back to sleep."

Andrea also had a history of migraine headaches. The two problems appeared to be related: really bad migraines tended to follow really bad nights of sleep, and she'd been seeing neurologists about the situation for years. In recent months her migraines had gotten worse.

"It was to the point where they were interfering with things I wanted to do," she said. "I'd have such severe pain that I wouldn't be able to move. I couldn't lay down because that hurt. Light and sound: all that was too painful."

Andrea finally agreed to take medication for the migraines. But she didn't like the idea of taking sleeping pills, so her doctor steered her to CBT-I. Participating in a group therapy program changed her life.

"I think I found it more helpful than anyone else in the class," Andrea said afterward. Before, she was taking a couple hours to fall asleep and waking up repeatedly for long stretches at night. Now, she falls asleep within minutes of getting in bed. She wakes up less in the middle of the night. When she does wake up, she falls quickly back to sleep. In the morning she's rested and ready to go. But the biggest impact the therapy had was on her headaches.

"Before, I had some form of a headache daily," she said. "I'd take ibuprofen every other day. Now I take it almost never. In the last six weeks I've only had two headaches. That's definitely the best outcome for me."

Andrea's experience will sound like a fairytale to many people with chronic insomnia. Yet she achieved what she did with guidance from psychologist Deirdre Conroy, clinical director of the Behavioral Sleep Medicine Program at the University of Michigan.

Four of us joined Andrea in a seven-week group therapy course in the winter of 2008. For an hour and a half on Tuesday evenings, we gathered around a table in a small conference room with a white-board on the wall. We were all seeking relief from insomnia. Yet there the similarity ended.

Elaine's trouble sleeping had begun the year before with the death of her husband. She'd tried prescription sleeping pills, but none really worked.

The rest of us were card-carrying members of the insomnia elite. Eric had woken up too early for over twenty years. The four or five hours' sleep he usually got just wasn't enough. Matt had suffered insomnia for twenty-five years and, a few years before, was diagnosed and treated for sleep apnea. But his insomnia was persistent, and he wanted relief from that, too. I was there to see if I could learn anything in group therapy beyond what I'd learned attempting CBT-I on my own four months before. In age we ranged from thirties to sixties.

Conroy spent a fair bit of time explaining the rationale behind the treatment we were about to undergo. It's important information, so here's a summary.

You might think, judging from the name, that CBT-I consists mainly of cognitive therapy with a dash of behavior mod tossed in for flavor. In fact, the opposite is true: The principles guiding treatment are mainly behavioral. In 1987, when psychologist Arthur Spielman laid out his theory explaining the development of chronic insomnia, his central claim was that insomnia becomes chronic due to *behaviors* people adopt to cope with poor sleep. Spielman's model serves as the basis for CBT-I today.

Psychophysiologic insomnia (psychofizz, old friend!) develops in a three-stage process, Spielman said.[4] First come attributes that make you vulnerable. You might have an overactive arousal system (jump out of your skin when startled, for example) or a sluggish homeostat. You might be a worrier, or inclined to ruminate. By themselves, these "predisposing factors" may never lead to insomnia. But they do increase the odds.

Situational factors—Spielman called them "precipitating factors"—trigger acute episodes of insomnia: shift work; emotional stressors like illness, divorce, or worries about losing your pension or your house; or the sedentary lifestyle you might suddenly adopt on retirement. Any one of these can give rise to insomnia, the second stage in the Spielman model. But acute insomnia does not spell doom. Sleep can—and, in many people, does—return to normal once the situational triggers for insomnia get resolved.

It's your response to poor sleep that determines whether the problem escalates to the third stage and becomes chronic, Spielman said. If concern about insomnia prompts you to spend more time in bed trying to recoup sleep you've lost, you start down the road to perdition. Go to bed too early, and you end up fighting your body clock; take naps or sleep late in the morning, and you reduce the build-up of sleep drive. These are some of the behaviors Spielman singled out as "perpetuating factors" in chronic insomnia.

Spielman's three-factor model of chronic insomnia has been modified in recent years by researchers whose neurocognitive model suggests a fourth factor in the process, namely, conditioned arousal of the cerebral cortex.[5] Long stretches of wakefulness in bed (Spielman's third factor) lead to worry and rumination, and to high-frequency EEG activity during sleep onset and non-REM sleep (the fourth factor in the neurocognitive model). Thus some insomniacs are prone to information processing and memory formation even as we sleep.

Now it might strike you as just a teensy bit unfair (and also may strain your credulity) that so much bad could come from merely spending extra time in bed. Chronic insomnia seems like a far worse punishment than the petty crime of extending sleep opportunity deserves! Indeed, said Michael Perlis, director of the Behavioral Sleep Medicine Program at University of Pennsylvania, "there's never been a natural study to say that people who are good sleepers who are subjected to an acute bout of insomnia and who compensate by extending time in bed are the ones that go chronic." (Researchers are exploring that issue now.) But what *is* clear, Perlis and other behavioral sleep experts claim, is that chronic insomnia involves a mismatch between sleep ability and sleep opportunity. Make a habit of going to bed early, or lie in bed in the morning hoping to fall back to sleep, and you keep the pot boiling. The elephant moves into your bedroom and stays.

The good news is that chronic insomnia is reversible, according to these behavioral models. And about this, Conroy was reassuring. We could all improve our sleep by changing our habits. This would be our goal in therapy.

Our first assignment was to keep daily sleep diaries. We were to record our time in bed, the time we slept, the length of any naps and our use of substances known to affect sleep: tobacco, caffeine, and alcohol. We were to refrain from taking sleeping pills. Keeping sleep diaries would be an ongoing task.

"Piece of cake" was the consensus when, at our second meeting, Conroy asked how we'd fared with the diaries. As for content, there were no surprises. We were behaving like typical insomniacs, with trouble falling asleep and staying asleep. Most of us were averaging three, four, and five hours' sleep a night. Andrea came in at the bottom of the pack, averaging a whopping hour and thirty-seven minutes.

All of us wanted more sleep. That's what we were there for, or so we thought.

But Conroy's talk that evening centered not on how to get more sleep but rather on the mismatch between how much time we were actually sleeping and how much time we spent in bed. Good sleep was efficient, she said. Most of the time good sleepers were in bed, they were asleep.

Poor sleep, on the other hand, was inefficient. An insomnia sufferer might spend eight hours in bed, but of those eight hours, he was sleeping only five. Here she drew a line with gaps—indicating periods of sleep interrupted by patches of wakefulness—above a timeline on the whiteboard. Did the broken line resemble a sleep pattern we were familiar with?

A few people nodded. Most of us had experienced nights of disrupted sleep.

The "sleep efficiency" (percent of time in bed actually spent sleeping) of this hypothetical insomniac was low, Conroy said. You could determine it by dividing his total sleep time (five hours) by his time in bed (eight hours), and multiplying by 100. It worked out to 63 percent. How, she asked, could he make his sleep efficiency go up?

"Go to bed earlier?" someone offered.

More time in bed would probably make his sleep efficiency go down.

It emerged that the only way this insomniac could improve his sleep efficiency would be to *reduce* the time he spent in bed. Then his sleep, rather than being broken by stretches of wakefulness, might begin to resemble something like a solid line. This was an important first step to getting better sleep and eventually more sleep. Here Conroy paused.

We too could start down the path to better sleep by simply spending less time in bed. Would we all agree to try it?

I looked around the table. My comrades' faces registered a mix of reactions, everything from polite interest to skepticism. But to Conroy's question we all said yes.

The week's marching orders were to restrict our time in bed to the average number of hours we were currently sleeping, according to our sleep diaries, but no fewer than five hours. Each of us chose a wake-up time and counted backward to arrive at a new bedtime. We were to stay up till then. Other rules were these: If after fifteen or twenty minutes we were still awake (by our estimate, since once we got in bed, looking at the clock was verboten), we should leave the bedroom and stay away until sleepy. Absolutely no naps unless we felt too sleepy to drive.

Andrea wasn't sleeping much anyway, so the idea of reducing her time in bed didn't faze her. In fact, the regularity of the protocol actually appealed.

"I'm kind of a rule follower," she said. "If you tell me not to do something or to do something—especially if it's for a medical reason—I'm going do exactly what you tell me to do."

But Matt was apprehensive. A radio announcer, he was concerned about his health. Would restricting his sleep lead to sickness? Would he be able to perform on five and a half hours' sleep a night, without the benefit of his usual naps? Conroy was confident about her method, but would it work for him?

Matt's doubts were tame compared to my first reaction to sleep restriction. When I came across the concept in the 1990s, I thought it was a joke. Sleep restriction for the sleepless, when we were already sleep deprived? Wasn't that like prescribing celibacy for the sex-starved? What sort of twisted mind had dreamed this up?!

I was tired of hearing that insomniacs must cut down, shape up, and regulate every corner of our lives. I was tired of the message that I was a "disordered sleeper,"[6] that bad habits were perpetuating my insomnia, and that the Rx was to peg my sleep strictly to the clock (and a narrow wedge on the clock face, at that). There was already plenty of structure to my days—work, chores, exercise, dinner preparation. The suggestion that I should impose a structure on my nights as well made me cross.

But my biggest objection to sleep restriction was this: I was sure it wouldn't work. Why should it work, when sleeping between the goalposts was a feat I'd never been able to achieve in all my life?

The last time I'd lived with a fixed bedtime was as an adolescent. And bedtime then had nothing to do with sleep. At 10:30 p.m. I turned out the lights and crawled dutifully under the covers, then waited for Mom's or Dad's footsteps on the stairs to fade and the rumblings of the TV. Then I turned on the wall light above my bed and read mysteries and biographies. Or in the darkness I planned tricks to play on my younger sister. Her tricks on me were better than mine on her, and I got plenty of mileage plotting how to reestablish the superiority I felt was my birthright.

As an adult, I'd never fared any better at fixing my bedtime, whether early or late. In fact, fixing a bedtime—getting in bed at a given time with the aim of falling asleep—was a surefire summons to insomnia.

The thought of fixing a wake-up time was even worse. Mornings were my catch-up time, especially when I was going through rocky periods with sleep. Over the years I'd adopted guerrilla tactics, plopping down at the first yawn. That could be as early as 10 p.m. Or it could be as late as 3 a.m. When that happened, I wasn't about to rise 'n' shine at 6 a.m.

Not only was the idea of restricting my time in bed to a set few hours distasteful; it was scary. Sleep was unpredictable. What if, during the designated hours, it went totally on the lam? I'd have to endure my sleeplessness and the anxieties it provoked on my own, without the assistance of my friendly pills. Did I have the courage and stamina to face this night after night? And what about the mental idiocy I'd experience during the daytime? Would it force me to take time off work? Do the trivial tasks I'd saved up for when I broke my hip: assemble photo albums, copy recipes, purge files?

Sleep experts for years were touting sleep restriction and CBT-I as the next best thing to organic vegetables. But it was not for me. I packed the idea away in a box, and there it stayed for over a decade.

In the Belly of the Beast

After a week of sleep restriction, the mood during our therapy session was subdued. Andrea reported better sleep. The rest of us did not fare as well.

"I hate this," Elaine whispered as we were sitting down for class.

Conroy, prescient, invited us to share our "horror stories."

Elaine's complaint was that she couldn't figure out what to do with herself until 2:30 a.m. On other nights, she had a hard time falling asleep even at that late hour. "I just don't feel sleepy," she said, adding that once she'd been awake nearly all night.

Matt was worried about the effects of sleep restriction on his days. He felt more tired than usual, he said. He wasn't on top of his game. Once he'd forgotten to cue up an announcement when he was on the air. At other times he was overwhelmed by the desire to nap. "There are certain times of day when I feel I should say to myself, 'I shouldn't be driving right now.' That's happened before, but I feel like now it's more pronounced."

Eric also complained of sleepiness during the daytime. "By the weekend I was just exhausted," he said. "Usually on weekends I take those Tylenol PMs and have a few beers, and then I'm gone for a good eight hours. That's like my catch-up time." So he chucked sleep restriction over the weekend and reverted to the familiar.

I'd come close to falling off the wagon myself. Lingering jet lag and a minor crisis at home were the ingredients for a perfect insomniac storm. To make matters worse, over the weekend I'd gone out of town to a party where control over where and when I went to bed was completely out of my hands. The couple hours' sleep I got that night left me cranky and sleep deprived for the next few days.

But the difficulties of this second go-round were nothing compared to what I'd experienced trying sleep restriction four months earlier on my own. Then, armed with only a medical guidebook, I walked myself through all the steps I would later repeat with Conroy. I kept a sleep diary, determined the average number of hours I was sleeping (four hours and forty minutes), and fixed my bed- and wake-up times (12:30 to 5:15 a.m.). I took the plunge not because I'd overcome my doubts about sleep restriction, but because I was in the midst of a terrific bout of insomnia and using too many pills, and none of the measures I usually took to regain control of my sleep was working. I was desperate and ready for anything.

Sleep restriction then brought me face to face with all my fears.

Going It Alone

First night of sleep restriction, September 24, 2007: Miles away from the bedroom and the perils lurking there, I commence the evening's vigil in the family room. I'm sitting in my favorite stuffed chair, surrounded by as many accouterments of comfort as I can assemble: an afghan, an ottoman, a glass of water, and a pile of newspapers and books.

I dive first into *The Science Times*, then pull out a biography. I'm counting on the controversy created by Father Coughlin and Huey Long to help while away the hours until I'm permitted to go to bed. It works for a while. Later when I feel my mind growing slack, I pick up a memoir. The story is quirky, the language, too. But as I read, I feel a familiar twinge in my stomach. Distracted, I raise my head and glimpse the clock. Already it's 1:45. Only three and a half hours until my wake-up time of 5:15. Yet I don't feel the least bit sleepy. My mind is dimming but my body's still aroused. This is not a good sign. My stomach clenches further, and moisture tickles my armpits. Suddenly I'm overheated.

I throw off the afghan, thinking coolness will calm me and help my concentration. But the tension in my stomach bleeds through the twists and turns in the memoirist's life. I lay the book aside, close my eyes and try deep breathing. "In, two, three, four, five six, out, two, three, four, five, six." I continue until I feel my tension start to fade. But no sooner do I stop counting than a malicious voice starts up: "You're going to feel lousy tomorrow. You're going to feel lousy all week."

A surge of electricity races down my arms and legs. I'm burning up and now I'm wired. Sitting is suddenly intolerable, I'm itching to move. But where to, and what to do? TV is unappealing, and I'm not up to doing work. I've spent too many hours on the computer to want to spend more. It's too late to call friends, and I don't feel safe walking outside. Balance my checkbook? Do light housework? Plan meals? Nothing appeals. I wander around the house and wind up at the digital piano in the living room.

There I raid my cache of golden oldies, thinking the ballads that once lulled me into drowsiness may work their magic again. I put on my earphones and play through the songs one by one. They're still comforting after all these years. When my vision starts to blur, I fumble some of the notes. "Misty" turns into a parody of the song I used to play so well. But I keep playing till the knot in my stomach has nearly disappeared. I try to relax further by talking to myself.

Maybe tonight I won't sleep at all. So what? I've survived all-nighters before, kept vigil with a book or on the Internet (more typically with a glass of wine at hand to dull the anxiety). At 3:30 or 4 a.m., when it's clear my "night" is over, I'll make a cup of coffee. The smell of the roasted grounds released by the heat will be soothing, the first sip, more so. And with the first pale gray stripes of light on the slatted blinds I'll crow: I've made it, I've survived intact. Daylight will release me from the trials of the night, bringing enough distractions to make me forget—temporarily—the sadness I feel at being unable to do what for most people is as easy as breathing air.

Tomorrow I will function. I'll put in six hours' work, do chores, meet friends, exercise. I don't renege on commitments, I've never collapsed. I do all I can to make the day as normal as possible: that, at least, allows me some control. Insomnia may wreck my nights, but I'll be damned if I let it wreck my days.

But I'll be running on empty. And the thought of having to push through that exhaustion, the dreariness, the lack of mental clarity is what keeps me burning through my insomniac nights.

Fear of sleeplessness and its consequences: I'm a textbook case. If they passed out awards I'd come first in my class. But naming what I have hasn't helped me overcome it. Nor has trying to reason it away, or the relaxation techniques proffered as cures. Thirty years have gone into its making. By now it's reflexive, like my startle response to loud noise.

"It will pass." I recall my husband's words of comfort, and on a rational level I know they're true. Even the worst bouts of insomnia always pass, after a week or two or four. Yet my gut feeling during bad nights is that my insomnia will be unending. I'll be trapped forever in a Twilight Zone where I'm neither sleeping nor fully awake.

Eventually I fall asleep. So far the CBT-I cure is worse than the disease.

Second night: The urge to sleep hits me at 10:30 p.m. . . . and I ignore it. Bedtime is not for another two hours. By 11, I'm yawning; by 11:15, my head is falling over my book. I keep having to jerk my head upward. I reread passages four and five times. By 11:45 I'm struggling keep my eyes open; I'm glancing at the clock every five minutes. Then a few minutes before 12:30, when I'm heading to the bedroom, fear ambushes me in the doorway. My stomach clenches up, and jitteriness courses through my arms and legs. For two hours I've fought off slumber. But now that the time for sleep has arrived, my malevolent double wishes me to stay up. I get in bed, but sleep is out of the question now. So I leave the bedroom fifteen minutes later per instructions in my guidebook, and return to reading. When I start nodding, I go back to bed. But once I'm there, fear seizes me a second time, and I get up again. Down, up. Up, down. How long can this torture go on?

Third night: A repeat of the second. And when the alarm wakes me in the morning, it feels like 2 a.m. I crave more sleep, I long for it with every fiber of my body. For a few minutes I lie still. I feel achy, beaten, spent. When finally I open my eyes, darkness stretches out all around me, with the palest moonlight streaming in from the window over the bed. I listen to the rhythmic breathing of my husband, whose sleep is undisturbed.

Am I really going to force myself to get up? I've done it before for early morning classes and jobs. Nervous energy usually comes to my rescue. But there's no hint of a rescue today. Eventually I push my legs off the bed, raise my torso, and stand up, only to succumb to enervation and sit down again.

There are other signs this will be no easy day. The kitchen light is too bright; the clatter of pots and pans, too loud. In slow motion I make my morning coffee and sit down at my computer. But the coffee has no impact. It is a molasses-brain day. When I start to rise, spots swirl at the periphery of my field of vision. I sit down and wait for the spinning to stop. Maybe I could crunch numbers; I could certainly paint walls. As for writing anything coherent or creative, today will be a wash. So I'll do some filing. Piles of articles clutter the room, waiting to be placed in folders. Five minutes into the operation, I realize even this is beyond me. I'll have to dedicate the day to folding clothes and paying bills. Resentment cuts through me like a sharp knife. Why am I having to pummel my body into doing what for others is second nature?

I page through my guidebook, looking for any scrap of encouragement I can find. This "initial sleep loss" is supposed to increase my homeostatic pressure for sleep. "What we're asking," the authors write, "requires a trade-off—'short-term pain for long-term gain.'"[7] OK. I understand delayed gratification. The tedious practice required to master a foreign language, the miles I've put in to get in shape for a long-distance cycling trip. But now I feel like I'm approaching the end of my tolerance. How much longer can I last?

Stubbornness was the main thing that kept me going during that first, self-guided experience with sleep restriction, a story I'll return to later. Now let's fast-forward to the story of the group.

Changing Negative Thoughts

Conroy did her best to urge us on. By staying the course with sleep restriction, leaving the bedroom if we were not sleeping, and observing the rules of sleep hygiene, we would all improve our sleep. Those of us whose sleep efficiency was at least 85 percent could spend fifteen minutes more in bed with each new week. (Some experts recommend that sleep efficiency be at 90 percent or above before increasing time in bed.[8])

The focus then shifted to the cognitive component of insomnia. So what were we thinking about before we went to sleep? Conroy asked. Each of us had filled out a questionnaire entitled "Dysfunctional Beliefs and Attitudes about Sleep," and this week's homework had involved the tedious task of writing down and analyzing any thoughts related to sleep.

Matt was worried that insomnia and sleep restriction might have serious consequences on his health. "I worry about being sleep deprived because I'm afraid I might get sick," he said. "And if I'm sick I can't use my voice, and without my voice I can't work."

Did Matt always get sick after a poor night's sleep? Conroy asked.

No.

How often did he get sick?

Once in a while. Not often.

So what would be a more realistic statement about what happens after a poor night's sleep?

I probably won't get sick.

Probably not. Conroy paused.

There was no one-to-one correspondence between insomnia and sickness or disease, she said, no evidence that insomnia made you sick. Also, sleep deprivation was not the same thing as insomnia. Sustained sleep deprivation could in the long run take a toll on health. But people with insomnia typically got *some* sleep—and perhaps more than we realized. The consequences of insomnia were not as dire as we might suppose.

I was far enough along in my research to know that correlations between chronic insomnia and diseases associated with aging were stacking up. But when I volunteered this information, Conroy reiterated her point that the correspondence was not one-to-one, and moved on to ask what other sleep-related thoughts we'd had. Evidently this was not to be a time for open-ended discussion.

Did we fear that a single bad night's sleep would trigger a series of bad nights?

In fact, she said, a short night's sleep would create a bigger sleep debt, which would help us sleep *better* the following night.

Did we worry about how insomnia would affect our ability to function the next day?

There was no evidence of a one-to-one correspondence between insomnia and performance. In fact, many things could have a negative impact on performance. The same stressors that could trigger insomnia—pressures at work, rocky relationships, poor health—could also interfere with daytime functioning. So we should shift our attention to these stressors and confront them directly, rather than blaming daytime difficulties on poor sleep.

Conroy's message was crystal clear. The fewer negative symptoms we attributed to insomnia, the less fraught with anxiety our nights would be. The fewer misconceptions we had about sleep, the more realistic our expectations would be. A positive mindset could help to improve sleep.

No doubt this was true. But it didn't speak much to the psychological component of my insomnia. The feelings I struggled with at night were certainly linked to negative thoughts and attitudes. Yet those fears and anxieties, thirty years in the making, felt more connected to my gut than to my head. Trying to chip away at them with reasoning and persuasion was like throwing darts at ceramic tiles.

But Matt felt otherwise. Conroy's talk about negative thoughts helped ease his anxieties. At our two-month follow-up, he reported worrying less about sickness, and that he'd stayed healthy through sleep restriction therapy. "I'm not sick," he said. "I'm not failing to do my job." Nor was he so concerned about fluctuations in his sleep. "If I sleep poorly one night, I know I'll sleep better the next."

Results

The five of us didn't enter therapy looking for a change in attitude, though; we came seeking tangible improvements in our sleep.

On that score Andrea hit the jackpot. I could imagine her featured in a glossy brochure. "That first week I was really tired," she said. "But the exhaustion, trying to stay up until midnight and being just exhausted, did it for me. I had to fight to stay awake, and then I'd go to bed and be asleep within minutes, and would not wake up until my alarm went off at 5:15.

"I won't say I sleep longer. But the quality of my sleep is better. That five hours I'm in bed, I'm asleep," she said, attributing her gains mostly to sleep restriction. "Now, after five, maybe six hours, I wake up and I'm ready to go."

Elaine's sleep was better, too: less interrupted by patches of wakefulness. "The main thing I got out of it was that I was going to bed too early," she said.

Matt's report on the improvements he made was more qualified. He was continuing to set a wake-up time, he was taking fewer naps, and, as a result, he said, "I've got my mornings back." But he didn't feel fully rested. "I feel like maybe I'm halfway there. I'm going to bed at 12:45 and getting up at 7:15. But I still feel like I need more sleep."

My sleep stayed in a holding pattern, regular but short, mainly because group therapy coincided with an unexpected stress. I'd stumbled upon another insomnia book soon to be released, and I wondered if after its publication there would be anything worthwhile left to say on the subject. It turned out there was not a huge amount of overlap in the content and tone of that book and mine, but I didn't know it at the time. I thought the years I'd devoted to my project might amount to years down the tube.

A truer picture of how I fared with CBT-I emerged during my first experience with sleep restriction.

A Different Kind of Night

Fourth night: Again my head starts bobbing a few hours before my scheduled sleep time. And at 12:30, as I approach the bedroom, my stomach clenches up. Here we go again, I think sourly. I'm in for another round of Pop Goes the Weasel. Step right up, ladies and gentleman. Prepare to watch this freak of nature sabotage her sleep.

I get in bed . . . and the next instant someone's shaking my shoulder. I swim into consciousness and open my eyes to my husband's moonlit face. The clock says 5:15. In the darkness I do a quick body check. I feel completely spent, like I've just woken up from the first sleep after jet lag. But there's no tension anywhere, no achy arms or legs. And I can barely remember getting in bed. I must have slept a full four hours and forty-five minutes. Shot cleanly through the goal posts without a moment's wakefulness.

I'm ready not to feel lousy, I think, sitting up. But, ready or not, I don't feel good. I sleepwalk through my morning routine, spilling coffee, dropping a dish. Mentally it takes a long time to rev up to speed. But I manage five hours' work at the computer, not brilliant, but passable. I run errands, do chores, call my mother, exercise, fix dinner . . . and wonder what the night will bring.

Sleep comes the minute my head touches the pillow, and in the morning I wake up to the alarm myself. I want more sleep. I want lots more sleep. But once I move into the day I feel OK. And—dare I admit this?—I feel hopeful. But hopefulness may queer the deal. I've tried so many things that have worked for a while only to fail me in the end. Wait and see, wait and see.

By the end of the first week I'm cautiously optimistic. I extend my sleep time by fifteen minutes per instructions in the guidebook, then by thirty minutes, then forty-five. At the beginning of the third week, it's clear my sleep has improved, and the improvement is holding. I don't always sleep a full night. Sometimes I wake up half an hour early; sometimes, at 1:30 a.m. But awakening then doesn't bollix the rest of the night. I'm able to fall back to sleep fairly quickly. I still have the yo-yo neck in the evening as I struggle over my book to stay awake. Sometimes I'm seized with panic, and the knot in my stomach returns. But not every night, not even most nights. And the panicky feeling is more apt to fade quickly, as I find myself feeling sleepy at about the same time every night. Often I fall asleep within ten minutes of lying down. And in these fifteen days only once have I taken a sleeping pill.

Outcomes

I have two motives for enrolling in group therapy four months later. One is to see if by placing myself in the hands of a professional and going through CBT-I in a group setting, I can improve my sleep still further. The other is to find out how other insomniacs respond to CBT-I, and what results they achieve.

On that score, our group fared about as well as statistics would predict. Four out of five of us felt we benefited from therapy. None of us made substantial gains in total sleep time. But the four of us agreed our sleep was better than before. It was easier to get to sleep and to fall back to sleep at night, and we felt more rested in the morning.

These are typical of gains made by insomniacs in CBT-I, research suggests. Increases in total sleep time will be modest. The average insomnia sufferer may get thirty minutes more sleep a night. Older people with insomnia may not make gains in total sleep time at all.[9]

But good sleep may have less to do with quantity than with quality. Sleep quality is associated in part with reduced wakefulness in bed; that is, sleep efficiency. Here, there's solid evidence that CBT-I gets results. The average insomniac can expect to cut her nocturnal wakefulness in half. She'll cut the time it takes to fall asleep by half; she'll cut the number of nighttime awakenings—and their duration—in half. Also, following CBT-I, patients' assessments of their sleep quality go up.[10] This subjective evaluation cannot be validated in the laboratory, as there is no objective measure of overall sleep quality. But what counts is not what a machine can measure but rather how you feel. If you think your sleep has improved, then it has.

As we saw in the last chapter, insomnia is sometimes associated with reduced slow-wave sleep (SWS). There hasn't been much investigation of the impact of CBT-I on sleep staging, but the results of two studies are encouraging. A team of French researchers found that after eight weeks of CBT-I, SWS durations were significantly increased in nine insomnia patients (average age 47).[11] In a Norwegian study of forty-six older insomniacs, subjects underwent one of three treatments: CBT-I, a sleeping pill (similar to Lunesta), or a pill placebo. Six months later, the sleep efficiency of the CBT-I group was up by 11 percent, and their SWS increased by 34 percent. In contrast, the sleep efficiency and SWS in the other subjects declined. Notably, subjects taking the sleeping pill experienced a 23 percent drop in SWS.[12] These results are "striking," say authors of the study, and I'll agree. Slow-wave sleep may not be the Holy Grail for all of us, but a therapy that enables more of it sure sounds good to me.

What about the effect of CBT-I on the daytime symptoms of insomnia—fatigue, low mood, mental lethargy? The results of older studies are mixed.[13] But in two recent studies, subjects who underwent CBT-I reported significant mood elevations and, in one, they also reported increased vitality and better social functioning. Another study showed that six weeks of CBT-I restored brain activity in areas of the prefrontal cortex that were underactive in insomnia patients, improving their performance on a verbal fluency task.[14]

So if you try CBT-I, there's a good chance the efficiency and quality of your sleep will improve, and a chance you'll feel better during the day. You may also make small gains in total sleep time, especially if you're young or middle-aged. A few studies tracking insomnia patients suggest that these improvements may continue for months and years after therapy ends.[15] And if you relapse, the experts advise revisiting the practices learned in therapy: stay out of the bedroom except when sleeping, and restrict your sleep for an hour or more for a few days until sleep is solid again.

But CBT-I does not have a 100 percent success rate. It was big disappointment for Eric. "I felt worse, " he told me later, when I asked about his experience with sleep restriction. "I got more irritated because I was more tired. I've tried staying up later, till 1, 2, or 3 in the morning. Still, I get three, four, or five hours of sleep. That's it." Nothing about CBT-I worked for him and he eventually dropped out of the course.

Sleep restriction does not suit everyone. When it was first tested twenty-five years ago, eight of the forty-nine insomniacs who signed up to participate withdrew "because of a mixture of discouragement and difficulty complying with the rigid schedule."[16] On average, Michael Perlis said, 25 percent of insomnia patients who try CBT-I drop out.

Is there a way to predict who's going to benefit and who won't? I asked Perlis.

"If you think insomnia is all about conditioned, persistent activation of wake-related assemblies," he said, "then stamping on the homeostat should force them to shut down and eventually lead to conditioning where they shut down all by themselves with less impetus, so CBT-I is fine for psychofizzers." As for people diagnosed with idiopathic insomnia (lifelong insomnia driven by biologic factors) or paradoxical insomnia (people whose EEGs register a full night's sleep but who may feel they're hardly getting any sleep at all), the benefits of CBT-I are not so clear. "I'm less confident that bringing homeostatic pressure to bear—particularly for paradoxical folks—is going to shut those assemblies down and make for a homogenous state of brain inactivity," Perlis said. In other words, while CBT-I is effective for people with psychophysiologic insomnia, it may not work so well for people with other types of insomnia. However, Perlis added, many people fall into more than one diagnostic category. We're mixed breeds, a percentage of our symptoms deriving from one set of factors, and another percentage, from another. Many insomnia sufferers should be able to benefit from CBT-I.

Whatever kind of insomniac I am, CBT-I has been part of the answer for me. For nearly five years now I've been practicing "sleep scheduling" (distasteful term!). The first year I worked my way up to six hours in bed. I stayed on that schedule about a year and a half, averaging about five hours and fifteen minutes' sleep a night. But I was still getting sleepy well before bedtime. The yo-yo head routine was frustrating. Bright light in the evening did nothing to help. Nor did moving my bed and wake times forward by half an hour. I simply had to work too hard to stay up till bedtime, and the effort was so arousing that by the time I got there, I was sometimes too wound up to sleep.

So I modified the routine. The key for me was, I felt, continuing to get up at the same time every day, rain or shine. Forcing myself out of bed after a bad night was a drag, the following day, never a picnic. But it was better to suffer a slowdown of a day or two rather than the meltdown I knew would occur if I allowed myself to sleep in.

Bedtime was a different matter. Pegging it strictly to the clock was creating anxiety, so I decided in the evening to turn all my clocks to the wall. I wouldn't go straight to bed at the first sign of sleepiness; that had gotten me in trouble before. Instead, at the first nod, I would earnestly apply myself to the task of staying up longer (just like good sleepers! or so the experts claim). I'd go through the yo-yo head routine and then, after three or four bouts of nodding, when I felt myself really tired, I'd head to bed. And that's where I am with it now. I don't know how much I'm sleeping; I'd guess I average five to five and a half hours. On rare nights I probably manage six.

If this gain sounds trifling, I assure you it doesn't feel that way. Sleep used to be unpredictable; that it comes now with any sort of regularity is amazing. I sometimes sleep right through the night, and more often I wake up feeling rested. Several months of sleep scheduling passed before I noticed consistent changes in my days. But now, with a boost from coffee and sunlight, my mood is better and my brain, more agile. Maybe I'm getting more sleep; maybe the quality of my sleep has improved. Maybe it's that I'm taking fewer sleeping pills.

But the biggest boon for me has been the lessening of fear. The clenching stomach that could occur at the sight of evening sunlight streaming through a window or the thought of darkness is mostly a thing of the past. And when fear does surprise me near bedtime, it's not quite the bogeyman it used to be. The sleepiness I normally feel as the evening progresses manages to trump it much of the time.

Psychologists would say I've essentially "extinguished" my fear, that new and positive experiences with sleep have led to a "rewiring" of my brain.[17] If so, I'm convinced that what enabled this rewiring was mainly my few weeks of sleep restriction and ongoing adherence to a fixed sleep schedule. Sloughing off fear has left me with new skin. And I like the feeling way too much to want to turn back.

I made these changes on my own; group therapy was basically a rerun. I hope this is encouraging for insomniacs who don't have health insurance or whose health insurance will not pay for therapy. What it requires is step-by-step instructions, available in self-help books and on the Internet, and ironclad discipline. It is not rocket science. Keep the sleep diary, make a few simple calculations, and enforce weekly bed- and wake times. Make sure your sleep efficiency stays at or above 85 (better yet, 90) percent. Two books that can guide you through the process are *The Insomnia Workbook*, by Stephanie Silberman and Charles Morin, and *The Insomnia Answer*, by Paul Glovinsky and Art Spielman. Online courses developed by experts in behavioral sleep medicine are available at these addresses: Cbtforinsomnia.com, Sleepio.com, and Shuti.me.

For those who prefer and can afford to work with a therapist face to face, there are advantages to doing so, as Matt was quick to point out. "Having somebody who's experienced with this telling me that, if I do this, there's a good chance everything will turn around is very inspiring," he said. Many therapists trained in behavioral sleep medicine treat patients one on one. Certified providers are listed online at Absm.org/BSMSpecialists.aspx and Behavioralsleep.org/findspecialist.aspx.

There are also benefits to working in a group. Everyone in my group had something positive to say about the camaraderie, including Eric. "I don't get as mad anymore now that I know it's not just me," he said.

Matt, too, found the group supportive. "I may have read about some of these things before," he said, "but having the opportunity to sit in a class with other people who are in the same boat—and the discipline of being in a class—makes it easier to do."

Empathy and support: they're available on blogs and in online forums, but otherwise for insomniacs they're pretty rare. "Who wants to hear how you slept last night?" demanded one frustrated insomniac. "I did pick up the vibe that 99.9 percent of the people I come into contact with could give a flying you-know-what about whether I slept last night. And when I thought about it, why should they?"

Yes, the savvy conversationalist learns to steer clear of talk about bad nights. And with so much unsolicited advice springing from the lips of the unencumbered—of the drink-warm-milk, get-a-better-mattress variety—who even feels like raising the topic at all? Yet in the presence of empathic listeners, insomniacs have a lot to say, and group therapy is a place where talk can happen. Nobody but another insomniac knows the challenges the sleepless face when we get together for family sleepovers; no normal sleeper will cluck quite so sympathetically at your wrenching dilemma over the guy who would be perfect except that he thrashes and snores. Other insomniacs may not have the answers. But you can rest assured they will not ask if you've seen that Ayurvedic doctor, or tried tapping seven times on the stress points all over your body. Small blessings can make all the difference in the world!

I enjoyed the people in my group. In short order they came to feel like fellow travelers, and I looked forward to hearing how they fared from week to week. But I wasn't completely at ease in my role as patient. Something felt Big Brother-ish about a therapist sifting through the details of my nights, monitoring substances I consumed and the hours I kept, on the lookout for "illicit" behavior. When I caught myself feeling guilty about taking a sleeping pill one night and hesitant to record it in my sleep diary, memories of all the negative experiences I'd had with doctors concerning my insomnia came flooding back. It didn't matter that this therapist was among the most empathic health professionals I'd ever met. It was hard to trust another to help when the solutions proposed were so exacting. I didn't fare as well during group therapy as I did before or have since. But that would not keep me from recommending the program to any other insomnia sufferer seeking help.

Even the most enthusiastic CBT-I proponents acknowledge that for all the benefits therapy affords, it does not change poor sleepers into really good sleepers. Of insomnia sufferers who achieve "clinically meaningful change," Canadian sleep investigator Charles Morin has written, many "reach a plateau and continue showing residual sleep disturbances after treatment and may remain at risk for relapse."[18]

This describes my situation to a T. The scaffolding my now more regular sleep is built on is not indestructible. Any change in routine—traveling, working or socializing at night, forgoing exercise—can trigger an episode of insomnia. Sleep scientist William Dement makes routine his credo: He habitually leaves parties early— even dinner parties at his own home!—so he can observe a routine conducive to his sleep. ("If I don't put sleep first, who will?" he tells his guests.)[19] That's not a trade-off I'd want to make. My body thrives on regularity; my spirit does not. In extraordinary times I head for the pills.

Even when I adhere to routine, my sleep is susceptible to influences that would not necessarily derail other people's sleep. A rough day at work, elation after a party, or anticipation of a trip can easily push me into overdrive. My body lights up like a radar screen detecting myriad flying objects. It stays this way for hours and hours.

In the daytime I can usually channel the extra energy into normal activities. But having to contend with the lit-up feeling at midnight is another matter. Then all bets are off when it comes to sleep. Which would not be such a burden if it didn't also open the floodgates to my fears. Then, anxious and sleepless, I'm back to square one. Insomnia redux.

So now it's time for a closer inspection of what's going on inside insomniacs' bodies and brains.

9

Lit Up Like a Christmas Tree

There's times I just don't sleep at all. I'm just too
wound up, too hyped up to sleep.

Brandie, an insomnia sufferer interviewed
for this book

Insomniacs sleep poorly and we slog through our days. At the
same time it can feel like there's triple espresso coursing through
our veins. No matter the fatigue and depletion, we just can't seem
to relax.

We've heard from experts who say this arousal is largely conditioned. It occurs mainly in the evening and at night, and can be
unlearned by pushing wakeful activities out of the bedroom and
restricting sleep.

But Michael Bonnet, clinical director of Kettering Sycamore
Sleep Disorders Center in Miamisburg, Ohio and professor at
Wright State University School of Medicine, disagrees.

"A lot of psychologists will tell you that insomnia stems from bad
behavior," Bonnet said in an interview at his clinic, "that because you

got sloppy and didn't behave very well, now you have an insomnia problem. I say you probably inherited a genetic predisposition to have a different underlying physiology, which is now causing you to have problems." These problems are not limited to sleep. Nor are they due to a lack of sleep.

"Insomnia is not a sleep problem," Bonnet said, adding that therapies focused solely on enhancing sleep are not the best type of treatment. The real issue is a hyperactive arousal system. "What you have," Bonnet tells his insomnia patients, "is a physiological problem where you're just turned on too much all of the time and can't really relax." The aim of treatment, he said, should be to down-regulate arousal.

We're going to delve further into the arousal connected to insomnia and explore how to tone it down. But first let's consider the other issue Bonnet raises: insomnia and genetic predisposition.

A Heritable Trait

Family and twin studies suggest that susceptibility to insomnia may indeed be programmed at birth. As we've seen, research shows sleep length and quality are under moderately strong genetic control, and the same can be said about insomnia. Investigators in a study of sibling pairs recently found that genetic factors account for about 37 percent of the variance in vulnerability to stress-related sleep disturbance. A much larger study of twins in Washington State put the heritability of insomnia even higher, at 57 percent. The risk for insomnia is nearly seven times greater among first-degree relatives of primary insomniacs, say researchers in France, than in the general population.[1]

Not many specific "insomnia genes" are known. But a research team in Germany recently found that a short variant of the serotonin transporter gene is significantly more common in insomniacs than good sleepers. While the gene should not be seen as *causing* insomnia, it "may generally predispose to disorders in which learned associations play a role, like primary insomnia, social phobia, and depression," say authors of the study. It may "predispose the individual to stress-related reactions in the context of a stressful life event."[2]

Even sleep scientists in the behavioral camp acknowledge that part of the problem must lie in the genes. "Given the ubiquitous nature of transient insomnia," Dieter Riemann, a sleep researcher at Freiburg University Medical Center, and colleagues have written, "it seems reasonable to assume that only those individuals with a certain genetic vulnerability for sustained hyperarousal are prone to develop chronic insomnia."[3] Despite the lack of specifics, the consensus seems to be that people with chronic insomnia are the way we are in part because of our constitutional make-up.

Arousal in the Driver's Seat

So what sort of arousal do insomniacs contend with? We'll explore this by first returning to Bonnet's provocative claim that insomnia is not a sleep problem.

This idea may strike some readers as farfetched. Any therapy that *really* gave insomniacs the sleep we crave would solve the problem, right? If we could just get rid of our lousy, patchy sleep, then everything else would fall into place. No more fatigue, no crappy moods. No concentration or memory problems, no dark circles under the eyes. We'd look and feel rested, we'd be set for life.

Yet experiments conducted by Bonnet and his wife and research partner, Donna Arand, suggest this might not be the case. "If insomnia really is just a sleep fragmentation disorder," Bonnet said, "then I ought to be able to produce all the symptoms that an insomnia patient has in a normal person by just giving them the same sleep pattern." But when Bonnet and Arand tried this, disrupting the sleep of normal sleepers every night for a week, their subjects only vaguely resembled insomniacs by the end of the experiment. Yes, they reported more fatigue and less vigor (symptoms of sleep deprivation), but there the similarity ended. Unlike insomniacs, these sleep-deprived normal sleepers came to experience *less* tension, *less* depression, and *lower* metabolic rates, and they fell asleep with increasing ease.[4] Apparently you can't turn gifted sleepers into insomniacs merely by fragmenting their sleep for a week.

Nor, in a second week-long experiment, did Bonnet and Arand succeed in making insomnia subjects feel worse by depriving them of 20 percent of *their* normal sleep. By the end of that week, some daytime symptoms in the insomniacs had actually *declined* in severity, while others remained unchanged. Importantly, the subjects did not report decreases in sleep quality, although their total sleep time was in fact curtailed.[5]

Bonnet interprets the results of these two experiments as proving his point. "Every sign I could see was saying, 'Hey, insomnia is not a sleep disorder,'" he said. "All these manipulations I've done to sleep haven't had the impact of causing insomnia or making insomnia worse. Insomnia is not sleep deprivation. It's another disorder altogether."

The closest Bonnet and Arand came to creating a human model of insomnia was in an earlier experiment where they took normal sleepers and dosed them heavily with caffeine, a central nervous system stimulant. The subjects in this study took sustained-release caffeine tablets—in the amount of 400 mg—three times a day for seven days. That's a heckuva lot of caffeine! The daily dose was equivalent to three Starbucks ventis (a venti holds twenty to twenty-four ounces of coffee).

As expected, the caffeine increased subjects' metabolic rate and arousal levels, particularly in the early stages. It also affected their sleep. Although by the last caffeinated day they were sleeping better than at first, still it took them longer to fall asleep and was harder to stay asleep, and they got less sleep (and less deep sleep) than normal. Tellingly, the caffeine strongly affected subjects' mood. Showing a steady increase over the week were feelings of fatigue, depression, anger, and confusion. The anxiety they felt moved significantly toward psychopathological levels.[6] Does this begin to sound like insomnia?

Bonnet thinks it does.

"If I want to give myself insomnia and feel like a real insomniac, basically I'll do the equivalent of drinking three or four cups of coffee," he said. "That's my internal model of insomnia, the feeling that you can't relax. You're always trying to go even though you don't necessarily want to go. You mainly just want to rest, but your body just won't let you. That's very, very fatiguing actually because it's like you're always walking uphill even though you're sitting still, and there's no way to escape."

Bonnet and Arand have concluded that sleep loss is at best a step-parent to the fatigue, irritability, and mental sluggishness insomniacs experience during the daytime. The true progenitor of both our sleep difficulties and our daytime symptoms, they argue, is excessive arousal—or "hyperarousal"—of the central nervous system.[7]

Hunting for Hyperarousal

The sensation will be familiar to many readers.

"Sleepstarved days," writes Gayle Greene in *Insomniac*, "days I'm on overdrive, those are the days I feel like a bundle of nerves, when I really might startle if a waiter drops a tray. I sigh a lot, I mutter to myself, and it all seems so overwhelming, my heart races and strains as though it has an appointment somewhere else. . . . Those are the nights when I get into bed and the system keeps on whirring. If you met me on a day like this, you'd say, That's one hyperaroused insomniac."[8]

Feeling all hyped up and short on sleep can be completely overwhelming. Yet scientists looking for evidence of hyperarousal in insomniacs' bodies have not produced overwhelming results. Detecting physiological differences between insomniacs and normal sleepers is a little like listening in on a guinea pig picnic: lots of squeaks but no big whoops.

Here's how we differ physiologically from our good sleeper peers:[9]

- Insomniacs have an elevated heart rate as bedtime approaches and during the night; two studies have documented higher heart rates during the daytime as well.

- Insomniacs have a higher whole-body metabolic rate around the clock, as demonstrated by the higher volume of oxygen we consume.

- Some insomniacs have lower heart rate variability (another measure of arousal).

- Elderly insomniacs tend to have a higher core-body temperature at night.

But not all studies indicate that insomnia is associated with excessive physiological arousal. The uneven results point to two big problems with insomnia research: The studies are often small, and insomnia subjects are not necessarily screened according to the same criteria from one study to the next. In the absence of consistent screening, it's hard to replicate results.

"I'm averaging together apples and oranges," Bonnet said, "and wondering why it doesn't look like an apple any more." Bonnet's claim is that insomnia patients with abnormal EEGs (recall that many insomniacs have EEGs that look quite normal) are the ones more likely to show significant physiological differences from normal sleepers.

Scientists have also looked at whether hyperarousal registers as higher levels of stress hormones floating around in our bodies and brains. Normally, stress hormones show up in full force in moments of crisis. Within seconds, the sympathetic nervous system has ramped up production of epinephrine and norepinephrine (a.k.a. adrenalin and noradrenalin). These chemical messengers are the body's first responders to stress, gearing us up to fight or flee. They can also become chronically elevated, as occurs when people are under persistent stress, or in people with anxiety disorders.[10] But the few researchers who have studied norepinephrine in insomniacs have come up with mixed results, some finding higher levels of norepinephrine and others, not.[11]

More effort has gone into examining the relationship between insomnia and the other limb of the stress system: the hypothalamic-pituitary-adrenal axis. Activation of the "HPA axis" results in the production of cortisol.

Cortisol, as mentioned before, is a key player in the sleep–wake system. It's one of those nice, domestic hormones secreted on a daily basis under orders from the circadian clock. It helps wake us up in the morning, and it exits the stage around bedtime. But in moments of crisis, it becomes a powerhouse of a stress hormone, the body's chemical equivalent of Clark Kent. Within minutes of sensing danger, the HPA axis is fully engaged. Cortisol production shoots upward, helping to mobilize stores of glucose, which rush toward our muscles to propel us into action. Then, even after we've got the situation under control, excess cortisol can remain in the bloodstream for several hours.[12]

Persistent stress can result in chronically elevated levels of cortisol, as can major depression. This is not a good thing. It interferes with learning, performance, and memory consolidation. Over the long haul, it puts people at higher risk for hypertension, cardiovascular disease, type 2 diabetes, and other stress-related illnesses.[13] Could insomnia, too, lead to elevated levels of cortisol and all the nasty fallout?

While short-term sleep deprivation causes a temporary elevation in cortisol levels in normal sleepers, the relationship between chronic insomnia and cortisol remains unclear. Some investigators have found higher levels of urinary or plasma cortisol in insomniacs than normal sleepers; others have not. A study presented at a 2010 conference did not find evidence of higher twenty-four-hour urinary cortisol in insomnia patients, yet it *did* show that the amount of cortisol and norepinephrine were significantly correlated, and that this correlation was greater in insomniacs than in good sleepers.[14]

Once again, mixed results underscore the need for research on a larger scale. Despite the uncertainty, though, most insomnia investigators are convinced that on this issue, where there's smoke, there's flame. Chronic insomnia likely involves alterations in HPA-axis activity that interfere with sleep and day-to-day functioning and may impact our long-term health. What's behind these alterations remains to be seen. Scientists are calling for further studies to sort out "whether it is the chronic (mostly minor) sleep loss of many insomniacs driving the cortisol abnormalities or whether a primarily hyperactive cortisol axis contributes to the development of insomnia."[15]

A Bedtime Story: Reading the Brain Waves

The study of insomnia and stress hormones is relatively new. But scientists have scrutinized our brain waves for decades, and it's here where the story on insomnia and hyperarousal comes into sharper focus. Electroencephalography is a lot more relevant to insomnia these days than it used to be.

You know the routine: Just as you're settling into bed or returning from the bathroom, a stray thought pops into your head. Suddenly you're replaying yesterday's argument blow by blow, what you said, what he said, what you could have said to *really* drive home your point. Or you're obsessing over work the next day, trying to figure out how to get everything done so you can cross the finish line in time to pick your daughter up at 6 p.m. Yes, insomniacs are prone to rumination and worry, especially at night.

But it's not just during spells of wakefulness that cogitating can compromise the night. The mental activity can continue even while we're sleeping.

"I've always been a very light sleeper," said Liz, a long-time insomnia sufferer, "one of those people who wake up at the slightest sound. When I first came to Canada I was married. I remember one night my husband said, 'My God, I think you can hear the grass grow!' I could hear a cat meowing three blocks away! I'm very sensitive to sound, especially an animal. If the cat was meowing outside, I'd hear it instantly and be up and letting him in."

When Liz went in for a sleep study, her EEG looked abnormal. "The thing they saw was that I never go into deep sleep," she said. "I'm always at the arousal level. It fits with what I always knew."

But in other instances—up to 50 percent of the time, you may recall—the EEGs of insomniacs who spend a night in the sleep lab look exactly the same as normal sleepers.[16] They show insomniacs sleeping about the same amount of time, and going through the same number of sleep cycles, as people who bounce out of bed like Energizer Bunnies. Yet like Liz, many insomniacs are disturbed at night by noises and sensations that good sleepers easily tune out. Our sleep feels shallow, broken, insufficient. Some insomniacs feel they hardly get any sleep at all.

What scientists now know about our brain waves does not stop with the standard EEG. Modern digital equipment captures a vast amount of information during overnight sleep studies, yet when this information is scored visually in standard fashion, a lot gets lost. Each 20- or 30-second sleep period (or epoch) is scored as one of four sleep stages: stage 1, stage 2, deep sleep, or REM. More than one wave pattern may be present in a 20- or 30-second epoch, yet only the dominant pattern gets scored.

"For visual scoring," sleep investigator Michael Perlis said, "the rule is, the majority rules. This is a great averaging technique, but if you're looking to explain why people dream during non-REM sleep, it's a bad way to do it." Sometimes low-pass filters are used to screen out the higher frequencies entirely, Perlis said. This makes it easier to single out the dominant wave formation in each epoch and score it accordingly.

But the standard EEG amounts to a gross simplification of neural activity occurring in the cerebral cortex at night. It "represents drastic data reduction, in that roughly four megabits of data is reduced to three bits of information." "Through data reduction," investigator Andrew Krystal said at a conference on sleep and sleep disorders, "we're throwing out the wheat with the chaff."[17]

So the usefulness of the standard EEG for many insomniacs will be next to nil. If you've ever wondered why your lousy night in the sleep lab wound up smelling like a rose to the lab tech who presented you with the fabulous news in the morning, this could be it!

The story changes, though, when scientists take all the signals captured in the EEG during sleep and perform something called a "power spectral analysis," or PSA. PSA is a mathematical technique used to deconstruct complex wave formations into the different frequencies they're composed of, and show how strongly represented each frequency is. It's similar to a color analysis of the designer paint on your kitchen wall. Complex colors are composed of many different colors, and if you want to match your wall color exactly, you have a paint chip analyzed to find out which colors the paint is composed of and how much of each color there is. Likewise, the neural activity in your brain at night consists of waves of slower and faster frequencies. At any given time, one waveform may predominate, yet others are present as well. Power spectral analysis reveals all of the frequencies and how much of each there is.

A PSA of normal sleep would show a lot of low-frequency neural activity (0.5 to 8 cycles per second), but there would not be much activity in the high-frequency bands. Beta waves (14 to 35 cycles per second) are abundant when people are alert and solving problems, but they're largely absent during sleep.

Not so in many insomniacs. A PSA of data captured during an overnight sleep study may reveal higher-than-normal levels of beta activity in the insomniac brain. Gamma activity—even faster waves associated with highly focused concentration—may show up as well.[18] It looks like our sensory antennae are attuned to the environment, and our brains engage in information processing, even as we sleep. Again, this high-frequency activity goes undetected in the standard EEG.

Some sleep scientists interpret excessive beta activity at night as evidence of hyperarousal. It makes it harder to fall asleep, and it compromises the sleep we get. It's also thought to explain why some insomniacs underestimate the time we sleep. "Enhanced information processing during non-REM sleep may blur the . . . distinction between sleep and wakefulness."[19] People who experience lots of this high-frequency activity at night are diagnosed with "paradoxical insomnia" (formerly known as "subjective insomnia," "sleep state misperception" and "pseudoinsomnia"). Overall the brain may be sleeping, but in several key areas, neurons continue firing away as they would if the sleeper were alert and taking in the sights on Broadway.[20]

The Insomniac Brain on Noise

Sleep studies are typically conducted in soundproof rooms, where no dripping faucet or flushing toilet can possibly interfere. But in recent years scientists have devised another way of measuring neural activity in the brain. Using equipment that introduces sounds—both regularly and randomly spaced—into the ear, they can study how the brain reacts to noise. The brain waves produced under these conditions are called "evoked response potentials," or ERPs.

Not many ERP studies comparing the reactions of insomniacs to those of normal sleepers have been conducted yet. But the technology enables exploration of a variety of issues. One question under investigation is this: Are insomniacs simply more sensitive to noise? Do our brains register more excitement at the sound of a beep or a click than the brains of normal sleepers? A few studies suggest this may well be the case.[21] What in most people's brains registers as a squeak may register in us as a squawk.

Scientists looking at ERPs can also see how hard the brain is working to block out noise, which typically occurs as people fall asleep and during sleep. Normal sleepers' brains are good at this. They "show compensatory mechanisms that allow them not to be so disturbed by stimuli and disengage from wake to sleep."[22] Insomniacs, on the other hand, appear to be C-minus students when it comes to blocking out noise. The few existing ERP studies to record brain waves during sleep onset and in the early minutes of sleep show that our brains have trouble inhibiting noise. Research also suggests that while good sleepers' brains easily tune out repetitive noises such as the ticking of a clock, insomniacs "may have difficulties closing channels to non-pertinent stimulation."[23]

As for whether this sensitivity to sound is mainly limited to the evening and the night (which would lend support to psychological and behavioral models of insomnia), or whether it's with us around the clock (which would be more in line with the hyperarousal model), the jury is still out.

"It's possible that they [people with insomnia] are hyper-attuned 24/7," Michael Perlis said, "that they're just like that all the time. During the day, it makes you a little light sensitive, gives you headaches, makes you a little sensitive to the din. But there's no real consequence, because it's not of a magnitude that creates a disorder during wakefulness. The problem is that during the night, it's got a consequence." And that consequence is disturbed sleep.

It's also possible that enhanced sensitivity to noise is mainly situational, occurring due to arousal occasioned by sleep-related worries and unsuccessful efforts to get more sleep. The question cannot be answered until more ERP studies are done, particularly studies at night.

This research fascinates me because it hits close to home. Sensitivity to noise is something I struggle with daily, and not just at night. At home and in the car, I'm forever turning music down. I stuff my ears with Kleenex at movies and concerts. My husband's loud sneezes set off mini rage attacks inside my head.

But when a housemate once described me as "finely tuned," I'm sure he was referring to more than my hypersensitivity to noise. The fact is that many strong stimuli cause me discomfort, including light and temperature extremes. My intolerance to heat is especially bad at night. Traveling in India in June, when no A/C was available, I tossed and turned all night. I'm sensitive to minor aches and pains and miserable with colds that others toss off in a few days. And when it comes to tactile sensations, I'm the queen of fussiness. Touch me lightly and that's too ticklish. Itches drive me crazy and I've got the scars to prove it. At night, I'm finicky about the covers around my neck. And the slightest jiggling of the mattress can send me through the roof.

Nobody has done ERP studies of insomnia and its relationship to these other sense modalities. But research is heading in that direction, Perlis said, adding, "We're going to a place where this third unseen rail is finally being addressed."

It may be that people with insomnia are "hyperproprioceptors," Perlis said. What a mouthful! "For whatever reasons, whether it's conditioned or lifelong, they [people with insomnia] hear a dripping faucet that most of us don't. They're potentially sensitive to light— although I doubt this—in a way that others are not.

"It's not going to be across-the-board, meaning every sense modality. I don't think it's going to be gustatory or olfactory. But I think it's probably going to be nociception—pain—and it's going to be audition, for sure. And it's going to be tactile, for sure."

Perlis hastened to add that these are just conjectures now. But ERP studies can be devised to test them. If it turns out that insomniacs' brains *are* more reactive to sensory stimuli (or have more trouble blocking them out), this will constitute further evidence that when it comes to CNS arousal, insomniacs are cranked up a notch too high. Still, this excess of arousal is not to the degree you'd feel if you came face to face with a masked intruder with a gun.

"Nobody can maintain levels of physiologic CNS excitation of a real fight/flight response," Perlis said. "We're simply not built for that. We'd burn out in a second." Rather, it would suggest that insomniacs are saddled with a vigilance and readiness to respond similar to that occurring in PTSD, Perlis said, and other disorders associated with a small but chronic elevation of stress hormones.

Alas, ERP studies are still few and far between, and the results, inconsistent. "But the bottom line is that it's an evolving story with a powerful technology," Perlis said. Stay tuned.

What a Picture Is Worth

Arguably the most striking evidence of excessive arousal in insomniacs comes from neuroimaging studies of the brain. We've seen that insomniacs' brain waves at night differ from normal sleepers'. Insomnia sufferers tend to experience more high-frequency activity in the cerebral cortex immediately before and during sleep. We've also seen that insomniacs' whole body metabolism tends to be higher than normal sleepers'. You'd expect this higher metabolic activity to show up in our brains as well, but a neuroimaging study in 2002 failed to affirm this premise.[24]

Then came another neuroimaging study that passed the "wow" test with flying colors. A group at the University of Pittsburgh School of Medicine used PET scans to assess glucose metabolism in the brains of insomniacs and good sleepers in the morning and as they were falling asleep at night. The results were presented as images, with quiet areas of the brain appearing in shades of gray and the regions metabolizing glucose showing up in a fiery orange-red.

What a difference between the brains of normal sleepers and insomniacs! Overall, both night and day, insomniacs' brains were burning brighter, metabolizing more glucose than the brains of good sleepers.

The contrast was particularly marked as subjects were moving from lighter to deeper stages of sleep. The metabolic lights went out quickly in the good sleepers. In short order, brain areas associated with arousal appeared in uniform gray. In contrast, those same areas in insomniacs' brains showed up as bright red. As insomniacs transition into slumber, it seems, a host of critical subcortical areas continue metabolizing glucose, stuck in the "on" position.[25]

"When people with primary insomnia tell us they can't shut their brains off, we think now that they really can't," said sleep researcher Gary Richardson in a conference presentation in 2009. "Metabolically, their brains seem to be working overtime. They're lit up like Christmas trees."[26]

Pictures this vivid are hard to argue against. Two years later, the group in Pittsburgh, again using PET scans, found in insomniacs a correlation between wakefulness and excessive glucose metabolism in the brain at night.[27]

These findings and others have led the Pittsburgh group to propose a neurobiological model of insomnia that incorporates the theory of sleep regulation set forward by James Krueger and colleagues (chapter 7). "Insomnia is characterized by simultaneous sleep and wake-like activation patterns in specific brain regions regulating sleep–wake state and self-awareness," they write.[28] Here again, insomnia is described as a hybrid state where we're neither fully sleeping nor fully awake. Especially noteworthy, says the Pittsburgh team, is heightened metabolism in an area of the cortex called the precuneus, which plays a role in memory, visual processing, and self-reflection. Metabolic activity here "may contribute to the subjective experience of self-awareness" at night. The authors also cite studies showing that glucose metabolism in the precuneus and various arousal centers is reduced following sleep restriction and treatment with the drug Lunesta (eszopiclone).

A Chemical Imbalance

A different sort of neuroimaging study also passed the "wow" test and suggests another possible biological explanation for the arousal associated with insomnia. A team of Harvard researchers led by

John Winkelman showed in 2008 that the brains of insomniacs were deficient in GABA, the brain's main inhibitory neurotransmitter.[29]

Sleep experts have long wondered if GABA is a culprit in insomnia. GABA neurons are found throughout the brain, and one of their main purposes is to shut down activity in areas associated with perception and thinking. Importantly, GABA is involved in the initiation and maintenance of slow-wave sleep.[30] Most sleeping pills on the market today—hypnotics such as Ambien (zolpidem) and Lunesta—work by increasing the activity of GABA neurons.

Winkelman and colleagues set out to study insomniacs and normal sleepers to find out if there were differences in the chemical make-up of their brains. They collected data using magnetic resonance spectroscopy (MRS).[31] Sixteen insomniacs and sixteen normal sleepers participated in the study and underwent MRS scans. The subjects remained in place for twenty minutes, positioned so the scanner could assess the relative concentrations of neurochemicals in a thick slab running through the center of their brains.

The study turned up one crucial difference between the brains of insomniacs and normal sleepers. Most chemical substances identified in the scans—choline, creatine, and glutamate, to name a few—were present in equal amounts. But average brain GABA levels in insomniacs were lower by nearly 30 percent! What's more, reduced GABA levels correlated strongly with poor sleep continuity, as reported by the subjects and as confirmed by polysomnogram. Winkelman's group is the first to offer evidence of a specific neurochemical abnormality associated with insomnia.

David T. Plante, a sleep researcher at the University of Wisconsin School of Medicine and Public Health, and colleagues conducted a second MRS study in which they measured levels of GABA in specific brain regions. This group compared twenty insomniacs and twenty healthy sleepers and found that the insomniacs had significantly less GABA in two areas of the brain: the occipital cortex and the anterior cingulate cortex.[32] Both studies suggest that reduced GABA may be a biomarker of insomnia. Reduced levels of GABA would upset the balance of excitatory and inhibitory influences in the brain, inclining the brain toward wakefulness. Thus it fits with the hyperarousal model of insomnia.

The hunt for hyperarousal in insomniacs goes on. While some studies point to significant differences between insomniacs and normal sleepers, lack of follow-up, and studies with conflicting results, have kept things inconclusive. But the more that excessive arousal can be documented, the more scientists can pinpoint the brain areas and substances involved, the closer they will be to identifying the biological mechanisms underlying our problems, and the easier it will be to formulate effective treatments.

This research should feel liberating to some readers. If for years you've shouldered the blame for your affliction, wondering if it's something psychological, why toeing the line in the sleep hygiene department is not the surefire fix it's said to be, or why your sleep gets thrown off by stressors that good sleepers can easily park at the bedroom door, here lie the beginnings of an answer. It's now pretty clear that parts of the insomniac brain have a hard time going and staying offline. It may even be that we're programmed for hyper-vigilance around the clock.

But this may also strike you as cold comfort. If behavioral treatments like sleep restriction and stimulus control fail to bring relief, or if stress continues to interfere with sleep, what next?

Relaxing into Sleep

Insomniacs don't have a good relaxation response, Michael Bonnet says. The parasympathetic nervous system, whose function is to help restore bodily equilibrium, isn't very good at wresting control away from the alarm system and calming us down. So it's time to look at treatments aimed at down-regulating arousal directly. Drugs are one possibility, and we'll explore hypnotics in the next two chapters. Here are some nonpharmacological alternatives you've probably heard about and may want to consider again.

Relaxation training. Several insomniacs I interviewed report that relaxation techniques help their sleep . . . sometimes. I can say the same. The rhythmic breathing I began in the early 1980s will occasionally come to my rescue when I'm on verge of sleep and just having trouble sliding over the hump.

The American Academy of Sleep Medicine recommends relaxation training as a standard "effective and recommended therapy" for insomnia—the highest stamp of approval the academy gives. Practices mentioned include progressive muscle relaxation and autogenic training (guided visualization). Yet in three of the four most recent studies this recommendation is based on, relaxation therapy, though it reduced insomnia symptoms, was far surpassed in efficacy by regimens that included some type of sleep restriction. Other studies of relaxation training have not found it to be effective for insomnia at all.[33]

I haven't heard anyone in the sleep community championing relaxation training as a stand-alone treatment for insomnia. But sometimes it's included as part of CBT-I.

Meditation. Jason found a path to better sleep through meditation. An engineer whose sporadic bouts of insomnia became chronic during a rocky relationship, he quickly chucked the Ambien his doctor prescribed and headed out to find a different cure. The cause of his sleep problem was "things that just run through my mind and that I just don't or can't stop thinking about," and it made more sense to him to address the chatter head-on rather than take a pill. He bought a book on meditation, which, together with changes in sleep hygiene, did more than anything else to help him get his sleep back on track.

"The thing to do is to relax your mind, and to focus on your breathing," he said. "Meditation has helped me learn how not to think. If I wake up in the middle of the night and just lay there and keep my mind from racing, then I can usually fall back to sleep."

Claims that meditation helps reduce arousal and promotes better sleep are legion. But scientific support is still slim. A recent pilot study combining mindfulness meditation with CBT-I showed that the combined treatment resulted in improved sleep for insomnia patients, and, the authors noted, "a significant correlation was found between the number of meditation sessions and changes on a trait measure of arousal." Most gains were maintained during a twelve-month follow-up period. But to my knowledge, only one randomized controlled trial has shown that mindfulness meditation training is effective for insomnia. In this study, eight weeks of mindfulness training was comparable to 3 mg of Lunesta taken nightly. The subjects made "large, significant improvements" in many aspects of sleep, including total sleep time and sleep quality.[34]

Tai Chi. This gentle Chinese martial art looks promising for older adults. Two RCTs have shown that six months of tai chi—a combination of meditation and movement—improved sleep quality and duration in older adults with moderate sleep complaints. The authors of one study speculate that the improvements came about because tai chi reduces arousal of the sympathetic nervous system as treatment progresses. Particularly in older adults whose insomnia is not yet chronic, they say, tai chi has the potential to "forestall the onset and progression of insomnia complaints to clinical severity."[35]

Yoga. Devotees claim it can do everything from straightening a crooked spine to curing yellow fever and worms! In fact the practice has been found to reduce stress and improve sleep in pregnant women, cancer patients, and disaster survivors. A small number of studies suggest it may do the same for insomniacs. For example, an RCT conducted on residents of an Indian home for the aged (most reporting sleep difficulties) found that sixty minutes of yoga practiced six days a week for six months led to a sixty-minute increase in reported sleep time, greater ease in falling asleep, and feeling more rested in the morning. In another RCT, postmenopausal women in Brazil who practiced yoga for four months reported reduced insomnia severity and greater resistance to stress than control subjects.[36]

Harvard Professor of Medicine Sat Bir Khalsa claims that yoga addresses aspects of insomnia that are not as well addressed in CBT-I. "Yoga works on inducing the relaxation response," he told me. It reduces activation of the stress system, altering the functioning of the autonomic nervous system and the hypothalamic pituitary axis. "Yoga and meditation also change the perception of stress," he said.

Khalsa conducted a pair of experiments on Boston-area insomniacs, finding in both cases that yoga led to "significant improvements" in sleep. In the second study, an RCT of sleep-onset insomniacs that Khalsa reported on at a conference in 2009, half of the subjects practiced daily yoga exercises involving simple arm postures, meditation, and slow breathing for forty-five minutes before bedtime. The other half received instruction in sleep hygiene. After eight weeks, the sleep of subjects in both groups had improved. But the yoga subjects' sleep had improved a lot more, the standout improvement being sizeable gains in reported sleep time.

Comparing the efficacy of yoga and other behavioral treatments for insomnia, Khalsa said that while "the yoga treatment is less effective than full CBT, yoga may address characteristics unaffected by CBT," promoting "a positive change in stress tolerance."[37] This sounds like a move in the right direction.

None of these mind–body practices is known to be efficacious as a stand-alone treatment for insomnia. But the literature suggests they may help insomniacs to down-regulate arousal. We insomniacs are a heterogeneous bunch. If you've got a runaway mind or a body buzz that never goes away, they're certainly worth checking out. Researchers now are promoting them as adjunct therapies to CBT-I.

Exercise

Every self-help book for insomniacs, every sidebar listing the ten steps to better sleep, touts the sleep-inducing benefits of exercise. "It is scientifically proven that exercise improves sleep," self-help guru Paul McKenna has written in a book on sleep. "You must tire your body if you hope to sleep well," said sleep expert Peter Hauri in his book, *No More Sleepless Nights*.[38] But is this bit of conventional wisdom true?

The idea that exercise facilitates sleep fits well with various theories about the purposes sleep serves in human beings. Do we sleep because of a periodic need to conserve energy? There's no activity that depletes our energy stores quite as much as exercise, which should help bring on sleep. Do we sleep because of a need to restore bodily tissue? There's no activity that causes quite so much breakdown of bodily tissue as exercise, which should also promote sleep. Or do we sleep to down-regulate body temperature? Again, there's nothing like exercise to elevate body temperature, which in turn should help to induce sleep.[39] Exercise *should* be more soporific than an all-night filibuster on the virtues of dental floss.

Bonnet is convinced that exercise is indeed the best path to better sleep. The core question for insomniacs, he said, is "How do I figure out how to get a good relaxation response?" The first thing he suggests to his insomnia patients is physical training.

Bonnet acknowledges that the suggestion is not well received. "Usually when I propose physical training to my patients, they don't like the idea," he said. "They're resistant to the idea of exercise, and this may have contributed to their sleep problems in the first place. A sedentary lifestyle may be one reason they are where they are today." But the patients who have heeded his advice and seriously pursued physical training have significantly improved their sleep.

In the past, research turned up little evidence for the sleep-enhancing benefits of exercise. Most early experimental studies were conducted on normal sleepers, whose sleep following various exercise regimens did not show significant improvement compared to the sleep of control subjects.[40] So when sleep is good to begin with, exercise probably won't make it any better.

But larger, epidemiological studies of the general population—which would include both good and poor sleepers—have typically found exercise to be moderately beneficial to sleep. Data from the National Sleep Foundation's 2013 *Sleep in America* poll show that

- Exercise correlates with better sleep quality. About 83 percent of the survey respondents who got vigorous exercise reported their sleep quality to be "very good" or "fairly good," as well as 76 to 77 percent of the respondents whose exercise was light to moderate. Only 56 percent of the non-exercisers reported good sleep quality.

- Exercise helps people fall asleep faster. Non-exercisers reported taking nearly twice as long to get to sleep as those who exercised vigorously.

- Exercise cuts down on feelings of sleepiness during the day. Nearly twice as many non-exercisers (24 percent) as exercisers (12 to 15 percent) experienced excessive daytime sleepiness.[41]

To date, studies of the effects of exercise on insomnia have been conducted only on poor sleepers middle-aged and older. The results suggest that exercise *is* at least somewhat beneficial to insomniacs in these age groups.[42] In a recent study of sedentary middle-aged insomniacs, for example, six months of moderate-intensity aerobic exercise three days a week significantly improved their sleep and quality of life. Polysomnography showed that exercise cut the time it took to fall asleep in half, and that wakefulness decreased by 37 percent. Subjects also reported better sleep quality and decreases in anxiety and depression. In two separate studies of elderly insomniacs, a sixteen-week course of aerobic exercise three or four times a week significantly improved subjects' sleep and reduced insomnia symptoms during the daytime. In one of the studies, the exercisers reported a net gain of forty-two minutes of sleep a night.[43]

Insomniacs prone to anxiety and depression may find that physical training is a twofer. Exercise has been shown to have a calming effect on anxiety, so if you're anxious *and* sleepless, there's double reason to believe exercise will help. Exercise has antidepressant effects for insomnia sufferers as well, according to the results of at least two studies.[44] It's quite possible that exercise will buoy your spirits as well as improve your sleep.

When it comes to the positive effects of exercise on sleep, I'm a true believer. But I didn't become a convert very early or very easily.

Not that I was ever a couch potato. I did a lot of hiking and bicycling on weekends (and still do). For a few years bicycling was also my means of transportation to work. But I didn't do either one out of concern for general fitness. Jogging was the most convenient way to see to that. A simple change of footwear and I was out the door. Jogging felt good; it got rid of whatever stress was left over from the day, and sometimes I got the celebrated endorphin high. For years I hit the pavement three days a week.

I didn't notice that jogging or any type of exercise affected my sleep one way or the other. But when my physician brother-in-law suggested I might be able to beat insomnia by physically exhausting myself, I started to look more closely. From what I could tell, sometimes I slept better after jogging, but not always. Anyway, I didn't want to do it more often. Jogging had its points, but the thought of stopping whatever else I was doing to lace up my Nikes at 5 p.m. every day did not appeal.

It was only when I began keeping a sleep diary that I noticed a consistent relationship between exercise and my sleep. Then the evidence was plain to see: overall, sleep came sooner, and was more solid, on days when I worked out on the elliptical trainer in the late afternoon. So with plenty of internal grousing (What? One more thing in the "have to do" column? Grrrrrr!), I moved to exercising every day.

Now I ride a bike in the summer and do my hamster-on-a-wheel routine in the winter, staving off boredom with recordings of Masterpiece Theater productions, movies, and news reports. On some days I'd rather be reading *The New York Times*, socializing with friends, or poking around in the garden. But with vigorous daily exercise I drop off more easily and sleep more soundly. Without it, I'm not as sleepy when my normal bedtime rolls around, and I wake up more frequently during the night. Somehow I try to fit the exercise in even when my schedule gets tight.

Been there, done that, and exercise hasn't worked for you? Here's where experimentation may be in order, guided by research suggesting that different strokes may work for different folks.

The type of exercise you do can make a difference. Typically recommended is aerobic exercise: vigorous, sustained activities that get you breathing deeply and your heart pumping faster. In most studies cited above, it was aerobic exercise that led to improvements in sleep. A 2010 study comparing the effects of three different types of exercise on insomniacs' sleep found that a single fifty-minute session of moderate-intensity aerobic exercise on a treadmill was far superior to three brief stints of high-intensity aerobic activity and also to a moderate-intensity strength training activity in improving sleep and reducing anxiety.[45]

As for duration and frequency of exercise, research has no definitive answers yet. In the long-term exercise studies cited above, subjects exercised anywhere from thirty to fifty minutes from three to seven days a week. That's quite a range! More exercise is probably better than less, but how much is enough is something insomniacs have to discover for ourselves.

For insomniacs wishing to start an exercise program, the overall goal should be to decrease their resting heart rate, Bonnet said. "Several studies have shown that there is a significant correlation between heart rate and sleep latency [the time it takes to fall asleep]. An acute effect of exercise is to increase heart rate, and if you exercise too much or too late," he said, the elevated heart rate may make it harder to fall asleep. "However, when you do training like jogging every day, your resting heart rate decreases. In general, a low basal heart rate is related to parasympathetic dominance [a better relaxation response]," which in turn should make it easier to fall asleep. Bonnet advises his patients to check their resting heart rate at the outset of physical training and strive to bring it down.

The timing of exercise can also make a difference. As mentioned before, one theory on the function of sleep holds that humans sleep to allow our bodies and brains to cool down. It follows that exercise, which increases body temperature, might enable more efficient temperature downregulation and so facilitate sleep. This supposition is based on a series of experiments conducted in the 1980s. Just as hot baths in the late afternoon and early evening raised subjects' core body temperature and at night led to increases in slow-wave sleep, so strenuous exercise four to eight hours prior to bedtime raised core body temperature in physically fit subjects and, subsequently, led to increases in slow-wave sleep.[46] Since then, the experts have promoted the benefits of exercise late in the afternoon or early in the evening. (The word on late-night exercise is not so consistent: some studies suggest it disrupts sleep and others show it does not, and that it may even enhance sleep.)[47]

There's one caveat to the advisability of exercise later in the day. Exercise, like light, entrains the circadian clock and can shift your cycle forward or backward. Evening exercise can delay circadian rhythms. So it may exacerbate the sleep problems of night owls, whose body clocks are already inclined to run late. Nocturnal types may find it's better to work out earlier in the day.[48]

For all the potential that physical training may hold for insomniacs, the scientific studies are few in number. Bonnet thinks this has partly to do with funding. "Nobody is going to pay for those things," he said, adding that the big money for research on insomnia treatments comes from pharmaceutical companies, whose aims lie elsewhere.

Another factor may be a lack of interest on the part of insomniacs. "Insomnia patients by and large hate exercise," Bonnet said. As clinical director of a sleep disorders center, he's certainly in a position to know this. But his clinic is in rural Ohio, and I wonder if the patients he sees are representative of insomniacs overall. Regardless, I'm sure the issue he raises will resonate with many insomnia sufferers. Exercise may well improve sleep, but how many insomniacs are ready to adopt a solution that requires ongoing practice? CBT-I calls for effort at the outset. But once you've gone through the first few weeks of treatment and adjusted your habits, all you do is observe the new routine. To benefit from yoga or meditation or exercise, on the other hand, you have to commit to *doing* something several times a week. Talk about behavioral treatments! These are the most demanding yet!

But for insomniacs who struggle with feelings of hyperarousal, who—for whatever reasons—are highly susceptible to stress-related sleep disturbance, treatments that do not target arousal head-on (such as sleep restriction and stimulus control) may be only halfway measures to better sleep. Relaxation techniques and physical training are specifically aimed at reducing arousal, and they're the main drug-free options on offer now.

These practices don't get much lip service at conferences these days. The lion's share of new research on nondrug treatments is devoted to CBT-I. I heard one expert dismiss physical training as irrelevant to the management of insomnia. Restrict sleep and get rid of conditioned arousal, he said, and insomnia patients will be good to go.

This may be exactly the right prescription for some insomniacs. (Again, it's important to remember that we're a heterogeneous bunch.) But the changes I made following CBT-I have only been *part* of the answer for me. Equally important is the exercise I do every day.

Would I give it up for a quicker fix that was risk free? I might.

So now we'll examine chemical solutions embraced by some insomniacs and mistrusted by others.

10

Perils of the Pill

Above all, do not try to dose yourself. The greatest evil that results from insomnia is the drug we may possibly take for it.

Victor Heiser, *Toughen Up, America!*, 1941

My friend Leslye used to be able to fall asleep on a dime. Now she uses sleeping pills.

"I have a crazy life," she told me recently. When Leslye isn't running conferences in far-flung parts of the globe, she puts in a long day at the office. Then she goes home to fix dinner and hang out with her husband until 10 or 11 p.m. Later, a few times a week, she heads upstairs to her computer to churn out reports until 2:30 or 3 a.m. "If my boss says it's due tomorrow, I don't have a choice." Leslye's not complaining; she loves her hectic life, and she's ready to burn the candle at both ends to hold things together. Her naturally high-octane energy level pumps her up during the daytime, and it used to be that when she finally lay down, she crashed. But now she can't sleep without Lunesta. "I couldn't function without my sleep," she said, "and my psychiatrist understands that."

About 8 percent of American adults take a hypnotic—a drug that induces sleep—at least a few nights a week, according to the National

Sleep Foundation's 2009 *Sleep in America* poll. "Notably," the report says, "the use of both sleep medication prescribed by a doctor and over-the-counter or store-bought sleep aids has increased significantly over the last few years." Statistics on prescription hypnotics bear this out. About sixty million prescriptions were dispensed in 2011, up about 20 percent since 2006, according to IMS, a health care information and market research company. Prescription sleep aids are also growing more popular among the young. An analysis by Thomson Reuters shows that the use of sleeping pills nearly tripled from 1998 to 2006 among students and other young adults ages eighteen to twenty-four.[1] These statistics suggest that the prescribing and use of hypnotics has grown more acceptable in recent years and may continue along this path.

The mass media in recent years have cited financial distress as a factor behind Americans' increasing use of sleeping pills. But the steep rise in use began before the economic downturn, with the regulatory change that occurred when the Food and Drug Administration approved Lunesta for the treatment of insomnia at the end of 2004. Before that, sleep medications were approved "for short-term treatment" only, based on concerns that long-term use could lead to the development of tolerance (the need to increase the dosage) and dependence. Doctors who wrote repeat prescriptions faced a "burden of therapeutic guilt" for prescribing in a manner deemed risky by the FDA.[2]

Clinical trials conducted by the pharmaceutical industry in the past decade and a half suggest the newer pills are safer than their chemical forebears, and the FDA has agreed. Lunesta (eszopiclone), Rozerem (ramelteon), Ambien CR (zolpidem), and Silenor (doxepin) have been approved for use without the short-term restriction. Doctors who write repeat prescriptions are now consistent with FDA guidelines. The availability of these newer, purportedly safer hypnotics "has undoubtedly reduced the stigma of prescribing sleeping pills."[3]

Promotional efforts by the pharmaceutical industry have also helped whet Americans' appetite for sleeping pills. In general, about 80 percent of the pharmaceutical marketing budget goes toward promoting drugs to physicians (that's $8,290 per physician!), but the rollout of new sleep meds from 2005 to 2007 also included a barrage of commercials that no TV viewer could miss. "Lunesta is non-narcotic and approved for long-term use," said the voiceover, as an iridescent luna moth glided in and out of windows dispensing sleep. "Ambien CR is a treatment option you and your healthcare provider can consider along with lifestyle changes," said the voiceover, as a giant time-release version of America's most popular hypnotic dissolved into granules over the body of a sleeper like dust from a fairy godmother's wand. Direct-to-consumer advertising worked well in the years immediately following these products' launch. The more the drug makers advertised their new sleep aids, the more we took their advice to "ask [our] doctor" if they were right for us, and the more we left the doctor's office with a prescription in hand.[4]

For insomniacs willing to entrust themselves to sleep meds, the past eight years have been good, at least in terms of accessibility. "My doctor is what I'd consider a reasonably conservative sort," wrote an insomniac I interviewed, "and has no trouble prescribing Ambien for me for continued use. So I'll probably be taking it for the rest of my life. A dependency? I suppose so. But I'm OK with it. Hey, I have a dependency on food."

Another insomniac shared with me a pill-and-alcohol regimen he'd devised for himself in order to get to sleep and keep pace with the demands of his job. "Being a pharmacologist, I'm not afraid of mixing and matching," he said, laying out a weekly menu that included Ambien, Imovane (the precursor of Lunesta), Sonata, and alcohol, on a rotating schedule. "I am incredibly totally dependent on the drugs six nights a week."

Sleeping pills are also accessible and attractive to people like Leslye, who don't think of themselves as insomniacs but who use hypnotics nevertheless. Data from a national survey of doctor's visits from 1993 to 2007 show that prescriptions for drugs like Ambien and Lunesta far outpace complaints of sleeplessness and insomnia diagnoses. In fact, prescriptions grew twenty-one times more rapidly than did sleeplessness complaints and five times more rapidly than did insomnia diagnoses. The data, say authors of the study cited above, suggest "that life problems are being treated with medical solutions, without benefit of formal complaint or diagnosis."[5]

There's no doubt that the regulatory change that occurred with the introduction of newer drugs like Lunesta has broadened their appeal. Interviews and informal conversations suggest that in some cases they're now being prescribed and used as performance-enhancing drugs. This is hinted at in a forecast published by the market research firm Piribo in 2009.[6] Piribo predicts the use of medications for sleep disorders will continue to grow in the United States and abroad. That growth will be driven by "an increase in the use of insomnia-alleviating and wake-promoting drugs in particular."

Doctors are divided in their attitudes toward sleeping pills. "You certainly find health care providers that are very comfortable prescribing medications long term for insomnia," said psychiatrist David Neubauer of the Johns Hopkins School of Medicine, an expert in sleep medications who spoke with me at a conference on sleep and sleep disorders. "On the other hand, there are those who as a practice never do because they don't believe in it." Despite the relaxed prescription guidelines and claims that current pills are safer than older pills, some doctors feel the risks outweigh the benefits, citing studies like the analysis published in 2012 by sleep investigator Daniel Kripke and colleagues, linking the use of sleeping pills to an increased risk of death.[7]

Insomniacs likewise are divided on the issue of sleeping pills. Some are passionate pill defenders who'd kill for Ambien. At the other extreme are insomniacs—even those with severe symptoms—who shun prescription hypnotics. Still other insomniacs stake out a middle ground, some content to pop pills intermittently, others using them with reservations.

This range in attitudes deserves exploration. By definition, hypnotics are drugs that induce sleep, yet for some people they have meaning beyond the function they perform. In my mind, for example, the bottle of Ambien has an aura of danger that the bottle of Prilosec does not. "Enter at your peril!" it says. A whiff of the unsavory clings to it, too, like cat pee to a mattress. No matter how the pharmaceutical companies try to sanitize their image, sleeping pills are morally suspect.

The writer Bill Hayes has expressed it this way: "I've been using Ambien on bad nights, two or three times a month, for a couple of years, and it works well, yet I still feel as if I'm doing something dishonest." The Ambien is "at the back of the pill shelf in the corner, where it belongs, I believe—there being a moral hierarchy for prescription drugs. It's not that sleeping pills are bad per se, but there is something disreputable about them. I wouldn't want the Ambien bottle to accidentally fall out of the cabinet in front of the pest control man."[8]

The pest control man? If we care what *he* thinks when the bottle of Ambien tumbles out of the cabinet, then sleeping pills must be tainted indeed.

We looked at physician attitudes toward sleep medications in chapter 4. But there's little research on the attitudes of people who might use them,[9] so the material that follows is drawn mostly from interviews conducted during my research.

A Bum Rap

About half of the insomniacs I contacted had no interest in using prescription hypnotics (although some found over-the-counter sleep meds acceptable). Their reasons were mixed. Some did not think of insomnia as a medical problem, preferring to address it through changes in lifestyle or psychotherapy rather than with drugs.

"I guess I'm wary of my body being chemically altered," Matt said, following seven weeks of CBT-I. "I have this gut feeling I should try to figure out what's wrong with my sleeping patterns on my own without relying on a pill."

"I'm more convinced the problem is psychological rather than physiological," Jon, a law student, said. "I'd prefer not to use anything for it. The first eight months of last year was the longest period of therapy I've been through. I wonder if that helped me deal with whatever the problems were that were causing the insomnia, and maybe it's sort of miraculously disappeared."

Other insomniacs opted to steer clear of sleeping pills because of negative feelings about medicine overall and about prescription hypnotics in particular. Jody, a social worker, had qualms about raising the issue of sleeping pills with her doctor and attributed her feelings to her mother's wide-ranging objection to drugs and a belief that the correct way to contend with most health problems was to tough them out.

"My mom's the kind of person who will get her tooth drilled without Novocain!" Jody said. She recalled a visit from her grandmother, who brought along several medications but declared, after Jody's mother threw some in the trash, that she felt better without them. So Jody regarded her wakefulness—unpleasant though it was—as a condition she should "deal with" on her own. It was a natural part of life that people were better off enduring sans medication.

"What will my doctor think of me if I ask for sleeping pills?" she asked herself. "God forbid I ask for something that I don't need!"

Laura, a student of physical therapy, also talked about the role her mother played in shaping her attitudes toward insomnia and sleeping pills. "My mother also has trouble sleeping," Laura said. "She takes that as a strike against her character. She is real old country, her parents are right off the boat from Ireland, and I'm only second generation. The way I was raised was, you don't even take aspirin, much less go to the doctor. I only sought out sleep meds starting six months ago. My husband has enlightened me to the fact that seeing a doctor and getting medicine isn't a weakness."

To regard insomnia as a character flaw is an onerous burden, as we've seen. We *should* be able to reverse the situation through better self-regulation, goes this line of thinking. So to throw up our hands and resort to sleeping pills is a further sign of weakness. Not only have we ushered the elephant into the bedroom; now we're admitting we're powerless to push him out. Taking pills turns us into even worse human beings than merely being stuck with the affliction.

Another strike against sleeping pills in the eyes of some insomniacs is that they're palliative rather than curative. If curative medications like antibiotics and antifungals are at the top of our moral hierarchy for prescription drugs, medications that only relieve symptoms would fall nearer the bottom, with hypnotics and other mind-altering meds falling lower still. Not only do sleeping pills serve merely to manage insomnia, but they also carry the same stigma as drugs associated with mood and other psychiatric disorders. Just as you wouldn't mention you're on lithium during chitchat at a cocktail party, so you wouldn't mention taking sleeping pills (unless you travel in the fast lane, in which case taking Ambien or Lunesta is possibly de rigueur). You might think twice about asking for them at the doctor's office.

"I was actually afraid to ask my doctor about sleeping pills because I kind of thought she'd probably think I was nuts," Liz said. "In a lot of articles I read, and things you watch on TV, this person or that was crazy, and was on sleeping pills, or was on antidepressants. I just think sleeping pills are getting such a bad rap now. If you say to somebody, 'I take sleeping pills,' they think you're somehow or other a little bit crazy."

It may be that sleeping pills carry more of a stigma than other mind meds, especially antidepressants. Physicians today are certainly quicker to prescribe mood-altering drugs than hypnotics. Compare the over $11 billion Americans spent on antidepressant medications in 2010 to the $2 billion spent on prescription hypnotics.[10] ("Do I think we give out sleep medications because they improve sleep randomly in all living human beings?" presenter Thomas Roth deadpanned at the 2011 meeting of the Associated Professional Sleep Societies. "No. We only do that with antidepressants.")[11]

This difference in physicians' prescribing preferences may be due to the fact that unlike hypnotics, antidepressants are unscheduled drugs (meaning, in the eyes of the US Drug Enforcement Administration, that they carry little risk of dependency or abuse). But other factors may also come into play. Among physicians and the general public, mood disorders like depression and anxiety are increasingly regarded as "chemical imbalances." This makes the idea of a chemical solution more acceptable.[12]

The notion that insomnia might be caused by some sort of chemical imbalance is not so widespread, and the use of hypnotics for insomnia is not so widely approved of. Sleep investigator Wallace Mendelson in 2003 made this observation about benzodiazepines, an older class of medications: they caused much less concern when their purpose was to calm anxiety or relax muscles than when the aim was to induce sleep.[13] To chemically alter human consciousness is apparently more acceptable than to block it out completely.

Yet another reason some insomniacs steer clear of prescription hypnotics has to do with perceptions about the way the drugs work.

Western poets for hundreds of years have described falling asleep as a gentle process: "The timely dew of sleep / Now falling with soft slumbrous weight inclines / Our eyelids," wrote John Milton. "Visit her, gentle Sleep! With wings of healing," wrote Samuel Taylor Coleridge. "Lay thy soft hand upon my brow and cheek / O peaceful Sleep!" Henry Wadsworth Longfellow wrote.

Some insomniacs regard the action of hypnotics as contrary to the notion of sleep as a gentle force. "I can't take any *hard-core* pharmaceuticals," an insomniac told me. "A mild antidepressant, that's something I'd consider. But I'm afraid of sleeping pills."

"My instinct is that to take stuff like that every day is not particularly good for you," said another. "It's like you *knock yourself out* and then you're dragging around the next day."

Yes, in a sense, sleeping pills are a "hard-core," knockout solution to insomnia: a chemical clobbering of the brain. Think of an army of GABA neurons suddenly empowered to paralyze the brain in one fell swoop. True enough, sleeping pills *do* act vigorously to facilitate the calming of the brain. But falling asleep naturally often involves a similarly swift disarming of consciousness, as we've seen. Once the forces of wakefulness are spent and sleep drive builds up high enough, the sleep switch is tripped, and—whoosh!—the whole alerting system shuts down and sleep rolls in like a wave.[14] Yet when the process occurs naturally, we experience it as gentle. Chemically assisted, it's regarded as excessively forceful, and this is a deal-breaker for some insomnia sufferers.

On the other hand, the chemical knockout solution is exactly what other insomniacs look for. And this is the sort of language used by medical professionals to describe what sleeping pills do. In 2009 I went to a conference presentation with the intriguing title, "When You Have a Hammer, Everything Looks Like a Nail." The two "hammers" the presenter talked about were CBT-I and hypnotic medications. The "nails"—I'll confess this only dawned on me a few minutes into the presentation—were insomniacs.[15] Ouch! Yet a remedy too potent for some insomniacs is precisely others' cup of tea.

These concerns may figure into decisions about whether or not to use sleeping pills. But the big concerns vis-à-vis hypnotics relate to tolerance, dependency, and side effects. Some insomniacs I interviewed cited fears based on personal experience.

Novelist Ella Leffland described what it felt like to be hooked on sleeping pills: "I felt so jittery and unlike myself, and as if a huge brick were pressing down on me all the time; plus other things, like the dry mouth and the taste in the mouth," she said. "The one thing that really was a very bad side effect was the fact that I did not dream. That's scary.

"The insomnia got so severe that I was doubling and tripling the doses. That's when I decided to give up sleeping pills forever. And I did."

Dale, a marketing executive, had a tragic story about sleeping pills to recount. "My mother actually got addicted to barbiturates and died from it," he said, "so I'm absolutely not interested in anything strong."

David Neubauer points to barbiturate drugs by way of explaining the stigma attached to the sleeping pill today. "Historically, there's been a generally negative attitude toward sleep medications," he said. "It probably dates back to the meds that were used earlier in the 1900s. The barbiturates and a few other meds that were used for sleep turned out to be rather dangerous. They were toxic and people became significantly dependent on them."

Michael Perlis and colleagues also have suggested that the negative attributes of older sleep meds have shaped some of our attitudes about sleeping pills today. "The first generation of hypnotics' [e.g., barbiturates'] potential for abuse, habituation, dose escalation, and adverse events from overdose," they write, "appears to be firmly embedded in the popular consciousness and has likely lead [sic] to the common belief that 'the cure is worse than the disease.'"[16]

But some of the taint may date from even further back in time. The gums, powders, and drowsy syrups proffered to the sleepless in the nineteenth century were even less safe than the barbiturates. And well-publicized tragedies involving sleeping pills in the past hundred years, and unprincipled practices of drug manufacturers as they sought approval for and went about marketing them, are cautionary tales. Our attitudes about sleeping pills are freighted with baggage from the past. The story of these older meds suggests a legitimate basis for our misgivings and is relevant yet today.

The Ghost of Sleep Aids Past

Opium was the nineteenth-century's cure-all for everything from fevers and dysentery to pain and sleeplessness. Praised as "God's own medicine," opium could be taken on its own or mixed with alcohol, water, and spices in laudanum. Opium was also the active ingredient in patent medicines sold as insomnia cures. Advertisements for these medicines—Dr. Greene's Nervura Nerve Tonic, Paine's Celery Compound, and Doctor Williams' Pink Pills—appeared regularly in newspapers from *The New York Times* to *Ohio Farmer*. Opium and opium-containing compounds were unregulated and available in all but the most remote locales. Doctors could prescribe them freely and the sleepless could dose themselves.[17]

Morphine, an opium extract administered as a painkiller to Civil War soldiers, became the insomniac's mainstay later in the century. Doctors made house calls to give morphine injections at night. Physician D.W. Cathell in 1882 complained humorously about having to perform these nocturnal ministrations.

"It is a real hardship," he wrote in a popular medical handbook reprinted several times, "after doing your day's work, that you must go and administer a hypodermic night-cap of morphia to the Rev. Mr. Cantsleep at eight o'clock p.m., to Mrs. Allnerves at nine, to Colonel Bigdrinker at ten, and to Miss Narywink at eleven o'clock, and probably be called from bed again to insert the sleep-giving needle for one or all of them before morning."[18] The sleepless could also administer the drug themselves. Morphine and do-it-yourself hypodermic kits were available to all at the local apothecary.

But the dirty little secret about opium and its derivatives soon emerged: They were addictive and often had dire consequences. Many users quickly developed tolerance, needing more and more to achieve the desired effect, and finally became dependent. Academic Horace B. Day's story about his struggle with morphine appeared in *Lippincott's Magazine* in 1868, detailing the drug's seductions and horrors.

"I first took opium, in the form of laudanum, nearly ten years ago, for insomnia, or sleeplessness, brought on by overwork at a European university," Day began. Not only was laudanum effective for sleep, but it also gave him "unparalleled energy," and his "capability for mental exertion all through this period was something incredible."

The following year, Day received an appointment in India and began using morphine. His tolerance to the drug mounted steadily, and he increased his daily dose from one grain to sixty grains. Physical dependency on the drug enslaved him: "Four hours' deprivation of the drug gave rise to a physical and mental prostration that no pen can adequately depict, no language convey: a horror unspeakable, a woe unutterable takes possession of the entire being; a clammy perspiration bedews the surface, the eye is stony and hard, the nose pointed, as in the hippocratic face preceding dissolution, the hands uncertain, the mind restless, the heart as ashes, the 'bones marrowless.'

"There is but one all-absorbing want, one engrossing desire . . . *morphia*.

"Let it be understood that after a certain time . . . the craving for opium is beyond the domain of the will."[19]

The image of the opium addict as spineless degenerate and walking corpse was a fixture in the popular imagination by the 1870s. Estimates of the number of American addicts in the final decades of the century ranged from 100,000 to 200,000 and sometimes higher.[20] Death by overdose of morphine and laudanum taken for insomnia was regularly reported in obituaries in the major newspapers of the era.

Drugs developed in nineteenth-century laboratories as remedies for the sleepless were not much safer. Bromide salts, introduced as sedatives in the 1850s, were popular through the end of the century and beyond. Neurologist William Hammond's favorite was potassium bromide, which he lauded as "the most deserving of the name of hypnotic." Physician F.D. Pierce praised the bromides, too: "With regard to soporific drugs, I think that the bromides are entitled to the first place in the treatment of this affection." But cases of bromide intoxication were not uncommon. The bromides have a long elimination half-life of twelve days, so they readily accumulate in the body. (Half-life is the time it takes for the drug in the blood plasma to decrease by half.) As the toxic dose is not much higher than the effective dose, it was easy to overdose, giving rise to hallucinations and delirium.[21]

Chloral hydrate, too, was touted in the last third of the nineteenth century as a wonder drug for the sleepless, "an agent which possesses the faculty of inducing sleep of a far sweeter and more tranquil character than opium or morphine procures." But woe to the harried businessman and neurasthenic housewife who lost their moorings and started down that path. Nightly users quickly developed tolerance and dependency. By the 1880s and 1890s doctors were castigating fellow professionals for turning so many insomnia sufferers into "chloral victims." Wrote William Rosser Cobbe in 1895, "Physicians insisted for years that a 'habit' was impossible for the chloral user, and there are some who still persist in the claim that one may take the drug indefinitely without harmful results; in the face of indisputable testimony that the country is full of chloral habitués. There is not one town or city in the United States that is free from slaves of the somnific, 'colorless, bitterish, caustic crystal.'"[22] Like morphine and laudanum, chloral hydrate not only destroyed the user's freedom of will but it also claimed lives through accidental overdose and suicide. Even so, the drug that took the life of the proud heroine in *House of Mirth*, and that induced paranoid delusions in Gilbert Pinfold, is still in use today, listed as a Schedule IV drug for the short-term treatment of insomnia.

The popular press in the final decades of the nineteenth century took a dim view of medicinal sleep aids, asserting that drugs did not induce natural sleep but rather "a counterfeit state of unconsciousness." They were poisonous agents of destruction. A physician writing in *Harper's Bazaar* lamented the numbers of women who, nervous, sleepless, or in pain, ended up more miserable still as addicts. "It matters little whether it be morphine, gum opium, laudanum, McMunn's Elixir, paregoric, chloral, chloroform, ether, or hashheesh," he declared, "the result is eventually the same—mental, moral, physical, and financial ruin, the sundering of family ties, the loss of self-respect, and to some, the most unfortunate, insanity, idiocy, suicide, theft, and murder."[23] The correct way to combat insomnia—in the eyes of pundits and journalists—was to eschew drugs and reform one's living habits.

The Barbiturates

Barbiturate drugs promised to be different. Introduced in the early twentieth century as the first sleep aids in tablet form, drugs like Veronal were touted as an "infallible cure for insomnia," producing sleep that was "wholly natural" and free of side effects. After World War I they became the insomniac's mainstay and remained popular until the early 1970s. Veronal and Luminal worked well and had fewer side effects than older drugs taken for sleep. They went down easily, put users to sleep quickly, and kept them sleeping through the night. Taken in prescribed doses, barbiturate drugs were comparatively safe.[24] They were also prescribed as daytime sedatives.

But by mid-century, there was evidence that barbiturates lent themselves to abuse. Like alcohol, barbiturates taken in high doses could intoxicate, turning heavy users into addicts whose stumbling inebriety made them look like alcoholics.

"The barbiturate addict presents a shocking spectacle," wrote novelist William Burroughs in *Naked Lunch*. "He cannot coordinate, he staggers, falls off bar stools, goes to sleep in the middle of a sentence, drops food out of his mouth. He is confused, quarrelsome and stupid. . . . Barbiturate users are looked down on in addict society: 'Goofball bums. They got no class to them.'"[25] Like their soporific forebears, the barbiturates turned incautious users into abusers stripped of willpower and self-control.

Shorter-acting barbiturates like Nembutal and Seconal were especially dangerous. The body built up tolerance to these drugs quickly, so users were prone to escalate the dosage. Barbiturates were sold over the counter in the United States until 1938, so it was easy to develop and sustain a habit, and many users did. Even in decades after that, when obtaining barbiturates required a prescription, users could return to the pharmacy or visit different pharmacies and have their prescriptions refilled time and time again. FDA inspectors after World War II found several cases like these: A barbiturate user hospitalized for an overdose had had a prescription for thirty capsules refilled sixteen times in three months. Another woman, who finally died of barbiturate poisoning, had had a prescription refilled for a total of 7,000 pills in five years. Tolerance to the barbiturates led to dependency and impaired judgment, increasing the risk of overdose. Abrupt withdrawal from high doses caused agitation, convulsions, delirium, and sometimes death. New York City health authorities estimated in the 1940s that one death from barbiturate poisoning was occurring every thirty-six hours.[26]

Prescription barbiturates were demonized in the popular press, as were their counterparts—"blue devils," "red birds," and "yellow jackets"—sold on the street. Commentators decried the sleep they induced as "unnatural" and inferior, and asserted that the urge to double and then quadruple the dose was irresistible. Titles of magazine articles written about sleeping pills from the late 1930s through the 1950s tell the story: "Dangerous Lullabies," "Lethal Lullaby," "Sleeping Pills Dangerous," "Sleeping Pills: Doorway to Doom," "Sleeping Pills Are Worse Than Dope," "The Menace of the Sleeping Pill Habit."[27] The poet Sara Teasdale died of a barbiturate overdose in 1933, followed in subsequent decades by Aimee Semple McPherson, Tommy Dorsey, Marilyn Monroe, Dinah Washington, Judy Garland, and Jimi Hendrix.

"Judy Garland's Death Ascribed to Long Use of Sleeping Drugs," the *Los Angeles Times* announced a few days after the actress died in June of 1969. The coroner said that Garland "already had such a high level of barbiturates in her blood stream that her body could not tolerate any more." Jimi Hendrix "died after swallowing nine times the normal dose of barbiturate tablets of suffocation due to barbiturate intoxication," the *Chicago Tribune* reported in September of 1970.[28] Readers of magazines and newspapers were well acquainted with the dangers posed by barbiturates.

At best, barbiturate sleeping pills were a "crutch" to be used temporarily, writers in the popular press allowed, and always under the strict supervision of a physician. The only effective long-term solutions to insomnia were to adopt regular and sensible habits and address the psychological factors that for a good part of the twentieth century were understood to be the real problem for insomniacs.[29]

Despite governmental restrictions on the sale of barbiturates in 1948 and 1951, the drugs continued to be prescribed for insomnia and anxiety through the 1970s. Some physicians claimed that barbiturates taken strictly as prescribed did not lead users to become physically dependent. But testimony presented in 1973 in Congressional hearings on barbiturate abuse in the United States suggests that many barbiturate users became addicts. The National Commission on Marihuana and Drug Abuse reported in 1972 that between 500,000 and 1,000,000 Americans were addicted to barbiturates. How many of these Americans were taking the drugs recreationally, and how many were taking them for sleep or other medical purposes, is unknown.[30]

In addition to fostering dependency and abuse, the barbiturates were found to suppress REM sleep. This reinforced the belief that chemically-induced sleep was dangerous. These drugs might be more effective and have fewer side effects than older soporifics, but they were similarly addictive and were best avoided.[31]

Thalidomide

Late in the 1950s another sleeping pill came on the world scene whose dangers dwarfed those of the barbiturates. Touted as a "wonder drug," a sedative that produced sleep without a hangover and was "completely safe" even for pregnant women and their unborn children, thalidomide led to the birth of some 8,000 grossly deformed children and many others that died. The harm did not occur because of overdose. Rather, a single dose taken in the second month of pregnancy could result in a child born with stumps for arms and legs, or without ears or internal organs. The thalidomide tragedy occurred mostly in Western Europe, Australia, and Canada, exacerbated because the drug's European manufacturers, even after being alerted to the dangers of thalidomide, waited four months to pull it off the market. That the catastrophe occurred mainly abroad was largely due to the vigilance of one FDA medical officer, Frances Kelsey. Her demands for more rigorous evidence of the drug's safety prevented it from gaining official approval in the United States.[32]

But lots of informal testing of thalidomide occurred in the United States. Before 1962, guidelines for testing drugs on human beings were lax. The marketing department of the drug's American distributor, Richardson-Merrell, sent sample tablets to 1,267 doctors, suggesting that they try it out on their patients and report the results. Over 20,000 Americans took thalidomide as part of these informal "clinical trials," some without being informed by their physicians who gave out samples. As a result, at least ten, and possibly sixteen or more, thalidomide babies were born in the United States.[33]

The news media pounced on the story and found evidence of foul play. Richardson-Merrell had received reports on how the drug worked from less than a quarter of the physicians who were allegedly testing it. According to *The Sunday Times of London*, Richardson-Merrell had told its sales force that the real objective of enlisting doctors to participate in the trials was "for the purpose of selling them on Kevadon" (the company's brand name for thalidomide). This led to charges that the company was commercializing the drug under the pretense of conducting clinical tests. (Richardson-Merrell at the time was also under investigation for another drug, a dangerous anticholesterol medication whose side effects included the development of cataracts, hair loss, and blood disease.)[34]

The thalidomide disaster shone a spotlight on myriad laxities in the American system for developing new drugs and bringing them to market. Journalists reported on physicians paid by drug companies to rig clinical tests, scientific articles ghostwritten by drug companies and reflecting company bias, drug companies pressuring FDA medical officers to approve new drugs, and top FDA officials more interested in befriending drug companies than ensuring that new drugs were properly vetted.[35] The take-home message was clear: an industry whose stated aim was to improve people's health (and the officials responsible for its regulation) was not averse to compromising its mission in pursuit of financial gain. Congress early in 1962 passed the Kefauver–Harris Drug Amendments, strengthening federal oversight of the pharmaceutical industry and protecting consumers from being used as unwitting guinea pigs.

The thalidomide story reinforced the belief that sleeping pills caused harm and should be avoided. It also exposed a lot of bad actors. Critics of barbiturates had complained that the drugs were too easy to obtain and railed against pharmacists who sold them by the bucketful. With thalidomide, the pharmaceutical industry came in for a hefty share of blame. The whole affair left a terrible taste in the mouth. By August 1962, New York City pharmacists were reporting a decline in sales of all tranquilizers, sleeping pills, and sedatives.[36]

Maligned though they were, sleeping pills for many insomniacs were not an expendable item in the medicine chest. Happily for these folk, drugs then in the pipeline would offer a safer route to better sleep.

The Benzodiazepines

Dalmane (flurazepam) arrived in 1970, but it was not the first benzodiazepine marketed in the United States. That distinction belongs to Librium (chlordiazepoxide) and Valium (diazepam), two drugs that gained renown for their tranquilizing effects in Jacqueline Susann's best-selling novel, *Valley of the Dolls,* and the Rolling Stones' song "Mother's Little Helper." All benzodiazepines calm the brain by facilitating the action of GABA, thereby decreasing arousal, relaxing muscles, and reducing anxiety.[37] But Dalmane was the first one specifically approved for sleep. The hypnotics Restoril (temazepam), Halcion (triazolam), and Doral (quazepam) followed in the 1980s; ProSom (estazolam), in 1990. All are still on the market for the short-term treatment of insomnia today. Other benzos sometimes used to treat insomnia are Ativan (lorazepam) and Xanax (alprazolam), approved for the treatment of anxiety.

The benzos in the early years were hailed as a godsend. They were at least as effective in sedating as the barbiturates, experts claimed, if not more so. Unlike barbiturates, they did not appear to suppress REM sleep. They were believed to carry minimal risk of addiction. And there was far less danger of fatal overdose. While ten to twenty times the prescribed dose of a short-acting barbiturate could kill, doctors Donald R. Wesson and David E. Smith testified before a Senate Health Committee in 1973, a mega-dose of a benzodiazepine would not. Dalmane was also touted as safe in the popular press. "Dalmane is extremely safe; one would-be suicide who took 7,500 milligrams of it, or 250 capsules, failed to kill himself," declared a writer in *Fortune* magazine.[38]

But by the end of the 1970s the benzodiazepines had lost some of their shine. One problem with Dalmane was its long half-life, from 48 to 120 hours. Dalmane was an effective hypnotic, but it left some users feeling groggy in the morning and could impair daytime performance through the early afternoon.[39] Also, some people became addicted.

Peter Ritson was one. He started on Dalmane while living in Spain. "During the early seventies," Ritson wrote in *Alive and Kicking*, "General Franco's regime was still in power. . . . A prescription was not necessary for most drugs, and practically anything could be bought over the local chemist's counter." One day he came away with a box of Dalmane (called Dormador in Spain) to help him sleep. Each night he took one capsule, and shortly he was hooked.

He then began to notice unwelcome changes. His tennis game started to suffer, and he lost interest in playing his guitar. He was avoiding contact with all but his most trusted friends. And he spent hours obsessing about underground shelters and nuclear war.

"It was during this time that I discovered even my sleeping tablet no longer offered me the oblivion I was seeking from my troubled thoughts, and I would occasionally be tempted to take a second. . . . This in turn led to whole days spent in a darkened bedroom, shutters closed against the bright sunlight," with stern requests that no one disturb him.

"I did vaguely associate my general malaise with the sleeping pills, because I had made a couple of efforts to stop taking them. But . . . five days was the limit I could stand." By then the withdrawal effects were so excruciating—extreme anxiety and temper tantrums—that Ritson would start on the sleeping pills again.

For the eleven years he was taking Dalmane, Ritson lived a "chemically lobotomized" life. Among the drug's adverse effects on him were kidney problems, continuous diarrhea, cuts that wouldn't heal, anxiety, suicidal depression, memory impairment, inability to concentrate, and loss of libido. Eventually kicking the habit forced him to endure symptoms that were more onerous still, including many sleepless nights. Ritson struggled through eighteen months of withdrawal before he was completely symptom free.[40]

Ritson's experience on Dalmane is a textbook case of benzodiazepine addiction and withdrawal. How common it is remains unknown. "We see all the failures," Peter Hauri, then director of the Mayo Clinic Insomnia Program and author of *No More Sleepless Nights*, said. "We don't see the thousands of people who take the standard 50 milligrams of Dalmane, or 100 milligrams of Seconal, or whatever, are satisfied with the pills, and live to be a ripe old age." The addictive properties of Dalmane's chemical cousin Valium were well documented and caused considerable alarm, especially in Britain.[41] But the main criticism of Dalmane was the length of time it remained in the body. Patients were wont to complain of morning grogginess.

By the end of the 1970s, replacement benzodiazepines were waiting in the wings. Restoril and Halcion, shorter-acting drugs, were expected to solve the problem of morning grogginess. Yet Halcion, with a very short half-life of two to four hours, posed different problems. Taken nightly for one to two weeks and then stopped, Halcion caused severe "rebound insomnia."[42] Subjects' sleep was worse for up to four nights after stopping the drug than it had been before. The temptation to restart the drug would thus be greater, researchers reasoned, as would the likelihood of getting hooked.

Other small studies showed that tolerance developed more quickly with shorter-acting benzos like Halcion. In subjects who took Halcion for eleven to eighteen days, the drug's efficacy was reduced by nearly half. A decline in effectiveness typically prompted users to increase the dose, which might lead to dependence. Moreover, in the Netherlands, where Halcion was sold at four times the strength being considered for use in the United States, doctors were reporting alarming side effects: amnesia, hallucinations, paranoia, and aggression.[43]

Shortcomings notwithstanding, Halcion was approved for short-term use in the United States in 1982. By the end of the decade it was the most popular sleeping pill in America, a must-have toiletry item for statesmen and business travelers.

Halcion was the first prescription hypnotic I ever knew. The sleeping pill that a Netherlands newspaper had branded as "worse than thalidomide" and that William Styron a few years later would describe as "indisputably monstrous" was for me the silver bullet I longed for. It put me to sleep and relieved the anxiety that gripped me during bouts of sleeplessness. In fact, the relief started from the moment I got the prescription in my hot little hands.

"You'd like to have them in the medicine cabinet just in case," the doctor said, repeating my words in an approving tone of voice and producing the slip of paper I believed would be my passport to better sleep. I was overwhelmed with gratitude. In a split second she'd made my request for sleeping pills sound reasonable (in contrast to the resident I'd asked about pills before, who reacted as though I'd asked for crack cocaine). The world was suddenly brighter and filled with possibility. My shoulders relaxed and I settled back in my chair. "Yes," I agreed, "it would be nice to have them there."

Every one of those thirty blue pills was a magic bullet. They shut me down at night and left me feeling refreshed in the morning. But I meted them out like a miser. Fear of dependency kept me from using more than a few each month. I was also concerned about getting another prescription. I knew Halcion would be hard to come by if I asked for a refill too soon. So I used the pills only as a last resort, on really bad nights when I was at the end of my wits and facing burnout. But they could not have been more welcome than elixir from Morpheus's flask.

For other Halcion users, though, the drug was a curse. By the end of the 1980s and the early 1990s, theirs were the stories making headlines.

"Halcion Nightmare: The Frightening Truth About America's Favorite Sleeping Pill" was the first in a pair of articles in 1988 documenting the destructive effects of Halcion on novelist Cindy Ehrlich.[44] Ehrlich's story began when she went to her psychiatrist complaining of sleep trouble and came away with a prescription for sleeping pills. After ten days on Halcion, she felt anxious and fearful. Whereupon the psychiatrist, not suspecting these symptoms to be drug related, prescribed the antianxiety drug Xanax on top of the Halcion. Ehrlich's situation went from bad to worse. She became emotional and weepy, she suffered memory lapses, and her thoughts veered toward "suicide, nuclear war, alien invasion and the meaning

of bumper stickers." Only when her two-year-old began reacting
to her breast milk, becoming unusually thirsty and unsteady on
her feet, did it dawn on Ehrlich that her symptoms might be drug
induced. (Apparently this never dawned on the psychiatrist.) After
six months Ehrlich stopped the Halcion and felt better, and, after
stopping all drugs, she felt better still. Halcion alone, she concluded,
was responsible for setting her on the path to perdition. It was a
dangerous drug whose use should be curtailed.

Another writer who suffered disastrous consequences while
using Halcion was William Styron. In an essay first published in
Vanity Fair in December 1989, Styron implicated Halcion in his
descent into madness (alcohol also was involved). The nightly use of
three times the normal dose of the hypnotic exacerbated the suicidal
thoughts that nearly claimed his life, he wrote.[45]

But it was the murders committed under Halcion's influence,
and subsequent allegations made about the drug's manufacturer,
that drew the most negative publicity and left the darkest stain on
Halcion.

- In 1989 Ilo Grundberg, who shot her mother eight times
  through the head, was released from prison because she
  was under the influence of Halcion, a "toxic agent" prescribed by her doctor, when she committed the murder
  and was therefore not responsible for her act. That same
  year, a psychiatrist on trial for attempting to murder his
  wife went free because the Halcion he was taking had made
  him "incapable of understanding the nature and quality of
  his actions."

- A Texas jury in 1992 awarded heavy damages to the family
  of a former assistant chief of police after a jury found he had
  shot his best friend while under the influence of Halcion.
  The damages were to be paid by the Upjohn Company, the
  drug's manufacturer.

- In 1993, a Michigan stockbroker convicted of murdering
  his wife was acquitted in a retrial because he was taking
  Halcion at the time of the killing.[46]

That Halcion could seemingly hijack a person's psyche and lead
him or her to commit a capital crime turned a popular sleeping pill

into a death-dealing scourge. Here was another hypnotic that robbed users of self-control and incited violent behavior. Other serious side effects reported by some users included anxiety, depression, and memory impairment.

Upjohn subsequently took steps to ensure that the drug was used safely, lowering the recommended dosage to 0.25 mg and strengthening warnings about possible side effects. But by then the damage was done. Halcion's link to violent behavior led to a dramatic plunge in sales. Between December 1991 and September 1992, sales fell by 55 percent. This was rather spectacular fallout for a drug prescribed in its heyday to 11 million Americans a year, the vast majority of whom did not engage in violent behavior or report serious side effects.[47]

The Grundberg case was particularly harmful to Halcion and to Upjohn. After Grundberg's release, she charged in a civil case that Halcion was a defective drug and that Upjohn had failed to warn the FDA and the public of its "severe and sometimes fatal adverse reactions." When the company settled out of court, the media smelled a cover-up. Journalists reported that in an early test of Halcion, Upjohn's summary of results failed to mention some of the psychotic events that test subjects experienced while taking the drug. Britain subsequently banned the drug. But it stayed on the market in the United States, and the debate about Halcion's safety and Upjohn's conduct raged on. Had the company willfully suppressed data, as critics charged, or did the omission merely reflect a "transcription error," as the company maintained?[48]

An FDA task force investigating Upjohn for possible misconduct turned up incriminating memos. One suggested that the company might have withheld data to gain approval for the drug for extended use. A two-week time limit on the use of Halcion, warned the memo writer, would cut drug sales in half.[49]

But the FDA never filed criminal charges. (FDA officials interviewed by a *Business Week* journalist a few years later acknowledged, however, that the evidence of misconduct had been strong enough to warrant turning the case over to the Department of Justice). Called on the carpet several times, Upjohn fought the allegations of misconduct and supplied the missing data. The company argued that the drug was safe and effective for users who took the 0.25 mg dose of Halcion exactly as prescribed. The FDA, after reanalyzing the data, accepted Upjohn's argument. Despite reservations about the company's conduct, the drug stayed on the market and it remains there today.[50]

The protracted tar-and-feathering of Halcion did a lot to reinforce negative stereotypes about sleeping pills and the companies that made them. Here was a drug that several medical researchers had serious reservations about, and whose potency was such that the "Halcion defense" could stand up in court in cases of murder. This fit right in with what the public knew about other sleeping pills: they were dangerous and better off avoided. And whether or not Upjohn was guilty of intentionally withholding clinical trial data from the FDA, the company's initial refusal to hand over documents—and the incriminating memos that eventually came to light—made it *look* like Upjohn had something to hide. Here was another sleeping pill manufacturer apparently willing to play fast and loose with the public welfare in order to increase its profits.

The hue and cry surrounding Halcion was enough to make President George H.W. Bush swear off his "little blue bombs."[51] But for many chronic insomniacs, it was a blip on the radar screen. They continued to seek medication as they always had. But with Halcion tainted, and researchers now claiming that all benzodiazepines could foster dependency and interfere with deep sleep, the pharmacopoeia for the sleepless was shrunken. What was a conscientious physician to do?

Some doctors simply refused to prescribe medication at all. The decade from 1987 to 1996 was leaner and meaner for drug-seeking insomniacs. Prescriptions for insomnia fell by 24 percent.[52]

The Antidepressant Solution

Other doctors reverted to default mode. Apart from barbiturates and benzodiazepines, no drugs were approved for the treatment of insomnia. But some antidepressants had sedative effects, blocking the action of key neurotransmitters active during wakefulness. Add to this the then commonly held belief that depression was actually the cause of insomnia, et voilà! A new class of sleep meds emerged overnight. Instead of prescribing Halcion and other benzodiazepines, physicians started offering sleep in the form of mood elevators such as trazodone and Elavil (amitriptyline). From 1987 to 1996, hypnotic prescriptions for insomnia declined by 54 percent, while antidepressant prescriptions for insomnia rose by 146 percent. In 1996 the sedating antidepressant trazodone was the most frequently prescribed drug for insomnia. This trend continued into the current century.[53]

Had clinical tests been done to ascertain the effectiveness of antidepressants in treating insomnia? No. Had antidepressants been approved for the treatment of insomnia by the FDA? No again. But physicians were free to prescribe them off-label (that is, for uses outside those approved by the FDA). This was an attractive option, in part because antidepressants were unscheduled drugs. Physicians felt they were safer than either benzodiazepines or barbiturates. Nor were there restrictions on how long antidepressants could be used. Physicians could prescribe unlimited refills without worrying about tolerance or dependency, and without feeling guilty about prescribing beyond recommended time limits set by the FDA.

Such a deal for the guys in the white coats! But was it such a deal for us? A few insomniacs I interviewed weighed in.

"When I first started taking trazodone," said Todd, a former sleep technician whose lifelong insomnia had driven him to experiment with several sleep medications, "it had the hangover effect in the morning. I had a headache, and I didn't feel real great. It hung with me a couple weeks. Since then there've been no side effects. It takes a bit longer to initiate sleep, usually thirty to forty-five minutes. But I get probably four to six hours a night. I've been real happy with it."

For Bill, who works in home maintenance and landscaping, antidepressants were a bust.

"The less said about what passes for antidepressants, the better," he told me. "I've tried them and they're worse than the affliction. I experimented with Prozac, and it was like a different form of speed. It just jazzed the hell out of me and made my insomnia worse.

"The antidepressants that are supposed to make you sleepy— trazodone and nefazodone—they were more like knock-out pills. Mirtazapine helped a little bit with sleep, but it caused restless legs syndrome." The "so-called antidepressant route" did not work for Bill.

Trazodone's ascendancy to number one on the list of drugs most prescribed for insomnia didn't sit well with everyone in the medical community, either. The drug hadn't risen to the top on its merits, critics pointed out. As of 1998, only two clinical trials of trazodone had been conducted on insomniacs. In neither study did it put subjects to sleep faster or increase their sleep time. (However, in one of the studies it reduced the time subjects were awake during the night.) Trazodone became king of the mountain by default, its detractors claimed. Hypnotics were far more effective, but none were deemed safe for long-term use by the FDA. This was regulatory rather than evidence-based medicine, they complained.[54]

Apparently, the evidence for trazodone as an effective treatment for insomnia came mainly from informal clinical observations. After all, the drug could not have gained such popularity if many patients hadn't been satisfied with how it worked. But it's unsettling that a drug so little tested for insomnia rose to the top of the best-seller chart for the sleepless and stayed there into the current millennium, especially given trazodone's nasty side effects: daytime sleepiness, cardiovascular complications, and erectile problems in men. Not to mention a troublesome finding that came to light in 2009 in the work of scientists studying the effects of trazodone on brain plasticity, the brain's ability to reorganize itself based on cues from the environment. Trazodone significantly impaired neural rewiring that would have occurred, under conditions in the experiment, during the normal sleep of young cats.[55] There may be downsides to the drug that in humans remain unknown.

Overall there's a dearth of clinical trials assessing the risks and benefits of antidepressants for insomnia. Apart from studies of doxepin, an antidepressant reviewed in the next chapter, the few existing studies show the positive effects of antidepressants on the sleep of insomniacs to be modest. No study (except the doxepin studies) has lasted more than four weeks.[56] Doctors in the 1980s and 1990s were keen to prescribe antidepressants in lieu of hypnotics because they viewed them as safer for long-term use. Yet no long-term studies of antidepressants as a treatment for insomnia had ever been done. To study only the short-term effects of a drug begs the question of what the risks and benefits would be to insomniacs taking it for months and years.

Physicians' readiness to jump on the antidepressant bandwagon without scientific data to back the practice up suggests a medical community clutching at straws, unsure of how to treat insomnia, and regarding it as a symptom of another disease. No wonder insomniacs a generation ago got such wildly different responses to our sleep complaints: from a few weeks' supply of a benzodiazepine to advice on relaxation, from unlimited refills on an antidepressant to nothing at all. In the eyes of many care providers, hypnotic sleeping pills were a medical bugaboo. They were tarnished by the tragic experiences of a small number of users and drug companies tempted to cut corners in the interest of earning a buck.

That tarnish still clings to the sleeping pill. Despite the pharmaceutical industry's efforts to clean up the pill's image, skeptics abound. Many sleep experts feel that CBT-I is a better form of treatment for insomnia in most cases; some take a "just say no" position toward drugs. Many insomniacs, too, believe the answer to their problem lies not in a bottle but in changes in behavior and mindset. Concerns about dependency and side effects continue to loom large, and they're justifiable in view of what we've seen. More recently, news reports of people sleepwalking, binge eating, and sleep driving on Ambien have added to the stain, as have new data suggesting that hypnotic use has an impact on mortality.[57] (We'll look at these issues in the next chapter.)

So do current sleeping pills meet a higher standard overall? Or would insomniacs do well to be more cautious of prescription pills used for sleep today?

A Caveat

Before addressing these questions, I'll offer a word of caution. Sleeping pill users can speak to a drug's benefits and drawbacks, as can doctors who prescribe hypnotics. But for a more objective and comprehensive look at what they do, we need studies assessing their effects on large numbers of people. Yet given the review system that exists today, in which the companies that will profit from a drug continue to sponsor most of the trials that determine its fate, we can never be sure that the results are truly objective. There's a fundamental conflict of interest when the company that stands to gain from a product is the only entity testing its safety and efficacy.

In fact the percentage of industry-sponsored trials is quite a bit higher for insomnia drugs than for drugs used in psychiatry and general medicine, says sleep investigator Daniel Kripke. A whopping

91 to 95 percent of the randomized, controlled trials of insomnia drugs cited in a recent meta-analysis were paid for by pharmaceutical companies. Contrast this with industry funding for 60 percent of the drug trials published in psychiatric journals and 52 percent of the drug trials for medicines used in gastroenterology.[58]

The problem with industry-funded studies is not that the research is conducted poorly, experts agree. It's that these studies tend to paint a more favorable picture of drugs than studies funded by disinterested parties like the government. A review group found that the results of industry-funded studies were 3.6 times more likely than others to favor the interests of drug manufacturers.[59]

There are several ways to burnish a new drug's image. It's true that pharmaceutical companies must submit the complete results of all drug trials to the FDA. It's illegal to withhold data, and companies suspected of doing so are prosecuted. But there are other perfectly legal ways of "stacking the deck," science writer Jim Giles has observed.[60]

One involves study design. To get a new drug approved, pharmaceutical companies need only to show that it works better than placebo. They're not required to demonstrate that it works better than other drugs on the market—a higher standard that is harder to meet. Industry-funded studies tend to use placebo comparators more often than do studies funded by disinterested parties, which are more likely to compare new drugs to existing drugs. So drugs in industry-sponsored studies more often look good.[61]

Another way of stacking the deck is to suppress the publication of negative or ambiguous results. While the results of all drug trials must be handed over to the FDA, there is no requirement that all trials be written up or published in medical journals. Drug companies commonly fund the write-ups. So most studies that find their way into journals, which is where physicians often read about new drugs, show medications in a favorable light.[62] Studies with ambiguous or negative results may appear after a drug has been on the market a while, funded by a disinterested party or by a rival drug company.

Write-ups of drug studies may subtly distort the picture in other ways, too. For example, they may omit or downplay some of the data. Writers may also contrive to put a positive spin on the results in the discussion section at the end. Add to these practices the possibility that journal editors may also be biased toward studies with positive results,[63] and the quest for the straight scoop on hypnotics may seem fraught indeed.

But to disregard the studies is to throw the baby out with the bathwater. What we're left with then are anecdotal testimonials, which are a part of the story and deserve inclusion. Yet alone they don't offer much help to insomniacs weighing whether or not to take a drug themselves. A drug that works for one insomniac is worthless to another; medical professionals have biases, too. It's to controlled studies that we have to turn in order to round out the picture of what today's drugs are more and less likely to do. So, in plain English, and using post-marketing studies and meta-analyses when possible, I'll use both science and testimonial to present the clearest picture I can of hypnotics available today and those in the pipeline.

11

The Insomniac's Pharmacopeia

This is something I've struggled with for so many decades now that if I can find something that will just help me sleep on a nightly basis, then that's OK.

Joan, a sleeping pill user interviewed for this book

It's easy to call up on the computer a blitz of information about sleeping pills. "Official" drug websites spout the company line on a drug's benefits. Medical sites are strong on warnings and side effects. PubMed provides access to published drug trials. Consumer sites offer personal testimonials, everything from "This drug saved my life!" to "Never will I take this again!"

Much of the information is useful. Yet it's easy to come away with unanswered questions: How do hypnotics compare from one to the next? Could I develop tolerance to the one I'm taking now, and is there a chance I'll become dependent? Will this drug affect my overall health?

Doctors are supposed to offer guidance here, and they're usually willing to spend a few minutes chatting about drugs. But insomniacs have good reason to want to become more knowledgeable about hypnotics ourselves. It's our bodies that absorb their impact. Our health and quality of life are at stake. A concise overview of hypnotics, including those in the pipeline, is what we need.

The first question every insomniac has about a sleeping pill is, will it work? The trend in recent years has been to develop drugs that are safer, but not necessarily more efficacious, than drugs that came before. Trending toward safety is good thing. But a drug that's ineffective at doing what you need it to do is worthless, no matter how risk free. Unfortunately, there's no way of knowing for sure if a drug will work for you or if you can tolerate the side effects until you try it out, as many insomniacs who've taken medication can attest.

But a little information can help you winnow the options. Insomniacs use hypnotics for different reasons, and a drug that works for someone who can't fall asleep may be a dud for a person who wakes up often in the middle of the night, and vice versa. Then, too, among hypnotics, there are a number of copycat drugs. Particularly if you're paying out of pocket, it's useful to know about the similarities among them. There might be a generic substitute available at a fraction of the cost you're paying for a branded drug. On the other hand, these "me too" drugs are not mere clones, if you believe the claims in the fine print. The minor differences among them may be important for some users. Ideally, there should be a match between your needs and the hard data showing what a drug does.

The next question for insomniacs is, are there hidden costs? Even diehard pill users suspect there's no free midnight snack. We take for granted that pills will put us to sleep sooner and keep us sleeping longer, but some of us also worry that pills may degrade the sleep we get. Pill sleep is better than no sleep, the thinking goes, but it doesn't measure up to the stuff we get when we're able to sleep soundly on our own. Commented one insomniac, "It's not restful, natural sleep; it is drug sleep. There is a difference." Where differences are noted in the literature, I'll point them out.

Hypnotics are notorious for their side effects as well. Complete lists of side effects are available on the Internet and package inserts; there's no need to duplicate them here. Instead, I'll focus on issues of concern to the insomniacs I interviewed, such as their impact on daily functioning and long-term health.

Last but not least, sleeping pills conjure up the specter of dependency. "Addiction is what most patients are afraid of," said Sonia Ancoli-Israel, professor of psychiatry at the University of California San Diego and Director of the Gillin Sleep and Chronobiology Research Center. "On the newer drugs, the studies have shown they're not addicting, and that they are in general safe. But they do all have side effects, and one does have to be careful. You have to use them correctly, which many patients don't. That's when you often run into trouble."

We'll consider the trouble some users run into with the newer sleeping pills and ways to avoid it.

Ambien Nation

Colin Powell's paean to Ambien rocketed through cyberspace in November of 2003: "So do you use sleeping tablets to organize yourself?" a reporter for a London-based Arabic newspaper asked.

"Yes," Powell replied. "Well, I wouldn't call them that. They're a wonderful medication—not medication. How would you call it? They're called Ambien, which is very good. You don't use Ambien? Everybody here uses Ambien."[1]

Well, not everybody. But by 2003 millions of Americans did. The events unleashed by 9/11 coincided with a little-remarked regime change here at home. It was then that the antidepressant trazodone, long the most frequently prescribed medication for insomnia, was deposed by Ambien. This new king of sleep meds spent nearly a decade rising to the top, but it finally got there and has dominated the hypnotics market ever since. The generic name for Ambien is zolpidem, and zolpidem in its many formulations is still the most frequently prescribed hypnotic.[2] It belongs to a class of hypnotics known as "Z-drugs," whose generic names begin with the letter *z*.

Ambien came on the scene in 1992 with barely a whisper. Direct-to-consumer promotion of drugs was not yet legal, and writers in the popular press mentioned Ambien in the same breath as Dalmane and Halcion, just one among many GABA-facilitating hypnotics approved for short-term treatment of insomnia. Who saw any magic in that?

But pharmacologists were heralding Ambien as a breakthrough in sleep therapy. Ambien achieves its soporific effect via the GABA system, as do the benzodiazepine drugs. All these drugs enhance the ability of GABA to do its job. They bind to $GABA_A$ receptor complexes on the receiving ends of nerve cells and, when GABA binds to these same receptor complexes, increase the flow of chloride ions moving into the cells. The cells are then inhibited from firing, which tranquilizes the brain.

But there are several kinds of $GABA_A$ receptor complexes. The benzodiazepines are not very discriminating about which kinds of complexes they consort with, binding to many. They produce an array of effects, including sedation, relaxation, protection against seizures, and—on the downside—amnesia, and other cognitive and motor impairments.[3]

In contrast, Ambien is much more selective in which receptor complexes it binds to. At standard doses it binds to fewer $GABA_A$ receptor complexes: only to those that have the alpha-1 subtype. Because of this, Ambien is more targeted in its pharmacologic action. It facilitates sleep and (less fortuitously) interferes with memory formation once the drug is taken. Early studies showed that compared to the benzos, Ambien produced fewer negative effects and was equally efficacious. In addition, the drug did not appear to interfere much with normal sleep staging. While the barbiturates were known to suppress REM sleep, and the benzodiazepines to suppress slow-wave sleep, quite a few studies suggested Ambien left slow-wave and REM sleep largely intact.[4] Plus it was short-acting, with a half-life of 1.5 to 2.4 hours. For these reasons, Ambien was touted as superior.

On the other hand, Ambien's short-acting nature was frustrating to insomniacs who needed something to keep them sleeping through the night. In response, Sanofi-Aventis, the drug's maker, launched a controlled-release (CR) version in October 2005. Ambien CR was the top-selling hypnotic in the United States through 2010.[5] A generic form of the drug, zolpidem extended-release, came on the market in October of 2010, produced by the pharmaceutical company Actavis.

Zolpidem in its many formulations has been a fixture for more than twenty years now: time enough to show plenty of warts. On the question of whether zolpidem-assisted sleep is really more "natural" than the sleep induced by older sleeping pills, the drug appears to have more of an impact on sleep staging than was first apparent. It tends to increase high-frequency brain activity and reduce slow-wave activity during non-REM sleep, but to a lesser degree than the benzodiazepines. Ambien has also been found to delay and decrease REM sleep in healthy subjects, but not to the same extent as barbiturates. So in terms of sleep staging, the sleep Ambien confers appears to be more natural than sleep bestowed by older drugs, but not quite the same as sleep unassisted. Whether and how much this matters is unknown.[6]

What about zolpidem's ability to preserve some of the functions that normally occur during sleep? A study published in 2010 suggests that the drug may slightly impair the learning of motor skills like operating a stick shift or playing the piano. Sleep typically improves the learning of motor skills, as we've seen. Researchers at Yale University showed that zolpidem interfered somewhat with subjects' ability to master the typing of a particular sequence of numbers on a computer keyboard; Halcion, however, interfered significantly more. Another recent experiment showed that in young cats, Ambien reduced sleep-dependent cortical plasticity by about 50 percent. Cortical plasticity is the brain's ability to successfully rewire itself in response to cues from the environment, which enables learning.[7] These two experiments suggest that zolpidem may interfere somewhat with important processes that occur during sleep. We won't know for sure until more evidence comes in.

Zolpidem has also given rise to scare stories. In 2006 a rash of reports about Ambien-induced sleep eating and sleep driving hit the newsstands, and stories have continued to surface ever since. Devin Dove, creator of Ambien Outrage, a website "designed to make the public aware of the dangers of Ambien," took 10 mg of Ambien one night, got in bed, and the next thing he knew he was in the hospital.

"What I'd done is the same exact thing that Tiger Woods did," he told me on the phone. "I got into my car and I drove, and I just smacked into my neighbors' yard. They have some big, flat rocks in their yard, and I high-centered on one of those rocks."

Dove has no memory of anything else that occurred that night: no memory of getting out of his car and knocking on the neighbors' door to ask that they call for help, no memory of being woken up by the police or of taking a breathalyzer test.

"It puts you in a zombie state," he said of Ambien. "People can talk to you and you'll respond—that's the funny thing—and you can get up and move around. But the next day you can't remember a thing."

At the hospital Dove tested negative for alcohol and narcotics, and the test for Ambien revealed only the amount his doctor had prescribed. Even so, he was charged with driving under the influence. He hired an attorney to fight the charge in court, but the jury found him guilty. "They don't care why you got in the situation you're in, they only care about what you did."

How commonly does Ambien induce parasomniac behaviors like Dove's, and why does this happen?

Two post-marketing studies suggest the incidence of Ambien-induced sleepwalking is low but not negligible. In one, seven out of 1,972 Swiss insomnia sufferers on Ambien developed sleepwalking (0.3 percent); in the other, one out of ninety-six French insomniacs developed sleepwalking (1 percent). But published case reports (doctors' reports on individual patients) are few. In a 2008 review of medical literature, sleep researchers Christian Dolder and Michael Nelson located reports on only fifteen patients who experienced sleepwalking, eating, talking, driving, sex, and shopping while under the influence of Ambien. The authors say the incidence of Ambien-induced wake-like behaviors is likely rare but that it "may be higher than reported in the published literature."[8]

Some of these complex behaviors have occurred in people taking Ambien in higher doses than prescribed. In fact, merely doubling the highest recommended dosage of 10 mg can be dangerous. (The recommended dosage for women is now 5 mg, based on reports showing that women take longer than men to metabolize the drug, which can cause morning drowsiness and impair driving.) Subjects who took 20 mg in the middle of the night and then tried to drive four hours later were more severely impaired than they would have been with a blood alcohol content of 1.0 g/L, which is higher than the legal driving limit.[9]

Taking too high a dose is just one factor behind these parasomniac behaviors. They can also occur as the result of drug–drug interactions. Devin Dove was on Paxil when the sleep driving incident with Ambien occurred, learning only later that "you should not mix it with certain other medications." Ambien-induced parasomnias are also more likely to occur in people prone to sleep eating, sleepwalking, or substance abuse, and in people with restless legs syndrome, sleep apnea, or a mood disorder. But in some cases there are no complicating factors; patients have taken the drug exactly as prescribed. So far there are only theories about why Ambien triggers these unconscious behaviors. It may have to do with the drug's particular binding affinity and an ability, in rare instances, to prompt users to engage in habitual actions like walking and driving.[10]

Whatever the mechanism, I'd be chary of Ambien if I were a sleepwalker or prone to midnight raids of the fridge. I'd be cautious if I had sleep apnea or took mood meds or other psychotropics. And exceeding the recommended dosage is always risky. The Substance Abuse and Mental Health Services Administration recently reported that emergency department visits caused by adverse reactions to zolpidem increased from over 6,000 visits in 2005 to over 19,000 visits in 2010.[11]

As troublesome as these stories are, of greater concern to insomniacs I interviewed was Ambien's potential to cause dependency. A few informants described themselves as dependent, and addiction stories loom large on the Internet. "A *Glamour* writer reveals how her secret addiction nearly killed her," reads the subtitle of an online article written by a former Ambien "junkie." Are we all vulnerable to sliding down the same slippery slope?

The literature is reassuring for intermittent users. In studies lasting eight, twelve, and twenty-four weeks, subjects were instructed to take a pill at least three times a week "as needed."[12] In none of the studies did Ambien lose effectiveness over time. Subjects did not increase the number of pills they were taking or escalate the dose. Nor was there evidence of rebound insomnia—worse sleep than before starting the drug—on non-pill nights or at the studies' end. This suggests a low risk of tolerance and dependence for users of Ambien on an as-needed basis.

It's nightly, long-term use where the issue gets cloudy. If you take Ambien or Ambien CR every night for just a few weeks, probably the only dependency-related symptom you might notice is that your sleep is worse on the night you stop the drug. But not much is known about the likelihood of tolerance or dependency developing over months and years of continuous use. Subjects in a six-month study were not required to take the drug every night.[13] Instead, they took a pill at least three and up to seven days a week. This begs the question if, over a six-month span of nightly use, symptoms associated with dependence would emerge. The authors hint at these concerns themselves. In their rationale for employing the "as needed" protocol, they note that "the costs and risks of adverse effects associated with taking a medication nightly become increasingly important considerations" the longer a drug is taken. It's hard not to draw some negative inferences about Ambien here. On the other hand, a smaller study of zolpidem taken every night for twelve months found that upon discontinuing the pills, subjects on Ambien did not suffer any more rebound insomnia or withdrawal symptoms than subjects taking a placebo.[14]

So can nightly users develop tolerance to Ambien? Case reports suggest that tolerance *may in some users* begin to develop within a few weeks. Can you become dependent? At least psychologically, it seems some users can. Stories of Ambien dependency are floating all over cyberspace, and medical literature has documented instances of tolerance, dose escalation, unsuccessful attempts to stop the drug, withdrawal symptoms upon discontinuation, and other hallmarks of drug dependency. Most reviewers in medical journals insist the risk of developing a dependency is small.[15] But as the television commercial for Ambien CR says, "Like most hypnotics, it has some risk of dependency." That's about as far as we can go.

Ambien aficionados may be interested in newer formulations of the drug, available at brand-name prices. Edluar is a sublingual pill that purportedly puts users to sleep a few minutes faster than the original, and Zolpimist is a spray that does the same thing. Their makers skipped doing safety studies, so they're approved only for short-term use. More recently, Purdue Pharma launched Intermezzo, a dissolvable zolpidem clone approved for use in the middle of the night. Insomniacs with Cadillac prescription coverage may want to try them; I'm sitting tight with the generic.

The Challengers: Sonata and Lunesta

"It's got a great name," a friend remarked as I was telling her about Sonata, a sleeping pill introduced in 1999. Many classical music lovers would agree: short of "Lullaby," more suitable for cranky infants, what better name could you come up with for a drug meant to lull insomniacs to sleep?

Like Ambien, Sonata has a strong binding affinity for alpha-1 $GABA_A$ receptors, and studies suggest the two are comparable in facilitating sleep. Sonata is arguably safer. With a half-life of just one hour, it loses potency quickly. This feature has its points. In trial after trial, subjects of all ages have woken up free of morning grogginess. Some researchers have suggested it's a good drug for elderly insomnia sufferers. Others have suggested it's even safe to take Sonata in the middle of the night.[16]

What's more, Sonata, a Z-drug whose generic name is zaleplon, does not seem to have any appreciable side effects. Its impact on sleep staging is negligible and it carries practically zero risk of dependency. The authors of three review articles concur: no tolerance to Sonata develops, and no rebound insomnia or withdrawal symptoms occur when the drug is stopped.[17]

But the drug has never achieved Ambien's popularity; it hasn't even come close. It may be that Sonata is long on safety but short on features that matter as much or more. In a toe-to-toe comparison of the two drugs, a majority of sleep-onset insomniacs preferred Ambien to Sonata. Ambien put them to sleep more easily, they said, and did more to improve their sleep quality.[18]

"Sonata is the weirdest of all of the Z-drugs," wrote Moss, a psychopharmacologist I quoted in the last chapter, in the online message board talkaboutsleep.com. "Some people swear by it and others, like me, have found it has virtually no effect at doses under 30 mg." That's three times the highest pill strength sold.

I couldn't get Sonata to work for me, either. The one time I took the pill at bedtime, I spent the entire night on the sofa paging through magazines and catalogs, bleary-eyed and awake. Also, the drug is useless for insomniacs whose problem is *staying* asleep, and for a majority of insomniacs this is the main complaint.

"Many prescribing physicians (and perhaps patients, as well) quickly became disillusioned with it when it was viewed as another 'all-purpose' hypnotic and failed to help people sleep through the night," said David Neubauer, a psychiatry professor and sleep medicine specialist at Johns Hopkins School of Medicine.

Sonata "is fine for what it should be able to do based upon its pharmacologic properties," Neubauer continued, namely, put people to sleep, and exit the system quickly. "The downside is that it doesn't last very long." Generic zaleplon is available, however, so it's inexpensive for those who find that it works.

Lunesta is a different story. This Z-drug (S-zopiclone, or eszopi-clone) came on like gangbusters in early 2005. Prior to the launch of Ambien CR later the same year, Sepracor, Lunesta's maker, had five months to lure prospective customers into the Lunesta fold. Company marketers took full advantage of their window of opportunity. An iridescent green moth fluttered seductively across TV screens throughout the nation, proffering goodies like no hypnotic before.

"Lunesta helps most people sleep *all through* the night and works quickly," said the voiceover. "Lunesta is non-narcotic and approved for *long-term* use."

Let's consider the regulatory issue first. The FDA's approval of Lunesta without the short-term restriction came about largely because the drug's maker was willing to sponsor long-term trials. Sepracor (now Sunovion Pharmaceuticals Inc.) was the first pharmaceutical company ever to fund a study in which subjects took a hypnotic every night for six months. The company's gamble paid off. The results of a key Lunesta study showed that compared to placebo, the drug put insomniacs to sleep faster, cut down on nocturnal awakenings, and gave users more than half an hour of extra sleep. There was "no evidence of tolerance" and "no evidence of significant withdrawal symptoms" in the run-out period.[19] High five! The main unpleasant side effect was a metallic taste the drug left in some users' mouths.

For some insomniacs, Lunesta's no-restrictions label eased concerns about prescription sleeping pills. Before it came on the market, Terry was leery of the hypnotics he was taking. "I use pills sporadically," he told me at our first meeting. "But I wouldn't want to take them every night. I'm afraid of becoming dependent or developing a tolerance." I asked him again about his insomnia a year later, and he was all smiles. "It's not a problem anymore," he said, "now that there's Lunesta."

What about the claims about Lunesta's effectiveness? How has the drug fared in the real world, and what do post-marketing studies say?

Retail sales data tell a part of the story. By this measure Lunesta has done fairly well. It was running neck and neck with Ambien CR in 2010, but sales of Lunesta fell off somewhat after the competitor drug went generic that same year.[20] An informal survey of online ratings by Lunesta users suggests satisfaction here as well. Lunesta has its share of detractors, to be sure, yet more reviewers sing its praises.

I was fifty when Lunesta came on the scene. By then, insomnia could strike at any time of the night: beginning, middle, or end. News of a drug that would knock me out and keep me out made it sound appealing, so I gave it a try and found it worked a lot like Ambien. Other than the metallic taste it left in my mouth, the only differences I could discern were that Lunesta took a little longer to take effect (forty to forty-five minutes, whereas with generic Ambien I could pretty much count on half an hour) and it kept me sleeping an hour longer. Sometimes I also woke up feeling calmer in the morning than I did after taking Ambien.

Lunesta *should* keep insomniacs sleeping longer than zolpidem. It's got a half-life of five to seven hours (vs. zolpidem's half-life of 1.5 to 2.4 hours). But to significantly reduce the time you spend awake during the night, studies suggest you may have to take 3 mg, the highest approved dosage. Lunesta also binds differently to the $GABA_A$ receptor complex than do zolpidem and zaleplon. So you'd expect it to have somewhat different effects. Unlike these older drugs, Lunesta appears to act predominantly through alpha-2 and alpha-3 receptors (and to a lesser extent, through alpha-1 receptors), say reviewers David Nutt and Stephen Stahl, which may give the drug some mood-regulating effects. For example, Lunesta in one study improved insomnia and symptoms of depression and anxiety associated with menopause.[21] But this property has yet to be fully investigated in clinical trials.

You'd think after a run of eight years, Lunesta's reputation would be a little worse for wear, but it isn't, at least in medical journals. Few post-marketing studies of Lunesta have appeared. But quite a bit is known about the downsides of zopiclone, Lunesta's parent drug. Lunesta contains only one form of the compound, S-zopiclone. But zopiclone, a drug sold in countries outside the United States since 1987, is composed of two: S-zopiclone and the less active R-zopiclone. Zopiclone has been found to decrease REM sleep, interfere with memory formation, and cause hangover effects. Tolerance to the drug can develop, and stopping it can result in rebound insomnia and anxiety. Zopiclone carries some risk of dependency, as documented in the World Health Organization's *Assessment of Zopiclone*, published in 2006.

Yet we can't assume that Lunesta produces these same effects. Both parent and offspring bind to $GABA_A$ receptors (and they are less selective than zolpidem and zaleplon in the numbers of receptors they bind to). But their impact on these receptors is different, laboratory studies have shown. So the two drugs would not be expected to produce identical effects in human beings.[22]

In drug trials to date, Lunesta has not altered slow-wave sleep or REM sleep. Nor have subjects reported grogginess or performance impairments in the morning. On the contrary, subjects have tended to report improvements in next-day functioning and alertness. Long-term users have not developed tolerance to the drug during six- and twelve-month trials; in only one study did subjects experience rebound insomnia the first night off the drug.[23]

Yet Lunesta carries some risk of dependency, the "official" drug website informs us. Warnings on the website and in a recent TV commercial suggest that Lunesta, like Ambien, can induce sleepwalking, sleep eating, sleep driving, and aggressive behavior in some users. Hair loss may be among the drug's rarer side effects, according to various online sources. How common these effects are awaits further documentation. Only time will tell whether for Lunesta the scorecard of benefits and risks stays weighted to the positive.

Other issues have surfaced in post-marketing studies of the Z-drugs as a class. Florendo Joya and colleagues at Scripps Clinic Sleep Center in La Jolla analyzed multiple studies of four popular hypnotics—the Zs and ramelteon, a medication we'll consider shortly—to ascertain whether taking them increased the risk of infection.[24] They found that while 4.6 percent of the subjects taking a placebo developed an infection, the rate of infection among hypnotics users was 6.9 percent. Ambien and Lunesta were the two main culprits. Taking these drugs may make us more vulnerable to sore throats, colds, fevers, and other types of infection.

Use of the Z-drugs may also increase the risk of depression. Daniel Kripke, a sleep investigator at Scripps Clinic, reviewed hundreds of FDA files with data from drug trials involving the Z-drugs and ramelteon. Data on 7,853 study participants were included. The incidence of depression was 0.9 percent among the subjects randomized to placebo and 2.0 percent among those randomized to hypnotics. So taking a hypnotic more than doubled the risk. Kripke concludes that "when there is a risk of depression, hypnotics may be contra-indicated."[25]

These issues have not gotten much coverage in the popular press. But Kripke and colleagues' recent finding—that use of the Z-drugs and other commonly used hypnotics were linked to a three-to fivefold increase in the risk of death—made a splash. It found its way into most major newspapers and online health magazines. "Sleeping Pills Called 'as Risky as Cigarettes,'" ran the headline at the top of a story dated February 27, 2012, on WebMD.com.

Kripke and his team reviewed the medical records of some 10,500 patients with sleeping pill prescriptions and some 23,700 patients without hypnotic prescriptions over a two-and-a-half-year period. Zolpidem was the most frequently prescribed hypnotic at the time, followed by temazepam (the generic name for Restoril). Sleeping pill users and nonusers were matched according to age, sex, ethnicity, marital status, body mass index, alcohol use, and smoking status. In addition, an attempt was made to compare users with nonusers who had similar health problems (excluding mental health problems: state law prevented the researchers from obtaining this information.). By the end of the study period, 638 patients with sleeping pill prescriptions and 295 patients without prescriptions had died. Crunching the numbers, the researchers found that patients prescribed as few as eighteen pills were 3.6 times as likely to die as patients without prescriptions. Death hazard ratios increased with the number of pills prescribed. Patients prescribed more than 132 doses had a 5.3-fold increased risk of dying.[26]

"We think these sleeping pills are very dangerous," Kripke said. "We think they cause death. We think they cause cancers. It is possible but not proven that reducing the use of these pills would lower the U.S. death rate."[27]

This is not the only study to show a relationship between the use of hypnotics and increased mortality.[28] But it *is* the first to suggest that taking even a small number of sleeping pills could have such a profoundly negative effect.

The study has limitations, though, that raise questions about the results. First, establishing an association between two things does not prove causality. Nor can a direction of causality be inferred. Just as the data can be interpreted to suggest that sleeping pills confer an increased risk of mortality, it could also suggest that patients at greater risk of dying are more likely to ask for hypnotic prescriptions. Moreover, in the case of slowly developing diseases such as cancer, causality cannot be established over a period of just two and a half years. Also, the data do not include information on the cause of death, which could help put the results in perspective. Were the additional deaths among the hypnotics users due to cancer, were they due to car crashes or sleepwalking incidents, or did they involve excessive amounts of and/or interactions between drugs? We don't know.

Perhaps the most serious limitation is that the study did not control for insomnia itself, which has recently been shown to correlate with increased mortality.[29] To ascertain the mortality risk of hypnotics in the people who typically use them, investigators would have to conduct a randomized clinical trial. Subjects would include both insomniacs who took hypnotics and insomniacs who took a placebo (Kripke's retrospective study did not include this second group). All other confounding variables would have to be controlled for, including mental health problems.

Kripke has dismissed the idea of an RCT as unethical, comparing it to "randomized trials of cigarettes and of skydiving without parachutes."[30] But short of such a trial, there's really no way to prove that using hypnotics hastens death or how much of a mortality risk these drugs confer. It can only be said that use of the Z-drugs and other hypnotic medications may have serious long-term consequences. But so does persistent insomnia, as we have seen.

A Super-Melatonin: Rozerem

Never mind the kooky commercials featuring Abe Lincoln and the talking beaver. Never mind the message that at long last there was a sleeping pill you could take without fear of getting hooked. What I wondered when I heard about Rozerem was this: why spend millions developing a drug that acts on the melatonin system when melatonin supplements for most insomniacs are such a bust?

Rozerem (the generic is ramelteon) purportedly behaves like a sort of super-melatonin. It binds to melatonin receptors on neurons in the suprachiasmatic nucleus, and its binding affinity is stronger than that of melatonin itself. Its elimination half-life (1 to 2.6 hours) is longer than melatonin's, and it produces a metabolite that lengthens its effects still further. The claim is that while melatonin may not work for insomniacs, Rozerem does.[31]

Short-term efficacy studies suggest the drug helps insomniacs fall asleep and sleep a little longer. However, a key six-month study showed the drug's only positive effect was to put insomniacs to sleep more quickly than placebo. (Rozerem in this study also had a small but significant effect on sleep staging, decreasing deep sleep and increasing stage 2.)[32] So the drug's main strength is the same as that of Ambien and Sonata.

Where Rozerem seems to have a leg up is in safety and tolerability. None of the hallmarks of dependency have shown up in studies—there's no rebound insomnia or withdrawal symptoms when the drug is stopped. The Drug Enforcement Agency has not listed it as a controlled substance, and the FDA has given it the green light for long-term use.[33]

Moreover, while in clinical trials some Z-drug users have reported morning grogginess, memory impairments, and the like, insomniacs have made it through trials of Rozerem largely side effect–free. The drug's impact was the same as that of placebo in studies where subjects took it and were awakened two hours later and tested for balance and mobility. In this respect Rozerem is superior to some of the Z-drugs and the benzodiazepines, which depress the central nervous system and can create mobility problems for people who are up and about at night.[34] Rozerem would thus be safe for older insomniacs and others who frequently get up to use the bathroom.

But since its launch in early 2006, sales of Rozerem have never approached those of Ambien and Lunesta. Nor have consumers expressed great satisfaction. Online review sites reveal a mix of supporters and detractors of all drugs, but with Rozerem, the detractors predominate, offering comments like these: "Worthless." "Felt like a sugar pill." "It just doesn't work." Some users complain of negative side effects, including bad dreams. (Maybe this is what inspired the commercial with the talking beaver!) Users who most consistently give the drug high marks tend to be night owls wanting to get to sleep earlier.

"Rozerem is effective for sleep onset insomnia," David Neubauer said, "especially when there's a phase delay." In fact, one study suggests that Rozerem could be effective in treating circadian rhythm disorders, specifically sleep phase delay.[35] But insomniacs expecting any more from this drug may well be waiting for Godot.

Antidepressant Redux: Silenor

Sleep maintenance insomniacs are the target of this newer kid on the block. If you wake up too many times at night, or if you tend to wake up too early, then Silenor might be worth a bid.

Silenor is actually not a new drug. The name for the generic is doxepin, a drug used for decades as an antidepressant. As an antidepressant it has a raft of unwanted side effects: dry mouth, headache, dizziness, daytime sedation, and weight gain. In the drug's reincarnation as Silenor, though, Somaxon Pharmaceuticals claims it's been stripped of all those nasties (and stripped of its mood-elevating effects as well). The one property it retains is its ability to sedate.

How could this be?

For doxepin to work as an antidepressant it has to be taken in megadoses: 150 to 300 mg. At this strength the drug comes with lots of baggage. But taken in miniscule doses—3 or 6 mg—doxepin becomes a different sort of drug. (At least, that's the claim, based on the clinical trials upon which Silenor gained FDA approval.)[36] The single property it retains is its ability to bind to particular histamine receptors, H-1 receptors, located in the posterior hypothalamus. There, Silenor blocks the transmission of histamine, thereby tamping down arousal.

Compared to the Z-drugs, Silenor is slower to move in and out of the body. It takes at least three hours to reach peak concentration; in clinical trials it has not been shown to help insomniacs fall sleep. But the drug appears to have staying power once it arrives. With a half-life of fifteen hours, Silenor has consistently helped insomniacs *stay* asleep. This effect did not diminish in adult subjects after five weeks of treatment or three months of treatment in elderly adults,[37] so tolerance doesn't seem to be an issue.

The drug's fifteen-hour half-life may raise a few eyebrows. But the early trials show little evidence of any residual sedation beyond seven or eight hours. This may true because low-dose doxepin does not directly interfere with the activation of other bodily arousal systems, says Stephen M. Stahl, a professor of psychiatry at the University of California–San Diego in La Jolla. These systems, which typically swing into gear at wake-up time, are still poised to go online as we're opening our eyes. Also, our bodies naturally produce more histamine during the daytime; that extra histamine may successfully compete with the action of the drug.[38]

Silenor is also purportedly safe for insomniacs who have to get up a lot at night. "Unlike drugs that enhance GABA inhibition or block multiple arousal systems," Stahl has written, "selective blockade of histamine does not appear to globally suppress arousability, thus potentially allowing patients to wake up as needed throughout the night without feeling 'drugged.'"

Will all these claims prove to be true? We won't know till Silenor's been on the market a while longer and the court of public opinion weighs in.

Sales have been sluggish since Silenor came on the market in 2010. Perhaps this is a reflection of consumer satisfaction, or perhaps some would-be consumers are opting to use the generic instead. Doxepin is currently available in 10 mg capsules, only 4 mg more than the highest-approved dosage of Silenor contains. (Remember, as an antidepressant doxepin is available in strengths of up to 300 mg.) If sleeping through the night were my particular problem and I had no prescription coverage (or I just plain resented the fact that a pharmaceutical company had repackaged an old drug and slapped a brand-name price on it), I'd talk to my doctor about trying the generic. It's sold at a fraction of the price.

Off Label and Barely Attainable

Two more drugs deserve mention before we move on to drugs in the "investigational" category. Neither is approved for the treatment of insomnia. But if you hang with the sleep crowd, you're bound to hear talk of their use.

The first is Xyrem, or sodium oxybate. This drug's active ingredient is one and the same as the infamous date rape drug GHB (gamma-hydroxybutyrate), made illegal in 1990 following several notorious cases of abuse. But at the behest of scientists convinced of its medicinal value, a company called Orphan Medical resurrected it. The drug reappeared in 2002 as Xyrem, approved for the treatment of narcolepsy, a disorder whose symptoms include excessive daytime sleepiness and cataplexy (the loss of muscle tone that causes sudden falls).

Narcoleptics also suffer from disrupted sleep. Studies have shown that Xyrem helps them maintain daytime alertness by improving their sleep at night. Specifically, it increases the amount of slow-wave sleep they get and cuts down on nocturnal awakenings. As a result, narcoleptics on Xyrem can function better during the daytime.[39] So it might occur to you to think this drug could be used to treat insomnia, and it is.

"There certainly is some prescribing of Xyrem for people with severe insomnia," David Neubauer told me. "A lot of people with insomnia have tried lots of different meds that haven't worked for them. And so the gamma-hydroxybutyrate—it makes sense that it might work for them because it's sedating, it's relatively short acting, which is an advantage, and there is the very clear enhancement of slow-wave sleep. [This] may improve sleep quality, sleep depth, and a sense of getting restorative sleep. So all of those qualities make it very attractive."

But unless your insomnia is so refractory that does not respond to any other form of treatment, you'll need to jump through hoops to get anywhere near this drug. Xyrem is a strictly controlled substance. It's a Schedule III drug, deemed as dangerous and easy to abuse as barbiturates. (Illicit GHB is a Schedule I drug, in the same class as heroin and LSD.) Repeated high doses lead to tolerance and dependence; discontinuation, to seizures and anxiety. In some cases users have ended up in a coma and a few have died.[40]

So a Xyrem surveillance program is in place to ensure that abuse does not occur. Prescribing physicians and patients must sign a registry, and the drug is dispensed from a single centralized pharmacy that tracks all shipments and permits delivery only to registered narcolepsy patients.

In cases of refractory insomnia, doctors may resort to off-label prescribing, Neubauer said. "But the fact that it's a Schedule III agent, that it's expensive, and that you have to go through this central pharmacy to get it makes the threshold for prescribing it much higher" than for some other hypnotic or off-label medicine currently used for insomnia.

Any chance that Xyrem might one day be approved for insomnia? I asked.

Not likely, Neubauer replied. Jazz Pharmaceuticals was unsuccessful in its bid to gain FDA approval for Xyrem in fibromyalgia patients, whose symptoms include fatigue and poor sleep. The drug's history would likewise be an obstacle to obtaining approval to use Xyrem for insomnia, Neubauer said. "It's clearly approved for narcolepsy because it works well and that's a unique condition that is quite severe. But it's different from insomnia, where there are a lot of other potential [treatment] options."

Ergo, unless your insomnia is resistant to every other form of treatment, forget this drug and put your eggs in some other basket.

Another unapproved-but-sometimes-used drug that deserves consideration here is modafinil. The brand name for this drug is Provigil. (It's manufactured by Cephalon, Inc., a company acquired by Teva Pharmaceutical Industries Ltd. in 2011.)

This wake-up drug—like armodafinil, or Nuvigil, a modified version of the drug—has the FDA's seal of approval only for excessive sleepiness in patients with narcolepsy, sleep apnea, and shift work disorder. But these users are small potatoes compared to the users who in 2011 lined Cephalon's coffers to the tune of $1.1 billion dollars. Between 80 and 90 percent of the company's earnings on Provigil have reportedly come from users in search of enhanced alertness and stamina: from students working on term papers to athletes, from frequent fliers to business executives striving to get ahead.[41] And there's talk of using it to treat the fatigue and sleepiness associated with insomnia.

"What?!" you may be thinking now. "Wouldn't that type of drug make insomnia worse?"

Clearly this was my doctor's line of thinking when I asked him to prescribe modafinil for me, for use on days when I felt wiped out and unable to cobble together a paragraph. I suggested it could serve as an alternative to my morning coffee, which sometimes irritates my bladder.

The withering look he shot my way spoke volumes. He then turned away (was he irritated? incredulous that I could suggest such a foolish thing? uncomfortable at having to turn me down?) and delivered his response to the wall. "No," he said, "I can't do that."

Is using modafinil to treat insomnia-related fatigue as crazy as it sounds?

David Neubauer, I discovered, takes a position similar to my doctor's. "I think most sleep specialists would argue that if somebody's not getting enough sleep and they're feeling fatigued and sleepy as a result," he said, "then the way to approach that is to help them get *more* sleep rather than having them take an agent that will help them stay awake and could sustain the sleep problem."

But Michael Perlis, director of the Behavioral Sleep Medicine Program at University of Pennsylvania, thinks otherwise. Perlis headed a team studying modafinil and cognitive-behavioral therapy for insomnia. Fatigue, if not outright sleepiness, is a common day-time symptom of insomnia, the authors note in their paper, and it typically worsens in the first several days of CBT-I. Their aim was to find out whether modafinil alone or combined with CBT-I would improve sleep continuity and reduce daytime fatigue.[42]

Alone, 100 mg of modafinil taken in the morning did nothing to improve subjects' sleep, but neither did it make their sleep worse. Nor did modafinil alter the sleep of subjects undergoing CBT-I. But the drug *did* significantly reduce daytime sleepiness in CBT subjects (as compared to CBT subjects taking a placebo) in the first week. That reduction in sleepiness continued throughout treatment.

Other investigators have concluded that modafinil taken in the morning or at midday enhances alertness but does not interfere with nighttime sleep. This might seem implausible, especially given that the drug's elimination half-life is twelve to fifteen hours. Yet there's a precipitous drop in blood plasma concentration anywhere from four to six hours after it is taken, suggesting that "the clinical effects of the medication may begin to wane after four to six hours." Modafinil is a stimulant that increases activity in wake-promoting neurons and decreases activity in neurons that promote sleep. It works dif-ferently from caffeine but its effects are similar.[43] And as a point of comparison, the elimination half-life of caffeine is five to six hours.

Well then, if fatigue and mental impairment are common symp-toms of insomnia, and if an appropriately timed dose of modafinil could ameliorate them without having a negative effect on sleep, why are physicians so leery of prescribing it? Do the drug's overall risks outweigh its benefits? Here again, studies assessing adverse events related to modafinil suggest otherwise. The most frequently reported side effect is headache, apparently varying with the dos-age taken. The only serious side effect—a life-threatening rash—is rare (exceeding the background incidence rate of one to two cases of serious rash per million person-years).[44]

What about the drug's potential for abuse? Most research has shown that the abuse potential of modafinil is low. However, like the Z-drugs, it is a Schedule IV controlled substance. A recent study utilizing PET scans to assess modafinil's effects on the human brain suggests the drug *does* increase levels of dopamine and could therefore give rise to abuse and dependency "in vulnerable populations."[45]

Perlis regards modafinil as a viable treatment option for insomniacs with debilitating fatigue. What to do when CBT patients complain that sleep restriction is turning them into zombies? "Modafinilize," he said. And he's an expert who puts his money where his mouth is. "When I sleep poorly," he told me, "I take modafinil, and force myself to double my activity the next day." He gets a lot done that way, and it may be that the increased activity leads to better sleep the following night.

But why not drink coffee—in moderation—instead? I asked.

Coffee is OK as tolerated, he replied. But modafinil comes without coffee's negative effects on the stomach.

That sounds like a big advantage to me.

But the use of modafinil for insomnia remains controversial, and it's easy to see why. If you think insomnia is all about poor or insufficient sleep, then you're bound to be suspicious of any drug that promotes wakefulness. But if you think of insomnia as more than just a sleep problem, then a drug like modafinil might begin to sound like a reasonable treatment option.

Whether modafinil would be an appropriate drug for most insomniacs is an open question. Large-scale clinical trials have never been mounted. But if you're interested in trying it (and can persuade your physician to prescribe off label), it's available now in generic form.

In the Pipeline

It's hard to say when we'll get the next Ambien. The vetting process is rigorous; even drugs that make it to Phase III clinical trials are not guaranteed of success. My file labeled "drug graveyard" is full of articles and hype on hypnotics that did not make it through the gestation phase and probably never will. The same thing that happened in 2009 to eplivanserin (abandoned because of safety concerns) happened to gaboxadol in 2007. And the window of opportunity for indiplon, a Z-drug projected to come on the market in 2007, closed because of problems with the extended-release version.

Here's the outlook for up-and-comers as of 2013. The buzz at the 2010 meeting of the Associated Professional Sleep Societies was about hypnotic medications called "orexin receptor antagonists." Unlike most other hypnotics, which work by enhancing the activity of sleep-promoting neurons, this new class of hypnotics works to suppress neurons that are active during wakefulness. The first of these novel compounds has already crashed and burned. But at least two others are still in the pipeline, one under review at the FDA when this book went to press.

Orexin neurons reside in that Grand Central Station of sleep and waking, the hypothalamus. They're active mainly when we're up and alert. In fact, their activity is crucial to our ability to stay awake. Anatomically, these orexin neurons are positioned near the sleep switch (described in chapter 7). They're believed to act like "a finger on the switch that might prevent unwanted transitions into sleep."[46] In insomniacs, the "finger" that prevents transitions to sleep may be too heavy. Excessive activity of the orexin neurons may contribute to heightened activity in the cerebral cortex and, in turn, to our problems falling and staying asleep. Even if this analysis isn't entirely accurate, blocking the action of orexin neurons may be an effective way to promote sleep.[47]

The backstory is interesting here. Orexins (a.k.a. hypocretins) were terra incognita until the end of the twentieth century. Not until 1998 were these neurotransmitters identified. Scientists studying obesity located a small cluster of neurons toward the rear of the hypothalamus that produced two unknown peptides. One team of researchers called them orexins; another team, hypocretins.[48] They observed that these orexin-producing neurons, well connected to subcortical arousal systems and to neurons in the cerebral cortex, were firing like mad during periods of wakefulness. But they were generally quiet during sleep.

Other scientists took the research a step further the following year. They found that dogs and mice deficient in the orexins and lacking orexin receptors exhibited symptoms of narcolepsy, succumbing to irresistible sleep attacks during the day. Scientists studying the brains of human narcoleptics then made a similar discovery. Examining the hypothalamus in their narcoleptic subjects, they noted a severe depletion of orexin neurons. The subjects' cerebrospinal fluid tested low for orexin-A as well. This, then, appeared to be the problem in narcoleptics: orexin deficiency.[49] The discovery of these important neuropeptides and the role they played in sleep and waking solved a mystery that had eluded understanding for over a hundred years.

Animal and human experiments have shown that blocking orexin receptors induces sleep, and at least two (and possibly three) pharmaceutical companies are currently at work on drugs that do this. Merck's new orexin receptor antagonist is called suvorexant, a drug now under review by the FDA. An advisory panel has endorsed the efficacy of suvorexant. But a majority on the panel expressed reservations about its safety at doses higher than 10 mg. In clinical trials, enough subjects suffered grogginess in the morning, impaired driving, thoughts of suicide, and "narcolepsy-like" symptoms that the panel recommended withholding approval of higher doses. Merck has not yet announced what the brand name for the drug will be should it get a thumbs-up from the FDA. Suvorexant will also have to pass muster with the Drug Enforcement Agency before coming on the market. Whether it will be classified as a controlled substance remains to be seen.

GlaxoSmithKline is also working on an orexin blocker for use in treating insomnia. Safety concerns led the company to abandon work on its original orexin receptor antagonist, almorexant, in January of 2011. The second drug, known now as SB-649868, is currently in Phase 2 trials.

Johnson & Johnson is developing an orexin receptor antagonist, too, according to a company representative I spoke with in September of 2012. But mum's the word on details.

Will these drugs ever hit the market? Will they be more effective and freer of side effects than the drugs that came before? We hope they will, but every drug has a price. Only one thing is certain: if orexin receptor antagonists do get the nod from the FDA, we can expect a lot of hype. Be sure to read the fine print before you try them out.

Parting Thoughts

The benefits of sleeping pills today look rather slim in the eyes of independent reviewers. A recent meta-analysis of the efficacy and safety of sleeping pills found that on average insomniacs who take a Z-drug will fall asleep 12.8 minutes faster than they would taking a placebo, and get 11.4 minutes more sleep.[50] In view of data like these and concerns about safety, it's easy to see why some physicians are reluctant to prescribe them.

But when an individual's health and quality of life is at stake, averages and objective measures don't have a lot of meaning. The nature and severity of sleep problems vary a lot from one insomniac to another, as does the ability to benefit from cognitive-behavioral changes, physical training, and mind–body therapies. When other sleep-promoting measures fail, medication can be a lifeline.

Said Larry, a lifelong insomniac whose sleep problem was minimally responsive to behavioral measures and exercise, "My insomnia has changed character since I started the Ambien/Zyprexa routine. Prior to these particular drugs, the insomnia was a rather grinding, continuous aspect of my life, with a lot of missed meetings, social events skipped due to fatigue and irritability. Now, I pretty much get seven to eight hours' sleep per night, right on cue. It's actually pretty amazing to decide at 11 p.m. to go to sleep, pop two pills, and be asleep at 11:15 or 11:30."

He contrasted his approach to that of his mother, who also suffered from insomnia. "My mother tended to stay up late and was rather melancholy," Larry said. "In those days, people tended to just suck it up and be sad and awake."

No insomniac today should be content to suck it up and be sad and awake. The strategies set forth in chapters 8 and 9 and the drugs reviewed here, imperfect though clearly they are, can help liberate us from that. And knowing enough about sleeping pills to be conversant with doctors can only help when we're deciding whether to use medication and which medication to use.

My take on sleeping pills hasn't changed over time. I still think the watchword should be caution, especially since nobody really knows the effects of hypnotics taken for years and years (which is how many chronic insomniacs actually use them). The best insurance policy against developing tolerance and habituation, or experiencing other negative effects, is to take them only as frequently as needed, and to use the lowest effective dose. I say this based in part on the assumption that sleeping pills are merely palliatives. They can't cure what ails us; they can only relieve symptoms.

But Michael Perlis and colleagues point out that this assumption has never truly been put to the test. "The traditional approach to chronic insomnia might be best likened to aspirin therapy for headache," they have written. Whatever the cause of a headache, we take aspirin as needed to relieve the pain. "What if, however, headache is not the appropriate analogy. What if chronic insomnia is more analogous to infection." In that case, they say, taking sleeping pills on an as-needed basis would not be expected to cure insomnia any more than antibiotics taken intermittently would likely cure an infection.[51] Just as to cure the infection you'd have to take a daily course of antibiotics for a long enough time, so sleeping pills might have curative powers if taken nightly for a long enough time.

This idea is at odds with everything I've ever heard or known about sleeping pills, so I pressed Perlis for an explanation. If hypnotics could actually cure insomnia, wouldn't lots more insomniacs be sleeping like logs?

It turns out that the idea that hypnotics could be curative depends a great deal on the *context* in which they're prescribed, and on behavioral theories of what insomnia is and how it develops. "The truth is," Perlis said, "it would be great if we could figure out a way to help physicians see that short-term use of hypnotics in the context of *acute* insomnia"—insomnia that presents during a stressful situation—"could be a potent tool to derail chronic insomnia." Instead, he continued, "when doctors *do* make a distinction between acute and chronic insomnia, what they do is unfortunate. If you come in with acute insomnia, instead of seeing that as an opportunity for prevention and cure, they see that as, 'come back when it's serious.' Unfortunately, they've missed the opportunity to get in when medication *might* cure. If you could stop people in their tracks from responding to the insomnia"—from going to bed early, from obsessing about sleep loss, from playing catch-up with naps—then it would stop the cascade leading to chronic insomnia, he said. Dysregulation of the circadian and homeostatic systems and the brain changes associated with insomnia might never occur.

It's an intriguing hypothesis, that hypnotics taken at the first presentation of insomnia might actually have curative powers if used nightly for a long enough time. Get on the ball, sleep mavens, and find out if and for whom this treatment strategy could work. The answer might be surprising.

But I doubt an extended course of hypnotics taken in my early twenties would have nipped my insomnia in the bud. That's because my sleep was never robust to begin with. My mother's reports about how easily noises woke me up as a sleeping infant, and her stories of the emotional struggles that kept me wakeful at night, suggest my fate as a fragile sleeper was sealed early on. Either I entered this world primed for arousal, or my early life experiences teamed up with my genes to assure that sleep would always be a challenge.

I believe, though, that with earlier access to sleeping pills, I might not have developed some of the sleep-related anxieties that later evolved, which doubtless made my insomnia worse. If on bad nights I'd had the comfort of knowing that sleep-in-a-bottle lay inside the medicine cabinet, it might have made a difference in how serious my problem became.

But a drug that could actually cure me, that could inoculate me against future encounters with insomnia? It would be a different sort of drug than is available now.

For now I'm pinning my hopes on a medication I could take as needed that does more than help me sleep. A drug that supplies some of the benefits good sleep affords: feeling rested and revitalized in the morning, with a mind that's thrumming and ready to meet the challenges ahead. A drug that comes without serious side effects or risks to my health. Something as benign as a statin or a beta blocker, so clean that even the likes of a Daniel Kripke would not trouble himself to find fault with it, much less conclude it would shorten my life.

Such a drug would be a pharmaceutical blockbuster ten times over. Build it, O pharmacologists, and we will come!

12

Destination Sleep

Oh, insomnia. I know a good cure for it—get plenty of sleep.

W.C. Fields, *Never Give a Sucker an Even Break*

Eight years ago I told an ophthalmologist friend about plans to write this book.

"Insomnia?" he said. "Aren't they close to finding a cure for that?"

"Not that I know," I shot back, thinking, "We should be so lucky!" and then, "Wait a minute. Is there a need for the book I'm envisioning if sleep-in-a-bottle lies just around the bend?"

Fat chance, that. One challenge of writing this book, I realized not long into the project, was that the word "cure" would not have a place within its pages. I could acquaint readers with treatments that might improve their sleep and reduce their symptoms—perhaps substantially—but no alchemy I was discovering could guarantee poor sleepers the golden eight hours so many desired. Nor would I be able to explain the causal mechanisms behind poor sleep. At best I could present theories based on accumulating evidence. Some research I could cite would be preliminary; sometimes the results would be mixed. Even so, though much about insomnia remains hidden, it's clear now that the disorder has too great an impact on quality of life and health to be dismissed as merely "a faulty state of mind."

So what's the next chapter in the insomnia story? Where is research headed, what novel treatments are in the offing? And what help can insomniacs get right now?

For a veteran insomniac like me, accustomed to doctors showing little interest in my problem, it's been heartening to speak with scientists who study sleep and insomnia. Many of these academics and physicians are strong advocates for our cause. Those whose work and words I've cited really "get" how important sleep is and how debilitating insomnia can become. They're as impassioned about uncovering its root causes, and developing more effective treatments, as I could wish them to be. (And no surprises here: some have confided that they or their spouse or mother suffer the affliction.) But a big constraint on their efforts to move ahead is a scarcity of funds.

About 10 percent of the population suffer recurring insomnia, so it's a more common sleep disorder than apnea, restless legs syndrome, or narcolepsy.[1] Insomnia is a causal factor in depression and a burden on society because of its role in absenteeism, reductions in productivity, and higher healthcare costs. It's associated with life-threatening ailments like high blood pressure and heart disease, and it impairs daily functioning and quality of life. Given these facts and that the causes of insomnia remain largely unknown, you'd think it would be a prime candidate for government funding. But it is not. The National Institutes of Health awarded $232 million to grant-funded sleep research in 2011, but only $8 million went to insomnia, or 3.4 percent.[2] Insomnia gets a beggar's slice of the pie.

Funders may be looking to the pharmaceutical industry to pick up the tab. There's logic in that, especially if you're convinced the solution lies in a pill. While pharmaceutical companies spend the lion's share of money promoting their products, they invest a lot in research and development, too. Major companies spend anywhere from $4 billion to $11 billion developing each new drug.[3] But only a handful of pharmaceutical companies are working on drugs for insomnia, as we've seen. Plus, no scientist I've interviewed believes the bulk of funding for insomnia *should* come from private sources.

"The drug companies fund a lot of insomnia research," said UC Davis sleep researcher Irwin Feinberg, "but then there's a conflict of interest issue. They're usually studying their own drugs. It's definitely a problem. If the NIH is assuming that the drug companies are going to fund this [the study of insomnia], it's not a really very satisfactory answer for a problem which is so pervasive and so expensive to society."

Attitudes held over from the past may keep insomnia from getting a larger share of public money. Decision makers may still regard insomnia as impacting only the night rather than also impairing daytime functioning, as "psychological" rather than multifactorial, as relatively harmless rather than consequential to our overall health, and as correctable through simple lifestyle changes or pills rather than deserving an investigative full-court press. Funding agencies have not yet recognized that insomnia is related to significant medical risks. So the exploration of the effects of insomnia on day-to-day functioning and overall health moves slowly.

Sleep scientists are pressing ahead with research in these important areas even so. Among the health consequences of poor sleep, one topic under investigation is how insomnia affects the immune system.

"Here's a place where we all believe heart and soul that if you don't sleep well, you are way more vulnerable to infection," Michael Perlis said. But the evidence is not solid yet. There is some research on insomnia and innate immunity, he said—the body's emergency response system that mounts a nonspecific inflammatory response when it detects a pathogen. So far this research is inconclusive.[4]

It's the second level of immunity—adaptive immunity—that Perlis suspects is compromised by insomnia. Adaptive immunity refers to the process by which the body, in response to an infectious agent (an antigen), produces antibodies to fight a specific virus or bacterium. "Not the first responders to a challenge," Perlis said, "but the rangers. The things that are tailored to a specific virus—*that* virus.

"If God said to me, 'You can get into heaven if you make a bet about something not known to humankind and you're right; otherwise, it's oblivion for you,'" Perlis said, "one of the guesses I might make would be that adaptive immunity is fundamentally compromised by insomnia."

The issue has yet to be put to the test. Scientists cannot infect human subjects to find out whether insomnia impairs their ability to mount an adaptive immune response or not. To work around this problem, investigators are now conducting studies where they're administering vaccines to good and poor sleepers and then comparing the results. Studies like these will help to determine whether and how insomnia compromises the body's readiness to fight infection.

Other scientists are probing further into the effects of insomnia on daytime functioning and performance. The question of insomnia's effects on memory, for example, is a hot topic. A recent meta-analysis concludes that insomniacs show "significant impairments of small to moderate magnitude" in tasks assessing the recall of factual information and events, and aspects of working memory. And results of a newer unpublished study affirm the perceptions of insomniacs who complain of memory problems. Insomnia subjects in this experiment were tested on a series of verbal learning tasks, and the insomniacs with memory complaints had significantly poorer recall of verbal information in long-term storage than the insomniacs without memory complaints.[5] Why only some insomniacs struggle with memory issues is unknown, but the evidence of a relationship between sleep problems and impaired memory is increasingly solid.

Causal Factors

Research on the causes of insomnia continues to move slowly, in part because of the funding issue and in part because there are so many horses in the race.

"Almost certainly there's more than one mechanism and probably there are myriad mechanisms associated with the syndrome of insomnia," sleep investigator Gary Richardson said at the 2009 meeting for the Associated Professional Sleep Societies.

The main culprit for some insomniacs may be the "sleep switch" itself (see chapter 7). If this important control center in the hypothalamus is weakened on either the sleep or the wake side of the circuit, so the theory goes, unwanted transitions between sleeping and waking are bound to occur frequently.[6] This could explain the situation of many elderly insomniacs, who are prone to middle-of-the-night and early morning awakenings and also apt to doze off during the day.

Other insomniacs may suffer from dysregulation of the sleep homeostat, also described in chapter 7. Precisely how the neurobiologic mechanisms associated with the homeostat interact to regulate sleep remains unknown. But various homeostatic sleep factors have been identified, adenosine chief among them. Daytime build-up of adenosine in the basal forebrain induces sleep, and a glitch in this process or related processes could be a main driver of insomnia.[7]

Alternatively or in addition, some insomniacs may—in key areas of the brain—suffer from reduced levels of GABA (chapter 9), the big kahuna when it comes to shutting down our neural circuitry at night. Two neuroimaging studies now suggest this may be the case.[8]

Yet another possibility is that insomnia could occur as the result of an overactive central nervous system, also discussed in chapter 9. Too many circulating stress hormones and too much activation of the HPA axis could interfere with sleep and incline us toward vigilance around the clock. An overabundance of orexin neurons in the hypothalamus—neurons that help keep us awake and alert—could have much the same result.[9]

Finally, a new theory of insomnia suggests that insomniacs whose problem is awakening frequently in the night may be suffering from "REM sleep instability." Analyses of data gathered on people with sleep maintenance insomnia show that, compared to normal sleepers, they get a reduced percentage of REM sleep and experience increased arousals and awakenings during REM sleep. Destabilization in the mix of arousing and calming activity that occurs in the brain during REM sleep could be the main factor behind nonrestorative sleep.[10]

"So is there a leading contender?" I ask at sleep conferences and everywhere I go.

None of the experts have an answer yet. Instead, pressed to explain the causes of insomnia, they talk in terms of possibilities that range over the entire biopsychosocial spectrum.

Insomnia, Perlis said, "is a multifactorial, multiply determined disorder, and you can find yourself with it for a number of reasons. You may be a GABA hypo-secretor—that'll probably get you there. You may be an orexin hyper-secretor, you may be wired for perceived threat. You may be highly conditionable, so that what takes other people a hundred trials of pairing takes you only five. You may be someone who's quick to compensate for perceived discomfort, and we can keep going for a while now. Every one of those things and more will make you someone with chronic insomnia sooner or later."

Presented with this smorgasbord of possibilities, I don't know whether to laugh or cry. It's hopeful that scientists are pursuing leads wherever they turn up. On the other hand, with so many suspects in the line-up, those of us waiting for answers may be in for a long wait indeed.

Researchers could speed the process up by getting smarter about how they conduct research. One problem with studying insomnia is that the symptoms are diverse and widely variable from one insomniac to the next. Some of us have problems falling asleep; others, staying asleep. Some are "short sleepers;" others are not. The forces driving our insomnia may be different depending on the symptoms we have. Yet insomniacs have often been studied as a homogeneous group. The consequence is a body of literature with conflicting results.

"If I average together people who have paradoxical insomnia [whose EEGs look normal] with people who have objective insomnia [whose EEGs look abnormal]," said Michael Bonnet, clinical director of Kettering Sycamore Sleep Disorders Center in Miamisburg, Ohio, "if I average together even their sleep values, it's going to look like they don't have abnormal sleep." The subjects under study have different problems, Bonnet said, and mixing them up does not produce meaningful results. Plus, he added, failing to screen subjects differentially makes it difficult for sleep scientists to replicate their colleagues' work.

Michael Perlis has a similar take on the problem. "It is remarkable to me that the fathers have thrice gone to the trouble of creating a classification system"—dividing insomniacs into types and subtypes—"and then gone on to ignore their children," failing to differentiate between them when they conduct research. "Why," Perlis said, "did you make this up if you're not going to use it in every study you do?"

I'm with Perlis, Bonnet, and others who call for taking account of distinctions between insomnia sufferers when conducting scientific research. Studying insomniacs as lumpenproletariat hasn't produced a lot of bang for the buck, and it's time to change course.

Divide and conquer is the way to win this battle, is how it looks to me.

Do Existing Treatments Work?

Many experts are also calling for a higher bar when evaluating the efficacy of insomnia treatments. "We talk so often about what goes wrong if you're not sleeping," said Sonia Ancoli-Israel of UC San Diego, "but what we don't know for sure yet is this: when we treat insomnia successfully, do those things get better? I think that's an area of research that's greatly in need. We know they [existing drug and cognitive-behavioral therapies] are effective in treating sleep, but what about the other consequences of not sleeping: the daytime consequences of insomnia, or health in general, and susceptibility to disease?" With treatment, she said, "does daytime performance improve? Is there less absenteeism once you fix someone's sleep?"

Consider sleeping pills. As noted in the last chapter, to gain approval from the FDA, hypnotic medications have to meet safety standards and be shown to improve sleep. But they are not required to reduce the incidence of depression or heart disease or any other health problem associated with insomnia, and some experts are calling for this to change.

Michael Bonnet is one. To prove that a drug is truly effective in combating insomnia, Bonnet said, "you have to do long-term studies to look at mortality and the development of depression over time. Because if a medication is effective, the people who take it are going to have a decreased incidence in the development of depression and a decreased incidence of mortality. They're not going to have the blood pressure problems or blood sugar problems" that insomniacs are vulnerable to now. The FDA should require that drugs for insomnia reduce the incidence of related health problems, Bonnet said.

Nor are drug companies currently required to demonstrate that hypnotics ameliorate the daytime symptoms of insomnia: fatigue, moodiness, impaired concentration, and the like. So not much is known about the daytime effects of sleeping pills. The results of studies mounted in recent years are mixed.[11]

Could the same pill that puts me to sleep also give me the daytime boost that a good night's sleep provides? By my lights that pill has yet to arrive. The little yellow tablets on my bedside table are dependable when it comes to knocking me out. If I didn't have them, if I were at the mercy of that "lit up" feeling that comes with arousal in the evening, I could be anxiously surfing the Net all night.

These pills get a C, though, for their next-day effects. Feelings on awakening? Slight malaise, and a whisper of anxiety. Energy level? Low, but rising as the morning wears on. Mental acuity? Passable. I can usually string sentences together, I can usually compose. As for my ability to grasp the big picture or come up with fresh ideas, more than likely, the day will be a bust. Is it asking for the moon to suggest that the pill I take to sleep afford more of the daytime benefits of a good night's sleep?

One approach to the issue would be to consider the functions sleep is believed to perform—the restoration of energy and alertness, the regulation of mood, the consolidation of memory—and require that drugs for insomnia help restore these functions, too. I heard something like this proposed at the 2011 meeting of the Associated Professional Sleep Societies. Thomas Roth, a sleep researcher with the Henry Ford Health System in Detroit, reacted with skepticism, saying that it would amount to putting the cart before the horse.

"We can't hold drug development people accountable to higher standards of improving functions which we haven't identified are impaired," Roth said. "You ask them to improve daytime functioning, and they ask, 'Well what do you want us to fix?'" The sleep community, he added, needs to go home and figure it out.

But Michael Perlis disagreed. "Sleep is not just about having the sensation and polysomnographically monitoring immobility and disconnection from the world," Perlis said. "Sleep *does* things. And the question is, when we get sleep continuity to look and feel approximately normal to the individual, what the hell happens to the rest of the stuff? We don't look at it because we don't know. And from where we do look at it, it looks like it's *not* normal. While hypnotics may confer much-improved sleep continuity," Perlis added, "they're not conferring normal sleep.

"The next generation of drugs should be held to a higher standard," Perlis continued. "The standard should be that we find these really reliable effects for memory consolidation by sleep. *That* should be one of the yardsticks that we measure treatment by, and there should be a set of things like that."

A sleeping pill that could actually restore the memory functions insomnia is believed to impair? That would be a different pill from the one I take now, bless its little amnesia-inducing soul. Yet as scientists home in on the functions sleep performs, and as they hone their understanding of the impairments and health problems associated with insomnia, it will become more feasible to ask for medications that improve sleep as well as daytime functioning and long-term health.

We need experts who are ready to acknowledge the shortcomings of the status quo and press for changes. Insomnia is not just a sleep problem, and general practitioners, sleep specialists, and professional associations need to pressure the FDA to make higher demands of the next generation of insomnia drugs. We who use medications can contribute to the effort by sharing our concerns about current drugs with our doctors. Otherwise, we'll never get anything that does much more than Ambien.

Nondrug treatments for insomnia should be held to higher standards as well. It's not enough to show that CBT-I hastens sleep onset and increases sleep efficiency. Researchers need to demonstrate that CBT-I is able to restore daytime functioning and reduce susceptibility to depression and heart problems as well.[12] If it cannot be shown to do these things, then other therapies need to be developed as adjuncts or replacements.

Nondrug Treatments in the Works

The majority of nondrug treatments under development today are variations on CBT-I.

Brief Behavioral Treatment for Insomnia (BBTI). This is CBT-I minus the "C," behavioral therapies like sleep restriction and stimulus control without the cognitive component targeting dysfunctional thoughts.

BBTI has improved the sleep of older insomnia subjects and may work for other age groups as well.[13] One of its virtues, as the name suggests, is its brevity.

"It's bloody brief," said Perlis. "There are four sessions, and the last two are on the phone. But it does produce equal outcomes, to my shock." The durability looks pretty good, too, Perlis added. Insomniacs interested in behavioral treatment who do not have the time (or money) to attend six to eight therapy sessions may find BBTI more doable.

The Sleep Spa. This, too, is an alternative form of CBT-I. Instead of having to confront your sleep demons on your own at home—where you might be tempted to break the rules—you do so in a supervised setting where creature comforts abound. High-end mattresses, eight-hundred-thread-count sheets. Pillows of different sizes and lofts, personalized bathrobes, private baths. A week or so in the lap of luxury in exchange for being hooked up to an EEG machine and observed by a friendly sleep monitor who sees you when you're sleeping and knows when you're awake. And knows if you're being bad or good. Try to pull a fast one—as in *lying awake in bed for more than 15 minutes*—and the phone at your bedside rings.

"Mrs. Jones," says a cheery voice, "I'm sorry, but you've got to get up! Come on down to the kitchen and have some nice warm milk. Oh, and remember to put on your slippers. You don't want to get cold feet."

Perlis conceded that sleep spas are an option only for the wealthy. But the option will be available in the not-too-distant future. "I'm looking forward to seeing what kind of good we can do in a week under a controlled environment," Perlis said. "And one that people will find pleasant."

Intensive Sleep Retraining (ISR). A sleep specialist I know has likened this treatment to waterboarding, but if you're in the market for a behavioral treatment that works in just twenty-five hours, this could be the answer. The premise behind ISR is that trouble falling asleep occurs mainly because of faulty conditioning (going to bed before you're sleepy, worrying about sleep loss, "trying" to sleep). The object of treatment is to undo that conditioning and teach you to fall asleep with ease. Experimental studies have shown that ISR is effective for insomniacs whose problem is falling asleep and who may also have trouble staying asleep.[14]

Here's how it works. You check in to a sleep lab in the evening, get wired up with electrodes, and go to bed around your normal bedtime. Then a day-long series of thirty-minute sleep trials begin. In each thirty-minute trial, you try to fall asleep. If you succeed, you're awakened after a few minutes and asked to finish off the session in a chair reading a book or watching a DVD. If you don't fall asleep, you're roused after twenty or twenty-five minutes and asked to remain awake for the few remaining minutes until the next trial begins.

People undergoing ISR tend to fall asleep more quickly as the night progresses. But you're never allowed more than a few minutes' sleep (and should you have trouble staying awake, a technician enters the room to keep you up with quiet conversation). Over the course of a twenty-five-hour period you get repeated exposure to what it feels like to fall asleep quickly. And by the end of that time, you're so sleep deprived that a good night's recovery sleep is virtually guaranteed!

Gains made by subjects who have gone through ISR—getting to sleep faster, spending less time awake in bed, and sleeping longer—have lasted up to six months, the research shows. But when this book went to press, ISR was not yet being offered in clinical settings.

Frontal Cerebral Thermal Transfer. The name is cumbersome, and the concept sounds like something from a science fiction novel, but here it is, the most novel treatment I've come across for the sleepless: a plastic cap designed to cool overactive brains at night and so improve sleep.

I was leery the minute I caught wind of it. My bedroom is cold in the winter, and I have to burrow under the covers for warmth. Now they're proposing to cure my insomnia by sticking the equivalent of an ice pack on my brain? Is there no end to the tortures these sleep scientists are capable of dreaming up?! (See sleep restriction and stimulus control.)

But University of Pittsburgh School of Medicine researcher Eric Nofzinger persuaded me not to dismiss the idea without a hearing. Nofzinger, who is working with colleague Daniel Buysse and with Cereve, Inc. to develop and test the device, said that insomnia subjects who have tried it have responded positively. "They describe it as sort of like a spa treatment," Nofzinger told me as we chatted during a poster presentation at the APSS Conference in 2011.

So what does wearing a polar cap have to do with combating insomnia?

"Insomniacs have too much metabolic activity in the frontal cortex," Nofzinger said. "It's very soothing to be able to settle that brain activity" by cooling down this region of the cortex. "It's as if your grandmother put a washcloth on your forehead."

Frontal cerebral thermal transfer entails wearing a soft plastic cap filled with circulating water at night. The temperature can be adjusted within a "comfortable" range of coolness, Nofzinger said.

In a recent study, wearing the caps helped insomnia subjects fall asleep more quickly and sleep more efficiently. Those who wore the device at the coolest setting got the greatest benefit. In fact, their sleep resembled that of healthy control subjects.[15]

A cap that would turn me into a normal sleeper? That would put me to sleep in ten or fifteen minutes? That would allow me to sleep through the night without wake-ups? It sounds too good to be true! Like those pie-in-the-sky claims for the dietary supplements and bath oils promoted on the Internet: "Designed to provide deep sleep and feelings of restoration in the morning. Results guaranteed."

Yet Nofzinger and Buysse are not your everyday entrepreneurs. They're highly respected medical researchers at the forefront of their field. Results of small clinical trials have been positive, but whether the device will work for large numbers of insomniacs remains to be seen. Over $1 million in grant money from the NIH will go toward settling this question. If the answer is yes, expect to see the device on the market in a few years.

Finding Help Now

One path to better sleep involves seeking professional help. Physicians certified as specialists in sleep medicine are knowledgeable about insomnia and qualified to provide treatments from A to Z. Psychologists and nurse practitioners certified in behavioral sleep medicine (CBSMs) are qualified to administer behavioral treatments like CBT-I. Again, lists of certified sleep medicine providers are available online at Absm.org/BSMSpecialists.aspx and Behavioralsleep.org/findspecialist.aspx.

When it comes to seeking professional help for insomnia, I'm biased in favor of the specialists. The pair I consulted—one an MD, and the other a psychologist—provided sound advice and were strong in empathy. (The empathy alone can count for a lot.)

But most people turn for help to primary care providers, and it's here where there's room for improvement. Some physicians I've had dealings with in recent years have seemed as clueless about insomnia as ever. And why should the situation be otherwise, when medical students receive no more than a few hours' training in sleep medicine, when the bulk of doctors' knowledge about insomnia comes from pharmaceutical companies, and when the solutions proposed by the pill purveyors may be seen as doing more harm than good?

This being the case, insomniacs need to be prepared to push for the care we deserve. What I'm proposing is something like an insomnia patient's Bill of Rights. Insomniacs who seek help should be able to expect that doctors

1.　Respond to complaints of poor sleep as attentively as they would to complaints of chest pain or diarrhea. Insomnia *can* be debilitating, and chronic insomnia *does* effect changes that compromise the quality of our lives and our health. Any doctor who dismisses it as trivial or unworthy of treatment is not the right doctor.

2.　Ask the sort of questions that will enable an accurate diagnosis. Gathering information about the duration, frequency, and severity of the problem, and whether it might signal the presence of an underlying condition, is crucial to arriving at an appropriate diagnosis and treatment. Doctors who don't have the time or the knowledge to ask such questions should steer us toward others who do.

3.　Lay out treatment options that are research based, and then involve *us* in coming up with a plan tailored to our individual needs. A prescription for sleeping pills is useless to a patient who has no intention of filling it. Likewise, CBT-I may not be viable for a single mother of a toddler attempting to hold down a full-time job. She can barely meet her daily obligations, never mind find time for therapy sessions or comply with a rigorous sleep restriction protocol. These points may sound obvious. Yet over half the insomniacs I interviewed who sought professional help either got no new ideas from their physicians or felt the solution proposed was unappealing or impractical. Treatment discussions should be dialogs, and doctors should encourage our participation.

We deserve no less. In the future, sleep problems may finally make it onto the systems checklist along with heart and respiratory problems. Primary care providers may someday be as proactive about identifying sleep problems as they are now about tracking cholesterol and bone loss. In the meantime, we're the ones who have to bring insomnia to the attention of our doctors and insist that it be addressed.

But placing yourself under the care of a physician is not the only way to go. You can accomplish a lot with knowledge of the biological systems controlling sleep and wake. To recap from earlier chapters:

- Brightening and dimming lights can have a big impact on the secretion of cortisol and melatonin and help to shift the timing of sleep.

- Curtailing time in bed and adopting a regular sleep schedule can enhance the homeostatic pressure to sleep, and may increase slow-wave sleep and restore neuronal activity in the prefrontal cortex during the daytime.

- Physical training can lower your resting heart rate and help to hasten sleep. Strenuous exercise also raises core body temperature and, if done in the late afternoon or early evening, can lead to increases in slow-wave sleep.

- Mind–body practices such as yoga and tai chi may also down-regulate arousal of the sympathetic nervous system and help build tolerance to stress, in turn enhancing sleep.

If these and other tricks in the behaviorist toolkit are insufficient, though, waste no time in seeking professional help.

My Journey to Better Sleep

People ask me if I've found a cure for my insomnia. They want to know if writing this book—beyond acquainting me with fascinating studies of the human brain, a cadre of inspired sleep scientists, and physicians from times past who were keen observers of the sleepless and recorded what they saw—has led to better sleep. It's a fair question. When I started my research I was not sure what I was going to find. I was obsessed with getting to the bottom of my insomnia, but I didn't know how much headway I was going to make. This could have turned into a very philosophical book.

It didn't, because in trying to find solutions to my own sleep demons I met with considerable success. Yet when I tell people this, something invariably gets lost in the telling. "You're doing daily workouts on the elliptical trainer? Waking up to your alarm clock at 5:30 every morning for a grand total of five to five and a half hours of sleep a night?" The raised eyebrows, the unspoken question: "So what's so great about that?"

The reply is that I'm light years beyond where I was before, but I realize that none but my closest confidantes have an inkling of how bad things used to be. How adolescent it felt to struggle with something as easy for others as eating and breathing; how debilitating it was to get by on a few hours' respite for nights on end, desperate for the catch-up night that finally came in a burst of dead-to-the-world sleep and dreaming; how exhausting to pretend to be energetic when I was crawling on empty; how infuriating it was to hear insomnia dismissed as "something psychological" and, at the same time, how embarrassing it was to admit to my fear of sleeplessness and know that the fear was making my insomnia worse; how powerless I felt at the mercy of forces in my brain that I did not understand. If I sought to downplay the effects of my insomnia then, it was because I was living in a kind of survival mode and denial was the best way to cope. I can admit to how bad things used to be only because my sleep and vitality are so much better today. If this doesn't qualify as improvement, I don't know what does.

The guerrilla sleeper I used to be, seizing my few winks at odd hours, is a person of the past. The fears that could steal over me near the end of the day have faded. When sleep *does* go on the lam, it's gone a few days and never more than a week. (Contrast this with the three- and four-week bouts of insomnia that once caused me such misery). When sleep plays coy, I head for the pills without a second thought.

My sleep is still on the fragile side of normal, though, which is a frustration. But I've come to see the problem in a larger context, and this in itself helps. I now view my insomnia as part of a predilection for vigilance throughout the twenty-four-hour day. And in me this predilection goes a long way back. My mother reports that as a toddler, I was afraid of gusting leaves. When they blew I cried and tried to run away. I was prone to detecting threats in my environment and responded with an exaggerated stress response.

I can now own this trait and admit that it has traveled with me all these many years.

It doesn't keep me on red alert all the time. When I'm surrounded by things familiar—sitting at my computer or on the back porch of my husband's cabin—I'm relaxed and can go with the flow. The vigilance kicks in anytime an unexpected challenge *could* come my way, aided by a keen pair of ears. My early warning system goes off at the least provocation and, once it's screaming, it's hard to turn down.

Sometimes this trait is useful—when I'm driving, for example. If I have to stop unexpectedly, I'm quick to check the rearview mirror and pull over onto the shoulder. Is that a police car ahead? I already hit the brake a few seconds ago. It's only at night when the vigilance becomes a problem.

I'm intrigued by the idea that wakeful proclivities like mine might once have been of use to humans after dark. Survival was a big issue for our ancestors at nightfall, and fire was a critical resource. Humans predisposed to vigilance had a role to play when a tribe's best defense against predators was to sleep communally around a flame. Those who kept watch while others slept, whose ears were attuned to the soft crackles and hisses of the flame and who awakened as easily to loud pops as to the absence of murmuring noise, performed a valuable service. So what if they weren't the fastest runners or the best hunters or the most resourceful problem solvers. They contributed to the communal welfare by tending to the fire at night.

If nocturnal vigilance was once adaptive, it follows that the trait might be conserved in some of us today. It might be the thing we call insomnia. And if wakefulness was as important to the survival of the species as sleep scientists now say, it stands to reason that it would show up in different forms and flavors. Not just as a propensity to keep vigil long into the night but, for some, as an inclination to awaken before sunrise. Not just as a lesser ability to sleep but, for some, as a tendency to wake up periodically or to be sensible of sounds and other sensory cues. "If indeed 'insomniacs' once were important for survival," write the authors of a paper on research challenges ahead, "then it is likely that insomnia should be a robust heterogeneous trait, solidly anchored in many different polymorphism profiles."[16] F. Scott Fitzgerald's observation—that every man's insomnia is as different from his neighbor's as are their daytime hopes and aspirations—may hold a grain of truth for reasons beyond those he imagined.[17]

Unfortunately, nocturnal wakefulness is not just a harmless vestigial trait, like tailbones and appendices. Sleep enables bodily functions that cannot occur while we're awake. These functions are not well understood, but sleep certainly does more than simply immobilizing us and helping keep us out of harm's way. It allows for the conservation of resources after periods of intense energy expenditure. Beyond that, sleep is restorative and likely has something to do with the capacity to respond to traumatic injury. Growth hormone is secreted during slow-wave sleep, enabling the knitting of bones and other types of tissue repair. Sleep also enables the generation of new neurons in the brain, which may affect memory and emotion.[18] Sleep facilitates the mastery of new skills and the acquisition of knowledge. It consolidates and stabilizes memory, and allows for the pruning of trivial information.[19] Sleep also regulates emotion, stripping memories of their negative charge and elevating mood. Sleep probably serves these functions and more. When it's compromised by persistent wakefulness, we lose out.

Sound sleep and daytime vitality are not beyond reach for people predisposed to wakefulness at night. Knowledge of the sleep–wake system, coupled with changes in habits and mindset, can be just the ingredients needed to achieve sound sleep and stamina fairly consistently. In addition, exercise and mind–body practices can lower stress and provide increased resilience to stress-related sleep disturbance. Sleeping pills can serve as stopgap measures in times of acute stress. And in people whose insomnia fails to respond otherwise, medication can become a long-term solution when judiciously prescribed.

These therapies are admittedly imperfect. Sleep scientists and the pharmaceutical industry should be working hard to come up with new and better options. At the same time, insomniacs should not dismiss the effectiveness of the tools on hand or allow older beliefs—that insomnia is a trivial problem, or that we ourselves are to blame for it—to interfere with seeking treatment.

The point of this book is not to suggest that every episode of insomnia should be cause for concern. On the contrary, simply ignoring transient insomnia can be the best idea for many people, especially those whose sleep is normally robust. "Do nothing," says Michael Perlis, "and the ship will right itself."

But for those of us who experience insomnia as a debilitating malady, or when insomnia threatens to become so, inaction is not the best approach. An unrelenting stream of sleepless nights and foggy days turns life into an obstacle course, and every day becomes a test of endurance. Beyond its negative effects on the quality of our lives, persistent insomnia sets the stage for chronic changes to occur in the brain, in turn making people vulnerable to depression and other major health problems.

There is no good reason for the perennially wakeful to take the affliction lying down. For insomniacs who haven't already done so, the time to act is now.

Acknowledgments

This book has been in the works for several years, and I'm grateful for the many forms of assistance I've received along the way. In the research phase, dozens of insomnia sufferers shared their experiences with me. These informants are too numerous to acknowledge by name (and many wish to remain anonymous), but I am beholden to each and every one for their affecting testimonials.

I'm indebted to the sleep specialists who shared up-to-the-minute information with me in interviews at conferences, clinics, and seminars; over the phone; and via e-mail. Especially generous with their time and counsel were Michael Bonnet, Michael Perlis, and David Neubauer, whose comments helped to shape this book and enliven its pages. I'm grateful to Irwin Feinberg, Sonia Ancoli-Israel, Jerome Sarris, James Krueger, and Charmane Eastman for the thought-provoking conversations we had about their research. Exchanges with Timothy Roehrs, Sat Bir Khalsa, Leon Lack, Eric Nofzinger, and Dane Anderson deepened my understanding of key topics. I owe special thanks to Deirdre Conroy, whose expert guidance in a group therapy program benefited me personally and furthered my research on cognitive-behavioral therapy. Finally, I'm grateful for the assistance I received from librarians at the University of Michigan's Taubman Health Sciences Library and William L. Clements Library, who provided access to rare books.

I could not have produced this book without the support I received from a small circle of critics during the writing phase of the project. Marlene Lee offered insightful comments on the early chapters, and Eric Burton, Ruth Maharg, and Geoffrey Biringer devoted countless hours to helping me organize the book and improve its readability. The technical nature of some chapters demanded close attention to accuracy, and I'm indebted to the experts who graciously consented to vet the science chapters: Michael Bonnet, David Neubauer, Irwin Feinberg, Deirdre Conroy, and Michael Grandner. I deeply appreciate the assistance of my editor, Sheila Buff, whose thoughtful comments led to a rounding out of content and a more polished book, and who was always available to step in when needed.

I'm fortunate to have had talented professionals to design and assist in promoting this work. On the production side, my thanks go to Helen Duval, Jordan Patchak, and Judy Seling for ably translating the verbal into the visual. My thanks to Nancy Elder as well, whose artistic savvy informed many decisions relating to the book's presentation. I'm indebted to Kathy Goss for the many weeks she spent laboring to create the online component of the book. I thank Sandra Beckwith for her work on publicity.

Moral support from Deb Kraus saw me through the early years of the project. My family and friends were also supportive, sending me relevant articles and gamely responding to my requests for input along the way. But I owe the greatest thanks to my husband, Eric Burton. In addition to being my first reader and sharpest critic, he encouraged me from the moment the idea for the book took shape through the later stages, when, seeing its potential, he pushed me beyond the bounds of comfort to produce the best book I possibly could.

Notes

Chapter 1: Sizing Up the Beast

1. Woods Hutchinson, "Sleep for the Sleepless," *Good Housekeeping*, May 1915.
2. Michael Bonnet and Donna Arand, "Hyperarousal and Insomnia: State of the Science," *Sleep Medicine Reviews* 14 (2010): 9-15.
3. Dieter Riemann et al., "The Hyperarousal Model of Insomnia," *Sleep Medicine Reviews* 14 (2010): 19-31; E.A. Nofzinger et al., "Functional Neuroimaging Evidence for Hyperarousal in Insomnia," *American Journal of Psychiatry* 161 (2004): 2126-8; E.A. Nofzinger et al., "Regional Cerebral Metabolic Correlates of WASO During NREM Sleep in Insomnia," *Journal of Clinical Sleep Medicine* 15 (2006): 316-22.
4. Willis G. Regier, "Cioran's Insomnia," *Modern Language Notes* 119 (2004): 994-1012.
5. Joyce Carol Oates, *Night Walks: A Bedside Companion* (Princeton: The Ontario Review Press, 1982), xiii.
6. Deborah Bishop and David Levy, *Hello Midnight: An Insomniac's Literary Bedside Companion* (New York: Touchstone Books, 2001), 65.
7. J.D. Edinger et al., "Insomnia and the Eye of the Beholder," *Journal of Consulting and Clinical Psychology* 68 (2000): 586-93; Teofilo Lee-Chiong, *Sleep Medicine: Essentials and Review* (New York: Oxford University Press, 2008), 75; D.J. Taylor et al., "Epidemiology of Insomnia, Depression, and Anxiety," *Sleep* 28 (2005): 1457-64; Les A. Gellis et al., "Socioeconomic Status and Insomnia," *Journal of Abnormal Psychology* 114 (2005): 111-8.
8. American Academy of Sleep Medicine, *International Classification of Sleep Disorders: Diagnostic and Coding Manual,* 2nd ed. (Westchester, IL: American Academy of Sleep Medicine, 2005); American Psychiatric Association, *Diagnostic and Statistical Manual of Mental Disorders,* 5th ed. (Arlington, VA: American Psychiatric Association, 2013); World Health Organization, *International Classification of Diseases,* 10th ed. (World Health Organization, 2010).

9. Michael L. Perlis et al., *Cognitive Behavioral Treatment of Insomnia: A Session-by-Session Guide* (New York: Springer, 2005), 3.

10. Sonia Ancoli-Israel and Thomas Roth, "Characteristics of Insomnia in the United States," *Sleep* 22, supplement 2 (1999): S347-53.

11. M.M. Ohayon, "Epidemiology of Insomnia: What We Know and What We Still Need to Learn," *Sleep Medicine Reviews* 6 (2002): 97-111.

12. C.E. Carney et al., "A Comparison of Rates of Residual Insomnia Symptoms Following Pharmacotherapy or Cognitive-Behavioral Therapy, *Journal of Clinical Psychiatry* 68 (2007): 254-60; R. Manber et al., "Cognitive Behavioral Therapy for Insomnia Enhances Depression Outcome in Patients with Comorbid Major Depressive Disorder and Insomnia," *Sleep* 31 (2008): 489-95.

13. Taylor et al., "Epidemiology of Insomnia," 1457-64; D. Neckelmann, A Mykletun, and A.A. Dahl, "Chronic Insomnia as a Risk Factor For Developing Anxiety and Depression," *Sleep* 30 (2007): 873-80; D.J. Taylor et al., "Comorbidity of Chronic Insomnia With Medical Problems," *Sleep* 30 (2007): 213-8; R.J. Ozminkowski, W. Wang, and J.K. Walsh, "The Direct and Indirect Costs of Untreated Insomnia in Adults in the United States," *Sleep* 30 (2007): 263-73; K. Sarsour et al., "The Association between Insomnia Severity and Healthcare and Productivity Costs in a Health Plan Sample," *Sleep* 34 (2011): 443-50.

Chapter 2: A Night at the Races

1. AASM, *International Classification of Sleep Disorders.*

2. Ibid.

3. National Sleep Foundation, *2008 Sleep in America Poll* (Washington, DC: National Sleep Foundation, 2008), 17-18; Sabrina Tavernise, "Day Care Centers Adapt to Round-the-Clock Demand," *The New York Times,* January 16, 2012; C.L. Drake et al., "Shift Work Sleep Disorder," *Sleep* 27 (2004): 1453-62.

4. Bonnet and Arand, "Hyperarousal and Insomnia," 9-15; Riemann et al., "The Hyperarousal Model of Insomnia," 19-31.

5. William C. Dement and Christopher Vaughan, *The Promise of Sleep* (New York: Delacorte Press, 1999), 101.

6. Christopher Dewdney, *Acquainted With the Night* (New York: Bloomsbury, 2004), 250.

7. "The Today Show," NBC, March 4, 2008.

8. Michael J. Thorpy and Jan Yager, *The Encyclopedia of Sleep and Sleep Disorders*, 2nd ed. (Facts on File, Inc., 2001), ix.

9. Eluned Summers-Bremner, *Insomnia: A Cultural History* (London: Reaktion Books Ltd, 2008), 50.

10. Jean Verdon, *Night in the Middle Ages*, trans. George Holoch (Notre Dame, IN: University of Notre Dame Press, 2002), 18, 47, 51.

11. Summers-Bremner, *Insomnia: A Cultural History*, 51-52.

12. Ken Dowden, "The Value of Sleep: Homer, Plinies, Posidonius, and Proclus," in *Sleep*, ed. Thomas Wiedemann and Ken Dowden (Bari: Levante, 2003), 146; Hippocrates, *The Aphorisms of Hippocrates, with a Translation into Latin, and English,* trans. Thomas Coar (Birmingham: The Classics of Medicine Library,

1982), II:3, VII:71, III:31; Hippocrates, *The Genuine Works of Hippocrates*, trans. Francis Adams (Birmingham: The Classics of Medicine Library, 1985), 47.

13. Aristotle, pseud., *Aristotle's Master-piece. Aristotle's Compleat Master Piece. Aristotle's Book of Problems* (New York: Garland Pub., 1986), 726, 1427-29.

14. Aretaeus, *Aretaeus, Consisting of Eight Books, on the Causes, Symptoms and Cure of Acute and Chronic Diseases*, trans. John Moffat (London, Logographic Press, 1785); Ernest Hartmann, *The Sleeping Pill* (New Haven: Yale University Press, 1978), 7; Aulus Cornelius Celsus, *De Medicina*, (Birmingham: The Classics of Medicine Library, 1989).

15. O. Cameron Gruner, *A Treatise on the Canon of Medicine of Avicenna* (London: Luzac and Co., 1930), 210-212, 271-274, 417-419.

16. Marsilio Ficino, *Three Books on Life*, trans. Carol V. Kaske and John R. Clark (Binghamton: State University of New York, 1989), 113-115, 157-159.

17. M. Andreas Laurentius, *A Discourse of the Preservations of the Sight: of Melancholike Diseases; of Rheumes, and of Old Age*, trans. Richard Surphlet (Oxford: Oxford University Press, 1938), 94-95.

18. Levinus Lemnius, *The Touchstone of Complexions*, trans. Thomas Newton (Ann Arbor: Early English Books Online Text Creation Partnership, 2005).

19. Ambroise Paré, *The Workes of That Famous Chirurgion Ambrose Parey*, trans. Thomas Johnson (Ann Arbor: Early English Books Online, 2006), 37.

20. Ibid., 850; Laurentius, *A Discourse of the Preservations*, 116; Robert Burton, *The Anatomy of Melancholy* (London: Chatto and Windus, 1927), 63.

21. Hartmann, *The Sleeping Pill*, 10.

22. Laurentius, *A Discourse of the Preservations*, 116.

23. Thomas Willis, *The London Practice of Physick* (Boston: Milford House, 1973), 412-17.

24. Carey Balaban, Johathon Erlen, and Richard Siderits, ed., *The Skilful Physician* (Harwood Academic Publishers, 1997), 6-9, 158-159; Louise Hill Curth, "The Medical Content of English Almanacs 1640-1700," *Journal of the History of Medicine and Allied Sciences* 60 (2005): 255-82.

25. A. Roger Ekirch, *At Day's Close: Night in Times Past* (New York: W.W. Norton and Company, 2005), 288-91; A. Roger Ekirch, "Sleep We Have Lost: Pre-Industrial Slumber in the British Isles," *American Historical Review* (2001): 343-86.

26. Ekirch, "Sleep We Have Lost," 356; Ekirch, *At Day's Close*, 271.

27. Edmund Burke, *A Philosophical Enquiry into the Origin of Our Ideas of the Sublime and Beautiful*, ed. James T. Boulton (London: Routledge and Kegan Paul, 2008), 143.

28. Michael Perlis, "Cognitive Behavioral Therapy for Insomnia," seminar held in Philadelphia, September 8-10, 2011.

29. A. Roger Ekirch, "Dreams Deferred," *The New York Times*, February 19, 2006.

Chapter 3: Running on Empty

1. Charles Andrew Czeisler, Orfeu M. Buxton, and Sat Bir Singh Khalsa, "The Human Circadian Timing System and Sleep-Wake Regulation," in *Principles and Practice of Sleep Medicine*, 4th ed., ed. Meir H. Kryger et al. (Philadelphia:

Elsevier/Saunders, 2005), 375-91; J.R. Schwartz and T. Roth, "Neurophysiology of Sleep and Wakefulness," *Current Neuropharmacology* 6 (2008): 367-78.

2. D. Kahneman et al., "A Survey Method for Characterizing Daily Life Experience," *Science* 306 (2004): 1776-80.

3. W.B. Mendelson, D. Garnett, and M. Linnoila, "Do Insomniacs Have Impaired Daytime Functioning?" *Biological Psychiatry* 19 (1984): 1261-4; W. F. Seidel et al., "Daytime Alertness in Relation to Mood, Performance, and Nocturnal Sleep in Chronic Insomniacs and Noncomplaining Sleepers," *Sleep* 7 (1984): 230-8; J.L. Sugerman, J.A. Stern, and J.K. Walsh, "Daytime Alertness in Subjective and Objective Insomnia," *Biological Psychiatry* 20 (1985): 741-50; D. Schneider-Helmert, "Twenty-Four-Hour Sleep-Wake Function and Personality Patterns in Chronic Insomniacs and Healthy Controls," *Sleep* 10 (1987): 452-62.

4. Schneider-Helmert, "Sleep-Wake Function," 452-62; E. Stepanski et al., "Daytime Alertness in Patients with Chronic Insomnia Compared with Asymptomatic Control Subjects," *Sleep* 11 (1988): 54-60; Michael Bonnet and Donna Arand, "We Are Chronically Sleep-Deprived, *Sleep* 18 (1995): 908-11.

5. K.L. Lichstein et al., "Daytime Sleepiness in Insomnia," *Sleep* 17 (1994): 693-702; Jim Horne, "Primary Insomnia: A Disorder of Sleep, or Primarily One of Wakefulness?" *Sleep Medicine Reviews* 14 (2010): 3-7; Bonnet and Arand, "Hyperarousal and Insomnia," 9-15; W.R. Pigeon and M.L. Perlis, "Sleep Homeostasis in Primary Insomnia," *Sleep Medicine Reviews* 10 (2006): 247-54.

6. J.D. Kloss, "Daytime Sequelae of Insomnia," in *Insomnia: Principles and Management*, ed. Martin P. Szuba et al., (Cambridge: Cambridge University Press, 2003), 23-41; J.L. Hossain et al., "Subjective Fatigue and Subjective Sleepiness," *Journal of Sleep Research* 14 (2005): 245-53; Simon D. Kyle, Colin A. Espie, and Kevin Morgan, "...Not Just a Minor Thing, It Is Something Major, Which Stops You From Functioning Daily: Quality of Life and Daytime Functioning in Insomnia," *Behavioral Sleep Medicine* 8 (2010): 123-40.

7. H.T. Hatoum et al., "Insomnia, Health-Related Quality of Life, and Healthcare Resource Consumption," *Pharmacoeconomics* 14 (1998): 629-37; S.D. Kyle, K. Morgan, and C.A. Espie, "Insomnia and Health-Related Quality of Life," *Sleep Medicine Reviews* 14 (2010): 69-82; K.L. Chien et al., "Habitual Sleep Duration and Insomnia and the Risk of Cardiovascular Events and All-Cause Death," *Sleep* 33 (2010): 177-84; C. Hublin et al., "Heritability and Mortality Risk of Insomnia-Related Symptoms," *Sleep* 34 (2011): 957-64; Kyle et al., "...Not Just a Minor Thing," 123-40; T.J. Carey et al., "Focusing on the Experience of Insomnia," *Behavioral Sleep Medicine* 3 (2005): 73-86.

8. Taylor et al., "Epidemiology of Insomnia," 1457-64.

9. Wilfred R. Pigeon and Michael L. Perlis, "Insomnia and Depression: Birds of a Feather?" *International Journal of Sleep Disorders* 1 (2007): 82-91.

10. D. Riemann and U. Voderholzer, "Primary Insomnia: A Risk Factor to Develop Depression?" *Journal of Affective Disorders* 76 (2003): 255-9; M. Fava, "Daytime Sleepiness and Insomnia as Correlates of Depression," *Journal of Clinical Psychiatry* 65, supplement 16 (2004): 27-32; F.W. Turek, "Insomnia and Depression: If It Looks and Walks Like a Duck," *Sleep* 28 (2005): 1362-3; C. Baglioni et al., "Insomnia as a Predictor of Depression," *Journal of Affective*

Disorders 135 (2011): 10-19; Pigeon and Perlis, "Birds of a Feather," 82-91; Kloss, "Daytime Sequelae of Insomnia," 23-41; Taylor et al., "Epidemiology of Insomnia," 1457-64; D.J. Buysse et al., "Daytime Symptoms of Primary Insomnia," *Sleep Medicine* 8 (2007): 198-208.

11. Rosalind Cartwright, *The Twenty-Four Hour Mind* (Oxford: Oxford University Press, 2010), 158.

12. Ibid., 25, 55-56.

13. Ibid., 41.

14. Ibid., 41-42.

15. Matthew P. Walker, "Sleep, Memory, and Emotion," in *Progress in Brain Research* 185, ed. G.A. Kerkhof and H.P.A. Van Dongen (Elsevier: 2010): 49-68.

16. D. Zohar et al., "The Effects of Sleep Loss on Medical Residents' Emotional Reactions to Work Events," *Sleep* 28 (2005): 10-19.

17. S.S. Yoo et al., "The Human Emotional Brain Without Sleep—a Prefrontal Amygdala Disconnect," *Current Biology* 17 (2007): R877-8.

18. Matthew Walker, "The Role of Sleep in Brain Function: Memory and Emotion," paper presented at the annual meeting for the Associated Professional Sleep Societies, San Antonio, Texas, June 5-9, 2010.

19. Kyle et al., "...Not Just a Minor Thing," 123-40.

20. J.D. Edinger et al., "Psychomotor Performance Deficits and Their Relation to Prior Nights' Sleep Among Individuals with Primary Insomnia, *Sleep* 31 (2008): 599-607; J. Backhaus et al., "Impaired Declarative Memory Consolidation During Sleep in Patients with Primary Insomnia," *Biological Psychiatry* 60 (2006): 1324-40.

21. Edinger et al., "Psychomotor Performance Deficits," 599-607.

22. E. Altena et al., "Prefrontal Hypoactivation and Recovery in Insomnia," *Sleep* 31 (2008): 1271-6.

23. D. Anderson et al., "Insomnia Severity Level Impacts Cerebral Activation During Working Memory, *Sleep* 34, abstract supplement (2011): A190-1.

24. Walker, "Sleep, Memory, and Emotion," 49-68; Y. Harrison and J.A. Horne, "Sleep Loss and Temporal Memory," *Quarterly Journal of Experimental Psychology* 53 (2000): 271-9; S.P. Drummond et al., "Altered Brain Response to Verbal Learning Following Sleep Deprivation," *Nature* 403 (2000): 655-7; Matthew P. Walker and Robert Stickgold, "Sleep, Memory, and Plasticity," *Annual Review of Psychology* 57 (2006): 139-66; Yoo et al., "The Human Emotional Brain," R877-8.

25. Walker and Stickgold, "Sleep, Memory, and Plasticity," 139-66.

26. M.P. Walker, "The Role of Slow Wave Sleep in Memory Processing," *Journal of Clinical Sleep Medicine* 5 (2009): S20-S26.

27. M.P. Walker et al., "Practice with Sleep Makes Perfect," *Neuron* 35 (2002): 205-11; S. Fischer et al., "Sleep Forms Memory for Finger Skills," *Proceedings of the National Academy of Science* 99 (2002): 11987-91; Walker, "Sleep, Memory, and Emotion," 49-68; S. Diekelmann and J. Born, "The Memory Function of Sleep," *Nature Reviews Neuroscience* 11 (2010): 114-26.

28. G. Ficca and P. Salzarulo, "What in Sleep Is for Memory," *Sleep Medicine* 5 (2004): 225-30; Walker and Stickgold, "Sleep, Memory, and Plasticity," 139-66; Walker, "Sleep, Memory, and Emotion," 49-68.

29. J.A. Shekleton, N.L. Fogers, and S.M. Rajaratnam, "Searching for the Daytime Impairments of Primary Insomnia," *Sleep Medicine Reviews* 14 (2010): 47-60.

30. C. Nissen et al., "Impaired Sleep-Related Memory Consolidation in Primary Insomnia," *Sleep* 29 (2006): 1068-73.

31. Backhaus et al., "Impaired Declarative Memory," 1324-30.

32. Perlis et al., *A Session-by-Session Guide*, 76; "The Buzz on Caffeine," *Time*, December 20, 2004.

33. D. Leger, M.A. Massuel, and A. Metlaine, "Professional Correlates of Insomnia," *Sleep* 29 (2006): 171-8; D. Leger et al., "Medical and Socio-professional Impact of Insomnia," *Sleep* 25 (2002): 625-9; Sarsour et al., "Insomnia Severity and Healthcare and Productivity Costs," 443-50.

34. D.J. Taylor et al., "Comorbidity of Chronic Insomnia," 213-8. Compared to normal sleepers, people with chronic insomnia report more heart disease (21.9% vs 9.5%), high blood pressure (43.1% vs 18.7%), neurologic disease (7.3% vs 1.2%), breathing problems (24.8% vs 5.7%), urinary problems (19.7% vs 9.5%), chronic pain (50.4% vs 18.2%), and gastrointestinal problems (33.6% vs 9.2%).

35. A.N. Vgontzas et al., "Insomnia with Objective Short Sleep Duration is Associated with a High Risk for Hypertension," *Sleep* 32 (2009): 491-7; A.N. Vgontzas et al., "Insomnia with Objective Short Sleep Duration is Associated with Type 2 Diabetes," *Diabetes Care* 32 (2009): 1980-5.

Chapter 4: Looking for Help

1. Michael J. Sateia, "Epidemiology, Consequences, and Evaluation of Insomnia," in *Sleep Medicine*, ed. Teofilo Lee-Chiong, Michael Sateia, and Mary A. Carskadon (Philadelphia: Hanley and Belfus, Inc., 2002), 151. For statistics showing that complaints of insomnia are on the rise, see Malread Eastin Moloney, Thomas R. Konrad, and Catherine R. Zimmer, "The Medicalization of Sleeplessness: A Public Health Concern," *American Journal of Public Health* 101 (2011): 1429-33.

2. Ancoli-Israel and Roth, "Characteristics of Insomnia," S349; Thomas Roth and Timothy Roehrs, "Efficacy and Safety of Sleep-Promoting Agents," *Sleep Medicine Clinics* 3 (2008): 175-87.

3. Glenn W. Most, trans., *Hesiod II: The Shield, Catalogue of Women, Other Fragments* (Cambridge: Harvard University Press, 2007), 257; Leo Duprée Sandgren, *The Shadow of God: Stories from Early Judaism* (Peabody, MA: Hendrickson Publishers, 2003), 301.

4. Christof Wirsung, *The General Practise of Physick* (Ann Arbor: University Microfilms International, 1980), 618; Salvatore P. Lucia, *A History of Wine as Therapy* (Philadelphia: Lippinco, 1963), 157, 165.

5. T. Roehrs et al., "Ethanol as a Hypnotic in Insomniacs," *Neuropsychopharmacology* 20 (1999): 279-86.

6. Ibid., 284.

7. J.T. Arnedt, D.A. Conroy, and K.J. Grower, "Treatment Options for Sleep Disturbances During Alcohol Recovery," *Journal of Addictive Diseases* 26 (2007):

41-54; M.M. Weissman et al., "The Morbidity of Insomnia Uncomplicated by Psychiatric Disorders," *General Hospital Psychiatry* 19 (1997): 245-50; R.M. Crum et al., "Sleep Disturbance and Risk for Alcohol-Related Problems," *American Journal of Psychiatry* 161 (2004): 1197-203; D.C. Vinson et al., "Alcohol and Sleep Problems in Primary Care Patients," *Annals of Family Medicine* 8 (2010): 484-92.

8. Maren Hyde, Timothy Roehrs, and Thomas Roth, "Alcohol, Alcoholism, and Sleep," in *Sleep: A Comprehensive Handbook,* ed. T. Lee-Chiong (John Wiley and Sons, Inc., 2006), 867-71.

9. T.A. Roehrs et al., "Insomnia as a Path to Alcoholism: Dose Escalation," *Sleep* 26, abstract supplement (2003): A307; T.A. Roehrs et al., "Tolerance to Hypnotic Effects of Ethanol in Insomniacs," *Sleep* 27, abstract supplement (2004): A52.

10. Suzanne Hegland, "I Wanna Be Sedated," *Huffington Post,* April 11, 2012, http://www.huffingtonpost.com/suzanne-hegland/sleeping-pills_b_1414148. html.

11. G.S. Richardson et al., "Tolerance to Daytime Sedative Effects of H1 Antihistamines," *Journal of Clinical Psychopharmacology* 22 (2002): 511-5.

12. C.M. Morin et al., "Valerian-Hops Combination and Diphenhydramine for Treating Insomnia," *Sleep* 28 (2005): 1465-71; J.R. Glass et al., "Effects of 2-week Treatment with Temazepam and Diphenhydramine in Elderly Insomniacs," *Journal of Clinical Psychopharmacology* 28 (2008): 182-8.

13. Hartmann, *The Sleeping Pill,* 6-9.

14. Jonathon R.T. Davidson and Kathryn M. Connor, *Herbs for the Mind* (New York: Guilford Press, 2000), 195.

15. John K. Crellin and J. Philpott, *Herbal Medicine Past and Present, II: A Reference Guide to Medicinal Plants* (Durham: Duke University Press, 1989), 247-9; Ida Macalpine and Richard Hunter, *George III and the Mad Business* (London: Allen Lane, 1969), 118, 146.

16. Amy Bess Miller, *Shaker Medicinal Herbs* (Pownal, VT: Storey Books, 1998), 153, 183.

17. Jerome Sarris et al., "Herbal Medicine for Depression, Anxiety and Insomnia," *European Neuropsychopharmacology* 21 (2011): 841-60.

18. J. Sarris and G.J. Byrne, "A Systematic Review of Insomnia and Complementary Medicine," *Sleep Medicine Reviews* 15 (2011): 99-106; A.D. Oxman et al., "A Televised, Web-Based Randomized Trial of an Herbal Remedy (Valerian) for Insomnia," *PloS One* 2 (2007): e1040; U. Koetter et al., "A Randomized, Double Blind, Placebo-Controlled, Prospective Clinical Study to Demonstrate Clinical Efficacy of a Fixed Valerian Hops Extract Combination," *Phytotherapy Research* 21 (2007): 847-51; G. Ziegler et al., "Efficacy and Tolerability of Valerian Extract LI 156 Compared with Oxazepam in the Treatment of Non-Organic Insomnia, *European Journal of Medical Research* 7 (2002): 480-6; P.D. Coxeter et al., "Valerian Does Not Appear to Reduce Symptoms for Patients with Chronic Insomnia in General Practice," *Complementary Therapies in Medicine* 11 (2003): 215-22; C.M. Morin et al., "Valerian-Hops Combination and Diphenhydramine for Treating Insomnia," *Sleep* 28 (2005): 1465-71.

19. S. Bent et al., " Valerian for Sleep: A Systematic Review and Meta-Analysis," *The American Journal of Medicine* 119 (2006): 1005-12; D.M. Taibi et al., "A Systematic Review of Valerian as a Sleep Aid: Safe but Not Effective," *Sleep Medicine Reviews* 11 (2007): 209-30; S. Taavoni et al., "Effect of Valerian on Sleep Quality in Postmenopausal Women," *Menopause* 18 (2011): 951-5.

20. J.D. Amsterdam et al., "A Randomized, Double-Blind, Placebo-Controlled Trial of Oral Maticaria Recutita (Chamomile) Extract Therapy for Generalized Anxiety Disorder," *Journal of Clinical Psychopharmacology* 29 (2009): 378-82.

21. Sarris and Byrne, "Insomnia and Complementary Medicine," 101.

22. K.L. Chien et al., "Habitual Sleep Duration and Insomnia and the Risk of Cardiovascular Events and All-Cause Death," *Sleep* 33 (2010): 177-84; C. Hublin et al., "Heritability and Mortality Risk of Insomnia-Related Symptoms," *Sleep* 34 (2011): 957-64.

23. Ancoli-Israel and Roth, "Characteristics of Insomnia," S350.

24. National Sleep Foundation, *Survey of Primary Care Physicians* (Washington, DC: National Sleep Foundation, 2000), 6; National Sleep Foundation, *2005 Sleep in America Poll* (Washington, DC: National Sleep Foundation, 2005), 34.

25. Harvey R. Colten and Bruce M. Altevogt, ed., *Sleep Disorders and Sleep Deprivation: An Unmet Public Health Problem* (Washington, DC: Institute of Medicine: National Academies Press, 2006), 75-8; J.A. Mindell et al., "Sleep Education in Medical School Curriculum: A Glimpse Across Countries," *Sleep Medicine* 12 (2011): 928-31.

26. E. Mai and D.J. Buysse, "Insomnia: Prevalence, Impact, Pathogenesis, Differential Diagnosis, and Evaluation," *Sleep Medicine Clinics* 3 (2008): 167-74.

27. M. Perlis, P. Gehrman, and D. Riemann, "Intermittent and Long-Term Use of Sedative Hypnotics," *Current Pharmaceutical Design* 14 (2008): 3456-65; NSF, *Survey of Primary Care Physicians*, 11: Asked what factors they consider when diagnosing insomnia, physicians cited lifestyle factors, 53 percent; sleep habits, 40 percent; health habits, 31 percent; and psychiatric problems, 31 percent.

28. T. Roth, J.A. Costa e Silva, and M.H. Chase, "Sleep and Health: Research and Clinical Perspectives," *Sleep* 23, supplement 3 (2000): S52; A.N. Vgontzas et al., "Chronic Insomnia Is Associated with Nyctohemeral Activation of the HPA Axis: Clinical Implications," *Journal of Clinical Endocrinology and Metabolism* 86 (2001): 3787-94; Perlis et al., "Intermittent and Long-Term Use," 3457.

29. C.M. Morin et al., "The Natural History of Insomnia," *Archives of Internal Medicine* 169 (2009): 447-53; J.G. Ellis et al., "Acute Insomnia: Current Conceptualizations and Future Directions," *Sleep Medicine Reviews* 16 (2012): 5-14; M. Vollrath, W. Wicki, and J. Angst, "The Zurich Study. VIII. Insomnia: Association with Depression, Anxiety, Somatic Syndromes, and Course of Insomnia," *European Archives of Psychiatry and Neurological Science* 239 (1989): 113-24; D.J. Buysse et al., "Prevalence, Course and Comorbidity of Insomnia and Depression in Young Adults," *Sleep* 31 (2008): 473-80.

30. C.E. Carney et al., "A Comparison of Rates of Residual Insomnia Symptoms Following Pharmacotherapy or Cognitive-Behavioral Therapy for Major Depressive Disorder, *Journal of Clinical Psychiatry* 68 (2007): 254-60; Manber et al., "Cognitive Behavioral Therapy for Insomnia," 489-95.

31. H. Gilbert Welch, Lisa Schwartz, and Steven Woloshin, "What's Making Us Sick Is an Epidemic of Diagnoses," *The New York Times*, January 2, 2007.
32. T. Morgenthaler et al., "Practice Parameters for the Psychological and Behavioral Treatment of Insomnia," *Sleep* 29 (2006): 1415-9; Perlis et al., "Intermittent and Long-Term Use," 3456.
33. A.D. Krystal and J.D. Edinger, "Measuring Sleep Quality," *Sleep Medicine* 9, supplement 1 (2008): S10-7.
34. New Choice Health: Medical Cost Comparison, accessed April 14, 2013, http://www.newchoicehealth.com/Directory/Procedure/51/Sleep Study (Polysomnography).

Chapter 5: All in the Head, and Other Ideas about Insomnia

1. Guenter B. Risse, "The Road to Twentieth-Century Therapeutics," in *The Inside Story of Medicines: A Symposium,* ed. Gregory J. Higby and Elaine C. Stroud (Madison: American Institute of the History of Pharmacy, 1997), 51-73.
2. Marsilio Ficino, *Three Books on Life,* 157.
3. William Cadogan, *A Dissertation on the Gout, and all Chronic Diseases* (Farmington Hills, MI: Cengage Gale, 2009); William Buchan, *Dr. Buchan's Family Medical Works: Containing Domestic Medicine* (Charleston: J. Hoff, 1816), preface.
4. "The Physician, No. II.—On Sleep," *The Atheneum; or, Spirit of the English Magazines*, January 1, 1823; "Time for Sleep," *Journal of Health*, November 11, 1829; Robert Macnish, *Philosophy of Sleep* (New York: D. Appleton and Co., 1834), 179; "Study and Sleep," *Trumpet and Universalist Magazine*, March 12, 1842.
5. Charles Rosenberg, "Body and Mind in Nineteenth-Century Medicine: Some Clinical Origins of the Neurosis Construct," *Bulletin of the History of Medicine* 63 (1989): 185-97.
6. Thomas Trotter, *A View of the Nervous Temperament* (Troy, NY: Wright, Goodenow and Stockwell, 1808); John Mason Good, *The Study of Medicine,* volume 3 (Philadelphia: U.C. Carey & I. Lea, 1825), 308-12; James Johnson, *A Treatise on Derangements of the Liver, Internal Organs, and the Nervous System* (Concord, NH: Horatio Hill and Co., 1832), 178-91; Thomas J. Graham, *Modern Domestic Medicine: A Popular Treatise* (London: Simpkin and Marshall, 1840), 598; Rosenberg, "Body and Mind," 191-2.
7. Trotter, *Nervous Temperament,* 331; Buchan, *Domestic Medicine,* preface; Good, *The Study of Medicine,* 309-12; Johnson, *Derangements of the Liver,* 191; Graham, *Modern Domestic Medicine,* 598; Charles E. Rosenberg, "The Therapeutic Revolution: Medicine, Meaning, and Social Change in Nineteenth-Century America," in *The Therapeutic Revolution: Essays in the Social History of American Medicine,* ed. Morris J. Vogel and Charles E. Rosenberg (Philadelphia: University of Pennsylvania Press, 1979), 5-6.
8. Macnish, *Philosophy of Sleep,* 178; "Sleep, Its Importance in Preventing Insanity," *American Journal of Insanity* (April, 1845): 319; Mary Ann Jimenez, *Changing Faces of Madness: Early American Attitudes and Treatment of the*

Insane (Hanover, NH: University Press of New England, 1987); Charles L. Dana, "Sleep and Sleeplessness," *Los Angeles Times*, March 7, 1901; Frederick Peterson, "An Exposition of Sleep," *Atlantic Monthly*, June 1914; "Insomnia as a Dread," *Medical Review of Reviews*, February 1917; Logan Clendening, "Insomnia Sufferers Usually Get Their Necessary Sleep," *The Washington Post*, January 10, 1939; "Many Beliefs about Insomnia Are Unfounded," *Hygeia*, November 1939.

9. "Sleeplessness," *Littell's Living Age*, September 1, 1866; Helen L. Bostwick, "Causes of Sleeplessness," *Ohio Farmer*, September 4, 1869; Charles N. Glaab and A. Theodore Brown, *A History of Urban America*, 3rd ed. (New York: Macmillan Publishing Co., 1983), 75; John H. Girdner, "To Abate the Plague of City Noises," in *City Life, 1865-1900: Views of Urban America*, ed. Ann Cook, Marilyn Gittell, and Herb Mack (New York: Praeger Publishers, 1973), 158-9.

10. Bonnie Ellen Blustein, "New York Neurologists and the Specialization of American Medicine," *Bulletin of the History of Medicine* 53 (1979): 170-83; William Hammond, *On Wakefulness* (Philadelphia: Lippincott, 1866), 40.

11. Hammond, *On Wakefulness*, 39; William Hammond, *Cerebral Hyperaemia* (New York: G.P. Putnam's Sons, 1878), 72.

12. Charles Rosenberg, *Our Present Complaint* (Baltimore: The Johns Hopkins University Press, 2007), 18, 19, 44; Rosenberg, "Body and Mind," 194-6; Charles Rosenberg, "The Place of George M. Beard in Nineteenth-Century Psychiatry," *Bulletin of the History of Medicine* 36 (1962): 245-59; Bonnie Ellen Blustein, "The Brief Career of 'Cerebral Hyperaemia': William A. Hammond and His Insomniac Patients, 1854-90," *The Journal of the History of Medicine and Allied Sciences* 41 (1986): 24-51.

13. Blustein, *The Brief Career*, 24-51; Hammond, *Cerebral Hyperaemia*, 18.

14. William Hammond, *Robert Severne, His Friends and His Enemies* (Philadelphia: J.B. Lippincott and Co., 1867), 45-56; Hammond, *On Wakefulness*, 39.

15. Hammond, *On Wakefulness*, 86-93; William Hammond, "Abstract of a Lecture on the Therapeutics of Wakefulness," *Boston Medical and Surgical Journal* 799 (1869): 349-50; Blustein, *The Brief Career*, 39.

16. William Hammond, *A Treatise on the Diseases of the Nervous System* (New York: D. Appleton and Co., 1871); Blustein, *The Brief Career*, 42.

17. George M. Beard, *American Nervousness, Its Causes and Consequences* (New York: G.P. Putnam's Sons, 1881), vi; Rosenberg, "The Place of George M. Beard," 248-9.

18. Beard, *American Nervousness*, 7; A.D. Rockwell, *Beard's Nervous Exhaustion* (1894), 235; George M. Beard, *A Practical Treatise on Nervous Exhaustion (Neurasthenia)* (New York: W. Wood and Co., 1880), 119.

19. Beard, *American Nervousness*, 96.

20. Ibid., 9-10, 26.

21. Beard, *Nervous Exhaustion*, 5-6, 121-124.

22. Rosenberg, "The Place of George M. Beard," 258.

23. Helen L. Manning, "Dealing With Insomnia," *Friends' Intelligencer*, November 11, 1893; "Overwork of Children," *The New York Times*, March 19, 1873.

24. "Terrell Suffered from Insomnia," *The New York Times*, June 14, 1896.

25. "Found Sleep of Death," *The Washington Post,* June 5, 1898.

26. "Insomnia Cause of Woman's Suicide," *The Washington Post,* April 11, 1899.

27. "Slumber Machines Needed," *The Washington Post,* March 4, 1898; Peterson, "An Exposition of Sleep," 769; "Insomnia as a Dread," 130.

28. "Insomnia and Its Therapeutics," *The Washington Post,* August 19, 1891; "The Mystery of Sleep," *The Spectator,* April 1, 1899; "Insomnia or Wakefulness," *Ohio Farmer,* July 1, 1882.

29. Francis G. Gosling, *Before Freud: Neurasthenia and the American Medical Community, 1870-1910* (Urbana: University of Illinois Press, 1987), 79-81.

30. Agnes H. Morton, "The Moral Aspect of Insomnia," *Chautauquan,* January 1901.

31. George M. Beard, "The Influence of the Mind in the Causation and Cure of Disease—the Potency of Definite Expectation," *Journal of Nervous and Mental Diseases* 1 (1876): 429-35; Nathan G. Hale, *Freud and the Americans* (New York: Oxford University Press, 1971), 66; Eric Caplan, *Mind Games: American Culture and the Birth of Psychotherapy* (Berkeley: University of California Press, 1998), 93-94.

32. Caplan, *Mind Games,* 65-72.

33. Ibid., 73-76.

34. Ibid., 95; Lewellys F. Barker, "Some Experiences with the Simpler Methods of Psycho-Therapy and Re-Education," *American Journal of the Medical Sciences* 132 (1906); Sheldon Leavitt, *Psychotherapy in the Practice of Medicine and Surgery,* 2nd ed. (Chicago: Magnum Bonum Company, 1907), 29.

35. Morton Prince, "Association Neuroses," in *Psychotherapy and Multiple Personality: Selected Essays,* ed. Nathan G. Hale (Cambridge: Harvard University Press, 1975); Morton Prince, "The Educational Treatment of Neurasthenia and Certain Hysterical States," *Boston Medical and Surgical Journal* 139 (1898): 332-7.

36. Elwood Worcester, Samuel McComb, and Isador Coriat, *Religion and Medicine: The Moral Control of Nervous Disorders* (New York: Moffat, Yard and Company, 1908), 48; Caplan, *Mind Games,* 117-52.

37. Samuel McComb, "Sleep and How To Get It," *Harper's Bazaar,* 1909, 848-50.

38. Samuel McComb, "Suggestion and Auto-Suggestion," *Good Housekeeping,* July-December 1908, 712-5; Samuel McComb, "Sleep and Sleeplessness, *Good Housekeeping,* July-December 1907, 50-1.

39. James J. Walsh, *Psychotherapy* (New York: D. Appleton and Company, 1912), 651; James J. Walsh, "Insomnia as a Dread," *International Clinics* (1916): 42-55.

40. H. Addington Bruce, *Sleep and Sleeplessness* (Boston: Little, Brown, and Company, 1920), 161.

41. Paul Dubois, *The Psychic Treatment of Nervous Disorders,* trans. Smith Ely Jelliffe and William A. White (New York: Funk and Wagnalls Company, 1905); Bruce, *Sleep and Sleeplessness,* 188-194.

42. "Insomnia Victim Leaps to Death," *The New York Times,* November 3, 1919; "Tried to Choke a Physician: Patient Insane from Insomnia Attacked Doctor Called to Attend Him," *The New York Times,* April 6, 1901; "Tragic Insomnia: Murderous Rage Caused by Lack of Sleep Proves Fatal to Two People," *Los Angeles Times,* July 16, 1904; "Long Sleep Brings Peace: Unfortunate Victim of

Insomnia Takes Own Life After Doctors Fail to Give Him Relief," *Los Angeles Times*, December 24, 1910.

43. Marie de Manaceine, *Sleep: Its Physiology, Pathology, Hygiene, and Psychology* (London: W. Scott, Ltd.: 1897), 65-6; Peterson, "An Exposition of Sleep," 769.

44. Dorothy Dunn, "Kellinger's Insomnia," *The Chicago Defender*, December 20, 1913.

45. Samuel McComb, "The Curse of Insomnia," *Everybody's Magazine*, 1911, 256.

46. Hutchinson, "Sleep for the Sleepless," 532.

47. Josephine A. Jackson, "Insomniacs I Have Known," *Woman's Home Companion*, March 1923.

48. R.D. Gillespie, *Sleep and the Treatment of Its Disorders* (New York: William Wood and Company, 1930), 117-23; Edwin Shorter, *From Paralysis to Fatigue* (New York: The Free Press, 1992), 232-4.

49. Sigmund Freud, *Introductory Lectures on Psychoanalysis*, trans. James Strachey (New York: Norton, 1977), 270-1.

50. I. Karacan and R.L. Williams, "Insomnia: Old Wine in a New Bottle," *The Psychiatric Quarterly* 45 (1971): 274-88; Otto Fenichel, "Symposium on Neurotic Disturbances of Sleep," *International Journal of Psycho-Analysis* 23 (1942): 49, 62-4; Leonard Gilman, "Insomnia in Relation to Guilt, Fear and Masochistic Intent," *Journal of Clinical Psychopathology* 11 (1950): 63-4; L.E. Wexberg, "Insomnia as Related to Anxiety and Ambition," *Journal of Clinical Psychopathology* 10 (1949): 373-4; P. Litvin, "Tension, Organic-Disease Phobia, Guilt, Competition and Insomnia," *Journal of Clinical Psychopathology* 11 (1950): 72-4; Philip Solomon, "Insomnia," *New England Journal of Medicine* 255 (1956): 755-60; Simon Rothenberg, "Psychoanalytic Insight into Insomnia," *The Psychoanalytic Review* 34 (1947): 141-68.

51. Jacob H. Conn, "Psychogenesis and Psychotherapy of Insomnia," *Journal of Clinical Psychopathology* 11 (1950): 85-91.

52. Karacan and Williams, "Old Wine," 277.

53. Edwin Diamond, "Long Day's Journey Into the Insomniac's Night," *New York Times Magazine*, October 1, 1967.

54. Iago Galdston, "Can Insomnia Conquer England?" *The American Mercury*, May 1, 1941; Victor G. Heiser, "When You Can't Sleep," *Science Digest*, August 1941; Don Eddy, "Rockaby Blues," *American Magazine*, January 1942; "Sleep Like a Baby," *Popular Mechanics*, December 1943; Irwin Shaw, "The Climate of Insomnia," *The New Yorker*, April 2, 1949.

55. Anne Harrington, *The Cure Within* (New York: W.W. Norton and Company, 2008), 158-61; Haynes Johnson, *The Age of Anxiety: McCarthyism to Terrorism* (Orlando: Harcourt, Inc., 2005).

56. D.A. Cozanitis, "One Hundred Years of Barbiturates and Their Saint," *Journal of the Royal Society of Medicine* 97 (2004): 594-8; Karacan and Williams, "Old Wine," 284.

57. Thorpy and Yager, *The Encyclopedia of Sleep and Sleep Disorders*, xxvi-xxvii; William Dement, "The Study of Human Sleep: A Historical Perspective," *Thorax* 53, supplement 3 (1998): S2-7.

58. Lawrence J. Monroe, "Psychological and Physiological Differences Between

Good and Poor Sleepers," *Journal of Abnormal Psychology* 72 (1967): 255-64.

59. S.C. Ribordy and D.R. Denney, "The Behavioral Treatment of Insomnia," *Behaviour Research and Therapy* 15 (1977): 39-50.

60. Carol Kahn, "Do You Dream (Perchance) of Sleeping?" *Family Health*, September 1977; Maggie Scarf, "Oh, for a Decent Night's Sleep!" *The New York Times*, October 21, 1973.

61. Scarf, "Decent Night's Sleep"; Kahn, "Do You Dream"; Mark Davidson and Nirmali Ponnamperuma, "Tossing and Turning All Night?" *Science Digest*, April 1977.

62. Hilary Rubinstein, *The Complete Insomniac* (London: Cape, 1974), 27-9; John Edward Putnam, "Insomnia: Nothing to Lose Sleep Over," *Working Woman*, November 1980.

63. Anthony Kales et al., "Hypnotics and Altered Sleep-Dream Patterns," *Archives of General Psychiatry* 23 (1970): 211-25; Karacan & Williams, "Old Wine," 283-4.

64. Anthony Kales et al., "Personality Patterns in Insomnia," *Archives of General Psychiatry* 33 (1976): 1128-34; Anthony Kales et al., "Biopsychobehavioral Correlates of Insomnia," *Psychosomatic Medicine* 45 (1983): 341-56.

65. Anthony Kales & Joyce Kales, *Evaluation and Treatment of Insomnia* (New York: Oxford University Press, 1984), 44-8, 94, 198-9.

66. Henry Kellerman, *Sleep Disorders: Insomnia and Narcolepsy* (New York: Brunner/Mazel, 1981), 150-51; Quentin R. Regestein, "Treating Insomnia," *Comprehensive Psychiatry* 17 (1976): 517-36; T. Roth, M. Kramer, and T. Lutz, "The Nature of Insomnia," *Comprehensive Psychiatry* 17 (1976): 217-20; E. Shevy Healey et al., "Onset of Insomnia: Role of Life-Stress Events," *Psychosomatic Medicine* 43 (1981): 439-51; E.J. Marchini et al., "What Do Insomniacs Do, Think, and Feel During the Day?" *Sleep* 6 (1983): 147-55.

67. Davidson and Ponnamperuma, "Tossing and Turning All Night," 17; Lawrence A. Mayer, "That Confounding Enemy of Sleep, *Fortune*, June 1975; Alice Kuhn Schwartz, *Somniquest* (New York: Harmony Books, 1979), 19; Putnam, "Insomnia: Nothing to Lose," 100; Ray Meddis, *The Sleep Instinct* (Boston: Routledge and K. Paul, 1977), 110; "Laying Insomnia to Rest," *Science Digest*, March 1985.

68. Valerie Moolman, *Forty Winks at the Drop of a Hat* (New York: Cornerstone Library, 1968), 53-4.

69. Schwartz, *Somniquest*, 182-3.

70. Gregg D. Jacobs, *Say Goodnight to Insomnia* (New York: Henry Holt, 1999), 28.

71. Richard Bootzin, "Stimulus Control Treatment for Insomnia," *Proceedings of the 80th Annual Convention of the American Psychological Association* (1972).

72. "Outline of Diagnostic Classification of Sleep and Arousal Disorders," *Sleep* 2 (1979): 17-31; Peter Hauri, "Childhood Onset Insomnia," *Sleep* 3 (1980): 59-65; Peter Hauri, " A Cluster Analysis of Insomnia," *Sleep* 6 (1983): 326-38; R.R. Freedman and H.L. Sattler, "Physiological and Psychological Factors in Sleep-Onset Insomnia," *Journal of Abnormal Psychology* 91 (1982): 380-9; K. Adam, M. Tomeny and I. Oswald, "Physiological and Psychological Differ-

ences Between Good and Poor Sleepers," *Journal of Psychiatric Research* 20 (1986): 301-16.

73.   J.D. Moriarty, "Insomnia: Often a Therapeutic Challenge," *Disorders of the Nervous System* 36 (1975): 279-80; J.L. Mathis, "Insomnia," *Journal of Family Practice* 6 (1978): 873-6; W. Dement, W. Seidel, and M. Carskadon, "Issues in the Diagnosis and Treatment of Insomnia," *Psychopharmacology Supplementum* 1 (1984): 11-43; J.D. Kales et al., "Biopsychobehavioral Correlates of Insomnia, V," *American Journal of Psychiatry* 141 (1984): 1371-6; B. Byerley and J.C. Gillin, "Diagnosis and Management of Insomnia," *The Psychiatric Clinics of North America* 7 (1984): 773-89; M.E. Giesecke, "The Symptom of Insomnia in University Students," *Journal of American College Health* 35 (1987): 215-21; P.J. Hauri and M.S. Esther, "Insomnia," *Mayo Clinic Proceedings* 65 (1990): 869-82; M.L. Perlis and P. Gehrman, "One More Step Towards Justifying Targeted Treatment for Insomnia," *Sleep* 34 (2011): 417-8.

74.   Michael L. Perlis, Michael T. Smith, and Wilfred R. Pigeon, "Etiology and Pathophysiology of Insomnia," in *Principles and Practice of Sleep Medicine,* 4th ed., ed. Meir H. Kryger et al. (Philadelphia: Elsevier/Saunders, 2005), 714-25.

75.   Colin Espie, "The Attention-Intention-Effort Pathway in the Development of Psychophysiologic Insomnia," *Sleep Medicine Reviews* 10 (2006): 215-45; Perlis et al., "Etiology and Pathophysiology," 723; D.J. Buysse et al., "A Neurobiological Model of Insomnia," *Drug Discovery Today: Disease Models* 8 (2011): 129-37; Hrayr P. Attarian and Catherine Schuman, *Clinical Handbook of Insomnia* (Totowa, NJ: Humana, 2010); Colten and Altevogt, *Sleep Disorders and Sleep Deprivation,* 75-8.

76.   Rosenberg, *Our Present Complaint,* 71.

77.   M.E. Moloney et al., "The Medicalization of Sleeplessness," 1429-31; Ancoli-Israel and Roth, "Characteristics of Insomnia," S350; R.C. Rosen, "Low Rates of Recognition of Sleep Disorders in Primary Care," *Sleep Medicine* 2 (2001): 47-55.

78.   Gayle Greene, *Insomniac* (Berkeley: University of California Press, 2008), 353.

Chapter 6: Battling the Body Clock

1.   George Dawes Green, "The Chains of Circadia," in *The Literary Insomniac,* ed. Elyse Cheney and Wendy Hubbert (New York: Doubleday, 1996), 63.

2.   E.R. Dodson and P.C. Zee, "Therapeutics for Circadian Rhythm Sleep Disorders," *Sleep Medicine Clinics* 5 (2010): 701-15; Jay C. Dunlap, Jennifer J Loros, and Patricia J. DeCoursey, ed., *Chronobiology: Biological Timekeeping* (Sunderland, MA: Sinauer Associates, 2004), 171; Czeisler et al., "The Human Circadian Timing System," 375-94; M. Okawa and M. Uchiyama, "Circadian Rhythm Sleep Disorders," *Sleep Medicine Reviews* 11 (2007): 485-96.

3.   Victoria Revell and Charmane Eastman, "Jet Lag and Its Prevention," in *Therapy in Sleep Medicine,* ed. Teri J. Barkoukis et al. (Philadelphia: Saunders, 2012), 390-401; C.A. Czeisler et al., "Exposure to Bright Light and Darkness to Treat Physiologic Maladaptation to Night Work," *The New England Journal of Medicine* 322 (1990): 1253-9.

4. Robert Y. Moore, "Biological Rhythms and Sleep," in *Sleep: A Comprehensive Handbook*, ed. T. Lee-Chiong (John Wiley & Sons, Inc., 2006), 25-9; Hans-Peter Landolt, "Genotype-dependent Differences in Sleep, Vigilance, and Response to Stimulants," *Current Pharmaceutical Design* 14 (2008): 3396-407; David K. Welsh and Louis J. Ptácek, "Circadian Rhythm Dysregulation in the Elderly: Advanced Sleep Phase Syndrome," in *Principles and Practice of Geriatric Sleep Medicine*, ed. S.R. Pandi-Perumal et al. (New York: Cambridge University Press, 2010), 134.

5. Benjamin Cheever, "The Door of Perception," in *The Literary Insomniac*, ed. Elyse Cheney and Wendy Hubbert (New York: Doubleday, 1996), 171-7.

6. Anne Fadiman, "Night Owl," *At Large and at Small* (New York: Ferrar, Straus and Giroux, 2007), 61-74.

7. AASM, *International Classification of Sleep Disorders*.

8. Dunlap et al., *Chronobiology: Biological Timekeeping*, 305.

9. John D. Palmer, *The Living Clock: The Orchestrator of Biological Rhythms*, (New York: Oxford University Press, 2002), 132-3.

10. Dunlap et al., *Chronobiology: Biological Timekeeping*, 171; Czeisler et. al., "The Human Circadian Timing System," 378-9.

11. Dunlap et al., *Chronobiology: Biological Timekeeping*, 172; Charles Czeisler and Kenneth Wright, "Influence of Light on Circadian Rhythmicity in Humans," in *Regulation of Sleep and Circadian Rhythms*, ed. Fred W. Turek and Phyllis C. Zee (New York: Marcel Dekker, 1999), 150.

12. Nathaniel Kleitman, *Sleep and Wakefulness* (Chicago: University of Chicago Press, 1939), 259-64; Nathaniel Kleitman, "Sleep," *Scientific American*, November 1952.

13. Kleitman, *Sleep and Wakefulness*, 264.

14. Michel Siffre, *Beyond Time*, trans. Herma Briffault (New York: McGraw-Hill, 1964).

15. Charles Czeisler et al., "Stability, Precision, and Near-24-Hour Period of the Human Circadian Pacemaker, *Science* 284 (1999): 2177-81.

16. Michel Siffre, "Six Months Alone in a Cave," *National Geographic*, March 1975.

17. Steven Strogatz, *Sync: The Emerging Science of Spontaneous Order* (New York: Theia, 2003), 75-6.

18. Ibid., 77-82

19. Ibid., 79-80, 84.

20. William Charney, ed., *Handbook of Modern Hospital Safety* (Boca Raton: Lewis, 1999), 805; Charles Lindbergh, *The Spirit of St. Louis* (St. Paul: Minnesota Historical Society Press, 1993), 360-7.

21. Leon C. Lack et al., "The Relationship Between Insomnia and Body Temperatures, *Sleep Medicine Reviews* 12 (2008): 307-17.

22. Strogatz, *Sync*, 92-3.

23. Peretz Lavie, " Ultrashort Sleep-Waking Schedule. III. 'Gates" and 'Forbidden Zones' for Sleep," *Electroencephalography and Clinical Neurophysiology* 63 (1986): 414-25; Lack et al., "Insomnia and Body Temperatures," 307-17.

24. M.A. Carskadon and W.C. Dement, "Sleepiness and Sleep State on a 90-Minute Schedule," *Psychophysiology* 14 (1977): 127-33.

25. L.C. Lack, J.D. Mercer, and H. Wright, "Circadian Rhythms of Early Morning Awakening Insomniacs," *Journal of Sleep Research* 5 (1996): 211-9; Leon Lack and Richard Bootzin, "Circadian Rhythm Factors in Insomnia and Their Treatment," in *Treating Sleep Disorders: Principles and Practice of Behavioral Sleep Medicine*, ed. Michael Perlis and Kenneth Lichstein (Hoboken: Wiley, 2003), 305-34.

26. Ehren Dodson and Phyllis Zee, "Therapeutics for Circadian Rhythm Sleep Disorders," *Sleep Medicine Clinics* 5 (2010): 701-15; J. Aschoff et al., "Re-Entrainment of Circadian Rhythms after Phase-Shifts of the Zeitgeber," *Chronobiologia* 2 (1975): 23-78; T.I. Morgenthaler et al., "Practice Parameters for the Clinical Evaluation and Treatment of Circadian Rhythm Sleep Disorders," *Sleep* 30 (2007): 1445-59.

27. Revell and Eastman, "Jet Lag and Its Prevention," 390-401.

28. N.E. Rosenthal et al., "Phase-Shifting Effects of Bright Morning Light as Treatment for Delayed Sleep Phase Syndrome," *Sleep* 13 (1990): 354-61; D.B. Boivin et al., "Dose-Response Relationships for Resetting of Human Circadian Clock by Light," *Nature* 379 (1996): 540-2; R.J. Cole et al., "Bright-Light Mask Treatment of Delayed Sleep Phase Syndrome," *Journal of Biological Rhythms* 17 (2002): 89-101; Leon Lack and Helen Wright, "The Effect of Evening Bright Light in Delaying the Circadian Rhythms," *Sleep* 16 (1993): 436-43; L. Lack et al., "The Treatment of Early-morning Awakening Insomnia with 2 Evenings of Bright Light," *Sleep* 28 (2005): 616; Daniel Kripke, *Brighten Your Life*, February 2012, http://www.brightenyourlife.info/ch6.html.

29. M.R. Smith, V.L. Revell, and C.I. Eastman, "Phase Advancing the Human Circadian Clock with Blue-Enriched Polychromatic Light," *Sleep Medicine* 10 (2009): 287-94; Lack et al., "Treatment of Early Morning Awakening," 616-23.

30. Kripke, *Brighten Your Life*, chapter 6.

31. Karuna Dewan et al., "Light-Induced Changes of the Circadian Clock of Humans," *Sleep* 34 (2011): 593-9; V.L. Revell and C.I. Eastman, "How to Trick Mother Nature into Letting You Fly Around or Stay Up All Night," *Journal of Biological Rhythms* 20 (2005): 353-65.

32. Boivin et al., "Dose-Response Relationships," 540-2; J.J. Gooley et al., "Exposure to Room Light Before Bedtime Suppresses Melatonin Onset," *Journal of Clinical Endocrinology and Metabolism* 96 (2011): E463-72.

33. Revell and Eastman, "Jet Lag and Its Prevention," 390-401.

34. Dodson and Zee, "Therapeutics for Circadian Rhythm Sleep Disorders," 701-15; Revell and Eastman, "How to Trick Mother Nature," 353-65.

35. I.M. van Geijlswijk et al., "The Use of Exogenous Melatonin in Delayed Sleep Phase Disorder," *Sleep* 33 (2010): 1605-14; M.A. Paul et al., "Phase Advance with Separate and Combined Melatonin and Light Treatment," *Psychopharmacology* 214 (2011): 515-23.

36. A.G. Wade et al., "Nightly Treatment of Primary Insomnia with Prolonged Release Melatonin for 6 Months," *BMC Medicine* 8 (2010): abstract.

37. Helen Burgess, "Human Phase Response Curves to Three Days of Daily Melatonin," *Journal of Clinical Endocrinology and Metabolism* 95 (2010): 3325-31.

38. Charmane Eastman, "Correcting Circadian Misalignment with Light and Melatonin: From Theory to Practice," paper presented at the annual meeting for the Associated Professional Sleep Societies, Minneapolis, Minnesota, June 11-15, 2011.

39. Revell and Eastman, "Jet Lag and Its Prevention," 398-9; M. Beaumont et al., " Caffeine or Melatonin Effects on Sleep and Sleepiness After Rapid Eastward Transmeridian Travel," *Journal of Applied Physiology* 96 (2004): 50-8.

40. Nina Buscemi et al., "The Efficacy and Safety of Exogenous Melatonin for Primary Sleep Disorders," *Journal of General Internal Medicine* 20 (2005): 1151-8.

Chapter 7: Waiting for the Big Wave

1. Alexander Borbély and Peter Achermann, "Sleep Homeostasis and Models of Sleep Regulation," in *Principles and Practice of Sleep Medicine*, 4th edition, ed. Meir H. Kryger et al. (Philadelphia: Elsevier/Saunders, 2005), 405-17.

2. Carol Worthman and Melissa Melby, "Toward a Comparative Developmental Ecology of Human Sleep," in *Adolescent Sleep Patterns*, ed. Mary Carskadon (Cambridge: Cambridge University Press, 2002), 69-117.

3. C.B. Saper, T.E. Scammell, and J. Lu, "Hypothalamic Regulation of Sleep and Circadian Rhythms," *Nature* 437 (2005): 1257-63; R. Szymusiak, I Gvilia and D. McGinty, "Hypothalamic Control of Sleep," *Sleep Medicine* 8 (2007): 291-301; Mircea Steriade and Robert W. McCarley, *Brain Control of Wakefulness and Sleep* (Boston: Kluwer Academic/Plenum Publishers, 2005).

4. John J. Ross, "Neurological Findings After Prolonged Sleep Deprivation," *Archives of Neurology* 12 (1965): 399-403.

5. Randy Gardner, "To Stay Awake for 11 Days," *Esquire*, August 2004.

6. George Gulevich, William Dement, and Laverne Johnson, "Psychiatric and EEG Observations of a Case of Prolonged (264 Hours) Wakefulness," *Archives of General Psychiatry* 15 (1966): 29-35; Laverne C. Johnson, Elaine S. Slye, and William Dement, "Electroencephalographic and Autonomic Activity During and After Prolonged Sleep Deprivation," *Psychosomatic Medicine* 27 (1965): 415-23; Ross, "Neurological Findings," 400-1.

7. The EEG recordings taken on the three nights following the experiment show that Gardner slept a total of about fifteen, ten and nine hours, respectively. That's about thirteen hours in excess of what he would otherwise have slept in that period. Unfortunately no EEG recordings were taken on nights 4 to 7 after the experiment, although by one week after the experiment, Gardner was sleeping seven-hour nights. Given the downward trend in total sleep time on the three nights following the experiment, it's safe to assume that the excess sleep he might have gotten on successive nights that week would not have been great. Assuming he got a little more sleep on nights 4 to 7, a total of fifteen or sixteen extra hours of sleep in the week following the experiment is somewhere in the ballpark of one-fifth of the eighty hours Gardner lost.

8. Alexander Borbély, *Secrets of Sleep*, trans. Deborah Schneider (New York: Basic Books, 1986), 162; Borbély and Achermann, "Models of Sleep Regulation," 406-7.

9. Mary Carskadon and William Dement, "Normal Human Sleep: An Overview," in *Principles and Practice of Sleep Medicine*, 4th edition, ed. Meir H. Kryger et al. (Philadelphia: Elsevier/Saunders, 2005), 19; M.M. Ohayon et al., "Meta-Analysis of Quantitative Sleep Parameters from Childhood to Old Age," *Sleep* 27 (2004): 1255-73.

10. Walker, "Sleep, Memory, and Emotion," 50-1; E.C. Landsness et al., "Sleep-Dependent Improvement in Visuomotor Learning," *Sleep* 32 (2009): 1273-84; D. Aeschbach, A.J. Cutler, and J.M. Ronda, "A Role for Non-Rapid-Eye-Movement Sleep Homeostasis in Perceptual Learning," *Journal of Neuroscience* 28 (2008): 2766-72; Thomas Roth and Derk-Jan Dijk, ed., *Slow-Wave Sleep: Beyond Insomnia* (Walters Kluwer, 2011), 3.

11. L. Maron, A. Rechtschaffen, and E.A. Wolpert, "Sleep Cycle During Napping," *Archives of General Psychiatry* 11 (1964): 503-8; I. Karacan et al., "Changes in Stage 1-REM and Stage 4 Sleep During Naps," *Biological Psychiatry* 2 (1970): 261-5; W.B. Webb and H.W. Agnew, "Sleep Cycling Within Twenty-Four Hour Periods," *Journal of Experimental Psychology* 74 (1967): 158-60.

12. Irwin Feinberg, "Changes in Sleep Cycle Patterns with Age," *Journal of Psychiatric Research* 10 (1974): 285-9.

13. Paul Glovinsky and Art Spielman, *The Insomnia Answer* (New York: Penguin Group, 2006), 40.

14. Karl H. Dannenfeldt, "Sleep: Theory and Practice in the Late Renaissance," *The Journal of the History of Medicine and Allied Sciences* 41 (1986): 415-41.

15. Philippe Martin, "Corps en repos ou corps en danger?" *Revue d'histoire et de philosophie religieuses* 80 (2000): 247-62.

16. J.J. Terrell, "Why Women Need Beauty Sleep," *Illustrated World*, January 1917; Letha O. Lile, "Sleep: How Much Do We Know About It?" *Today's Health*, December 1951; T.F. James, "How Much Sleep Do You Really Need?" *Cosmopolitan*, April 1959.

17. De Manaceine, *Sleep: Its Physiology, pathology, hygiene, and Psychology*, 60, 156; Elwood Worcester and Samuel McComb, *Body, Mind and Spirit* (New York: Scribner's Sons, 1932), 113.

18. Nathaniel Kleitman, *Sleep and Wakefulness*, 178.

19. Helen Jameson, "Be a Follower of Lady Hygeia," *Atlanta Daily World*, January 23, 1941; Irving S. Cutter, "How to Keep Well—Recharging the Batteries of Health," *Chicago Daily Tribune*, July 13, 1941; William Brady, "Here's to Health!" *Los Angeles Times*, December 28, 1942; James F. Bender, "Odd Facts About Sleep, *Science Digest*, November 1947; James F. Bender, "Sweet Sleep," *American Magazine*, August 1948; John E. Gibson, "Masterful Key to Restful Slumber," *Hygeia*, April 1949; Theodore R. Van Dellen, "How to Keep Well," *The Washington Post*, August 12, 1964.

20. D.F. Kripke et al., "Mortality Associated with Sleep Duration and Insomnia," *Archives of General Psychiatry* 59 (2002): 131-6.

21. K.L. Knutson et al., "Trends in the Prevalence of Short Sleepers in the USA," *Sleep* 33 (2010): 37-45.

22. F.P. Cappuccio et al., "Sleep Duration and All-Cause Mortality," *Sleep* 33 (2010): 585-92.

23. Cotton Mather, *Vigilius. Or, The Awakener* (Boston, J. Franklin, 1719); John Wesley, *The Duty and Advantage of Early Rising* (London: J. Paramore, 1786); Fred W. Eastman, "The Chemistry of Sleep," *Atlantic Monthly*, January 1, 1911.

24. Stanley Coren, *Sleep Thieves* (New York: Free Press, 1996), 278-80.

25. Verdon, *Night in the Middle Ages*, 164.

26. "The Early Rising Precept," *Scientific American*, February 1, 1896.

27. "Edison: The Greatest of All Living Inventors," *Los Angeles Times*, November 4, 1894.

28. S.M. Rajaratnam and J. Arendt, "Health in a 24-Hour Society," *Lancet* 358 (2001): 999-1005; Walker and Stickgold, "Sleep, Memory, and Plasticity," 140-4.

29. M. Partinen et al., "Genetic and Environmental Determination of Human Sleep," *Sleep* 6 (1983): 179-85; A.C. Heath et al., "Evidence for Genetic Influences on Sleep Disturbance and Sleep Pattern in Twins," *Sleep* 13 (1990): 318-35; Paul Linkowski, "EEG Sleep Patterns in Twins," *Journal of Sleep Research* 8, supplement 1 (1999): 11-3; Hyun Hor and Mehdi Tafti, "Physiology. How Much Sleep Do We Need?" *Science* 325 (2009): 825-6.

30. Y. He et al., "The Transcriptional Repressor DEC2 Regulates Sleep Length in Mammals," *Science* 325 (2009): 866-70.

31. K.V. Allebrandt et al., " A K(ATP) Channel Gene Effect on Sleep Duration," *Molecular Psychiatry* 18 (2011): 122-32; "Researchers Identify a Genetic Factor that Regulates How Long We Sleep," National Sleep Foundation, December 19, 2011, http://www.sleepfoundation.org/alert/researchers-identify-genetic-factor-regulates-how-long-we-sleep.

32. Schwartz and Roth, "Neurophysiology of Sleep and Wakefulness," 367-78.

33. Glovinsky and Spielman, *The Insomnia Answer*, 50.

34. B.L. Frankel et al., "Recorded and Reported Sleep in Chronic Primary Insomnia," *Archives of General Psychiatry* 33 (1976): 615-23; J.M. Gaillard, "Is Insomnia a Disease of Slow-Wave Sleep?" *European Neurology* 14 (1976): 473-84; J.M. Gaillard, "Chronic Primary Insomnia: Possible Physiopathological Involvement of Slow-Wave Sleep Deficiency," *Sleep* 1 (1978): 133-47; H. Merica, R. Blois, and J.M. Gaillard, "Spectral Characteristics of Sleep EEG in Chronic Insomnia," *European Journal of Neuroscience* 10 (1998): 1826-34; A.D. Krystal et al., "NREM Sleep EEG Frequency Spectral Correlates of Sleep Complaints in Primary Insomnia Subtypes," *Sleep* 25 (2002): 630-40.

35. Pigeon and Perlis, "Sleep Homeostasis in Primary Insomnia," 248.

36. Bonnet and Arand, "Hyperarousal and Insomnia," 9-15; Pigeon and Perlis, "Sleep Homeostasis in Primary Insomnia," 249.

37. E. Stepanski et al., "Effects of Sleep Deprivation on Daytime Sleepiness in Primary Insomnia," *Sleep* 23 (2000): 215-9; A. Besset et al., "Homeostatic Process and Sleep Spindles in Patients with Sleep-Maintenance Insomnia," *Electroencephalography and Clinical Neurophysiology* 107 (1998): 122-32.

38. T. Porkka Heiskanen et al., "Adenosine: A Mediator of the Sleep-Inducing Effects of Prolonged Wakefulness," *Science* 276 (1997): 1265-8; T. Porkka-Heiskanen, R.E. Strecker, and R.W. McCarley, "Brain Site-Specificity of Extracellular Adenosine Concentration Changes During Sleep Deprivation," *Neuroscience* 99 (2000): 507-17; Robert McCarley, "Neurobiology of REM and

NREM Sleep," *Sleep Medicine* 8 (2007): 302-30; R. Basheer et al., "Adenosine and Sleep-wake Regulation," *Progress in Neurobiology* 73 (2004): 379-96.

39. J.V. Rétey et al., "A Functional Genetic Variation of Adenosine Deaminase Affects the Duration and Intensity of Deep Sleep in Humans," *Proceedings of the National Academy of Sciences of the United States of America* 102 (2005): 15676-81; J.V. Rétey et al., "Adenosinergic Mechanisms Contribute to Individual Differences in Sleep Deprivation-Induced Changes," *The Journal of Neuroscience* 26 (2006): 10472-9.

40. James M. Krueger et al., "Sleep as a Fundamental Property of Neuronal Assemblies," *Nature Reviews Neuroscience* 9 (2008): 4.

41. Saper et al., "Hypothalamic Regulation of Sleep," 1257-63.

42. Krueger et al., "Neuronal Assemblies," 3.

43. Ibid., 1.

Chapter 8: Aligning the Powers That Be

1.   "National Institutes of Health State of the Science Conference Statement: Manifestations and Management of Chronic Insomnia in Adults," *Sleep* 28 (2005): 1049-54; C.M. Morin et al., "Psychological and Behavioral Treatment of Insomnia: Update of the Recent Evidence (1998-2004)," *Sleep* 29 (2006): 1398-414.

2.   Richard Bootzin, "Stimulus Control Treatment for Insomnia."

3.   C.M. Morin et al., "Nonpharmacologic Treatment of Chronic Insomnia," *Sleep* 22 (1999): 1134-56.

4.   A.J. Spielman, L.S. Caruso, and P.B. Glovinsky, "A Behavioral Perspective on Insomnia Treatment," *The Psychiatric Clinics of North America* 10 (1986): 541-53.

5.   M.L. Perlis et al., "Psychophysiological Insomnia: The Behavioural Model and a Neurocognitive Perspective," *Journal of Sleep Research* 6 (1997): 179-188.

6.   Daniel Goleman, "Why Did the Caveman Sleep?" *Psychology Today*, March 1982.

7.   Michael L. Perlis et al., *Cognitive Behavioral Treatment of Insomnia: A Session-by-Session Guide* (Springer, 2005), 67.

8.   Michael Perlis, "Cognitive Behavioral Therapy for Insomnia," seminar held September 8-10, 2011, Philadelphia.

9.   Morin et al., "Nonpharmacologic Treatment of Chronic Insomnia,"1137-9; M.R. Irwin, J.C. Cole, and P.M. Nicassio, "Comparative Meta-Analysis of Behavioral Interventions for Insomnia and Their Efficacy," *Health Psychology* 25 (2006): 3-14.

10. Ibid.

11. K. Cervena et al., "Effect of Cognitive Behavioural Therapy for Insomnia on Sleep Architecture and Sleep EEG Power Spectra," *Journal of Sleep Research* 13 (2004): 385-93.

12. Borge Sivertsen et al., "Cognitive Behavioral Therapy vs Zopiclone for Treatment of Chronic Primary Insomnia in Older Adults," *Journal of the American Medical Association* 295 (2006): 2851-8.

13. K.L. Lichstein, "Relaxation and Sleep Compression for Late-Life Insomnia," *Journal of Consulting and Clinical Psychology* 69 (2001): 227-39; G.D. Jacobs et al., "Cognitive Behavior Therapy and Pharmacotherapy for Insomnia," *Archives of Internal Medicine* 164 (2004): 1888-96; C.M. Morin et al., "Randomized Clinical Trial of Supervised Tapering and Cognitive Behavior Therapy," *American Journal of Psychiatry* 161 (2004): 332-42.

14. M.M. Sanchez-Ortuno et al., "Are the Effects of Insomnia Treatment on Daytime Measures Clinically Important?" *Sleep* 32, abstract supplement (2009): A252; V. Castronovo et al., "Clinical Outcomes of Group Cognitive-Behavioral Therapy for Insomnia," *Sleep* 32, abstract supplement (2009): A254; Altena et al., "Prefrontal Hypoactivation and Recovery," 1271-6.

15. "National Institutes of Health State of the Science Conference Statement," 1052; C.M. Morin et al., "Psychological and Behavioral Treatment," 1409.

16. A.J. Spielman, P. Saskin, and M.J. Thorpy, "Treatment of Chronic Insomnia by Restriction of Time in Bed," *Sleep* 10 (1987): 45-56.

17. Michelle G. Craske, Dirk Hermans, and Debora Vansteenwegen, ed., *Fear and Learning* (Washington, DC: American Psychological Association, 2006).

18. Morin et al., "Psychological and Behavioral Treatment," 1411.

19. Dement and Vaughan, *The Promise of Sleep,* 424.

Chapter 9: Lit Up Like a Christmas Tree

1. C.L. Drake, H. Scofield, and T. Roth, "Vulnerability to Insomnia: The Role of Familial Aggregation," *Sleep Medicine* 9 (2008): 297-302; N.F. Watson et al., "Genetic and Environmental Influences on Insomnia, Daytime Sleepiness, and Obesity in Twins," *Sleep* 29 (2006): 645-9; Y. Dauvilliers et al., "Family Studies in Insomnia," *Journal of Psychosomatic Research* 58 (2005): 271-8.

2. M. Deuschle et al., "Association Between a Serotonin Transporter Length Polymorphism and Primary Insomnia," *Sleep* 33 (2010): 343-7.

3. Riemann et al., "The Hyperarousal Model of Insomnia," 28.

4. M.H. Bonnet and D.L. Arand, "The Consequences of a Week of Insomnia," *Sleep* 19 (1996): 453-61.

5. M.H. Bonnet and D.L. Arand, "The Consequences of a Week of Insomnia. II: Patients with Insomnia," *Sleep* 21 (1998): 359-68.

6. M.H. Bonnet and D.L. Arand, "Hyperarousal and Insomnia," *Sleep Medicine Reviews* 1 (1997): 97-108.

7. Bonnet and Arand, "Hyperarousal and Insomnia: State of the Science," 9-15.

8. Greene, *Insomniac,* 152.

9. M.H. Bonnet and D.L. Arand, "Heart Rate Variability in Insomniacs and Matched Normal Sleepers," *Psychosomatic Medicine* 60 (1998): 610-5; M.H. Bonnet and D.L. Arand, "24-Hour Metabolic Rate in Insomniacs and Matched Normal Sleepers," *Sleep* 18 (1995): 581-8; M.H. Bonnet and D.L. Arand, "Physiological Activation in Patients with Sleep State Misperception," *Psychosomatic Medicine* 59 (1997): 533-40; K. Spiegelhalder et al., "Heart Rate and Heart Rate Variability in Subjectively Reported Insomnia," *Journal of Sleep Research* 20 (2011): 137-45; K. Lushington, D. Dawson, and L. Lack, "Core Body Tempera-

ture Is Elevated During Constant Wakefulness in Elderly Poor Sleepers," *Sleep* 23 (2000): 504-10.

10. Robert Sapolsky, *Why Zebras Don't Get Ulcers* (New York: Times Books, 2004), 319.

11. In the following two studies, analyses of urine and blood samples showed higher levels of norepinephrine in insomniacs at night: A.N. Vgontzas et al., "Chronic Insomnia and Activity of the Stress System," *Journal of Psychosomatic Research* 45 (1998): 21-31; M. Irwin et al., "Nocturnal Catecholamines and Immune Function in Insomniacs, Depressed Patients, and Control Subjects," *Brain, Behavior, and Immunity* 17 (2003): 365-72. But Gary Richardson, reporting on a study of 95 insomniacs and 110 normal sleepers in a presentation at the annual meeting of the Associated Professional Sleep Societies in June 2010, found no significant elevation of urinary norepinephrine in insomniacs over a 24-hour period.

12. Sapolsky, *Why Zebras Don't Get Ulcers,* 31, 73.

13. B.K. Lee et al., "Associations of Salivary Cortisol with Cognitive Function in the Baltimore Memory Study," *Archives of General Psychiatry* 64 (2007): 810-8; U. Wagner and J. Born, "Memory Consolidation During Sleep: Interactive Effects of Sleep Stages and HPA Regulation," *Stress* 11 (2008): 28-41; Backhaus et al., "Impaired Declarative Memory," 1324-30; Sapolsky, *Why Zebras Don't Get Ulcers*, 13, 215-23.

14. R. Leproult et al., "Sleep Loss Results in an Elevation of Cortisol Levels the Next Evening," *Sleep* 20 (1997): 865-70; F. Chapotot et al., "Hypothalamo-Pituitary-Adrenal Axis Activity Is Related to the Level of Central Arousal," *Neuroendocrinology* 73 (2001): 312-21; K. Spiegel, R. Leproult, and E. Van Cauter, "Impact of Sleep Debt on Metabolic and Endocrine Function," *Lancet* 354 (1999): 1435-9; E. Spath-Schwalbe et al., "Sleep Disruption Alters Nocturnal ACTH and Cortisol Secretory Patterns," *Biological Psychiatry* 29 (1991): 575-84; M. Ekstedt, T Akerstedt, and M. Söderström, "Microarousals During Sleep Are Associated with Increased Levels of Lipids, Cortisol, and Blood Pressure," *Psychosomatic Medicine* 66 (2004): 925-31; Vgontzas et al., "Insomnia and Activity of the Stress System," 21-31; Vgontzas et al., "Nyctohemeral Activation of the HPA Axis," 3787-94; A. Rodenbeck et al., "Interactions Between Evening and Nocturnal Cortisol Secretion and Sleep Parameters," *Neuroscience Letters* 324 (2002): 159-63; D. Riemann et al., "Nocturnal Cortisol and Melatonin Secretion in Primary Insomnia," *Psychiatry Research* 113 (2002): 17-27; M. Varkevisser, H.P. Van Dongen, and G.A. Kerkhof, "Physiologic Indexes in Chronic Insomnia During a Constant Routine," *Sleep* 28 (2005): 1588-96; J. Backhaus, K Junghanns, and F. Hohagen, "Sleep Disturbances Are Correlated with Decreased Morning Awakening Salivary Cortisol," *Psychoneuroendocrinology* 29 (2004): 1184-91; Gary Richardson, "Correlation Between Urine Norepinephrine and Cortisol in Insomnia: Evidence for Central Dysregulation," paper presented at the annual meeting for the Associated Professional Sleep Societies, San Antonio, Texas, June 5-9, 2010.

15. Pigeon and Perlis, "Insomnia and Depression," 82-91; T. Roth, M. Franklin, and T.J. Bramley, "The State of Insomnia and Emerging Trends," *The American*

Journal of Managed Care 13 (2007): S117-20; Bonnet and Arand, "Hyper-arousal and Insomnia," 9-15; Dieter Riemann et al., "The Hyperarousal Model of Insomnia," 25.

16. A.D. Krystal and J.D. Edinger, "Measuring Sleep Quality," *Sleep Medicine* 9, supplement 1 (2008): S10-7.

17. Krystal and Edinger, "Measuring Sleep Quality," S11; Andrew Krystal, "Poly-somnography in Insomnia," paper presented at the annual meeting for the Associated Professional Sleep Societies, Seattle, Washington, June 6-11, 2009.

18. H. Merica et al., "Spectral Characteristics of Sleep EEG," 1826-34; M. Hall et al., "Symptoms of Stress and Depression as Correlates of Sleep in Primary Insomnia," *Psychosomatic Medicine* 62 (2000): 227-30; Krystal and Edinger, "Measuring Sleep Quality," S10-7; M.L. Perlis et al., "Beta/Gamma EEG Activity in Patients with Primary and Secondary Insomnia and Good Sleeper Controls," *Sleep* 24 (2001): 110-7; D.J. Buysse et al., "EEG Spectral Analysis in Primary Insomnia," *Sleep* 31 (2008): 1673-82.

19. C.H. Bastien and M. H. Bonnet, "Do Increases in Beta EEG Activity Uniquely Reflect Insomnia?" *Sleep Medicine Reviews* 5 (2001): 375-7; A. Cortoos, E. Ver-straeten, and R. Cluydts, "Neurophysiological Aspects of Primary Insomnia," *Sleep Medicine Reviews* 10 (2006): 255-66; Bonnet and Arand, "Hyperarousal and Insomnia," 9-15; Perlis et al., "Etiology and Pathophysiology of Insomnia," 720.

20. Hyperarousal of the central nervous system is not the only explanation for high-frequency neural activity at night. As stated in chapter 7, the failure of the brain to completely disengage could signal a problem with the sleep homeostat. Also, rather than reflecting a trait-level hyperarousal, the high-frequency activity in insomniacs' brains at night could reflect a conditioned arousal amenable to change through CBT-I, as noted in chapter 8.

21. Q.R. Regestein et al., "Daytime Alertness in Patients with Primary Insomnia," *The American Journal of Psychiatry* 150 (1993): 1529-34; C.M. Yang and H.S. Lo, "ERP Evidence of Enhanced Excitatory and Reduced Inhibitory Processes of Auditory Stimuli During Sleep," *Sleep* 30 (2007): 585-92; C.H. Bastien et al., "Chronic Psychophysiological Insomnia: Hyperarousal and/or Inhibition Deficits?" *Sleep* 31 (2008): 887-98.

22. Bastien et al., "Chronic Psychophysiological Insomnia," 895.

23. Ibid., 895; Yang and Lo, "ERP Evidence," 590.

24. M.T. Smith et al., "Neuroimaging of NREM Sleep in Primary Insomnia," *Sleep* 25 (2002): 325-35.

25. E.A. Nofzinger et al., "Functional Neuroimaging Evidence for Hyperarousal in Insomnia," *The American Journal of Psychiatry* 161 (2004): 2126-8. Another notable finding of this study was that in the morning, there was reduced metabolism in one key area of insomniacs' brains: the prefrontal cortex. This suggests, in the words of study authors, "that these patients are chronically sleep-deprived, perhaps from inefficient sleep."

26. Gary Richardson, "Neuroendocrine and Autonomic Physiology of Insomnia," paper presented at the annual meeting for the Associated Professional Sleep Societies, Seattle, Washington, June 6-11, 2009.

27. E.A. Nofzinger et al., "Regional Cerebral Metabolic Correlates of WASO During NREM Sleep in Insomnia," *Journal of Clinical Sleep Medicine* 2 (2006): 316-22.

28. Daniel J. Buysse et al., "A Neurobiological Model of Insomnia," *Drug Discovery Today: Disease Models* 8 (2011): 129-37. Specifically, this persistent wake-like activity is seen in cortical regions (prefrontal and parietal areas, and the precuneus), regions of the paralimbic cortex, the thalamus, and hypothalamic/brainstem arousal centers.

29. J.W. Winkelman et al., "Reduced Brain GABA in Primary Insomnia," *Sleep* 31 (2008): 1499-506.

30. Barbara Jones, "Basic Mechanisms of Sleep-Wake States," in *Principles and Practice of Sleep Medicine,* 4th ed., ed. Meir H. Kryger et al. (Philadelphia: Elsevier/Saunders, 2005), 136-53.

31. Similar to magnetic resonance imaging (MRI), magnetic resonance spectroscopy (MRS) involves use of a powerful magnetic field. But unlike MRI, MRS can determine the concentration of various chemical substances in the brain. The machine emits waves in a range of radio frequencies, which knock hydrogen atoms out of alignment. The signals they then give off reveal which substances are present and in what concentrations.

32. David T. Plante et al., "Reduced GABA in Occipital and Anterior Cingulate Cortices in Primary Insomnia," *Neuropsychopharmacology* 37 (2012): 1548-57.

33. T. Morgenthaler et al., "Practice Parameters for the Psychological and Behavioral Treatment of Insomnia: An Update." *Sleep* 29 (2006): 1415-9; Irwin et al, "Comparative Meta-Analysis of Behavioral Interventions," 3-14.

34. N.Y. Winbush, C.R. Gross, and J.J. Kreitzer, "The Effects of Mindfulness-Based Stress Reduction on Sleep Disturbance," *Explore* 3 (2007): 585-91. This review of literature on mindfulness meditation shows that participants in four of seven studies improved on measures of sleep quality and sleep length. But in the three controlled studies, there were no significant differences in outcome between the groups that received mindfulness training and the groups that did not. J.C. Ong, S.L. Shapiro, and R. Manber, "Combining Mindfulness Meditation with Cognitive-Behavior Therapy for Insomnia," *Behavior Therapy* 39 (2008): 171-82; J.C. Ong, S.L. Shapiro and R. Manber, "Mindfulness Meditation and Cognitive Behavioral Therapy for Insomnia," *Explore* 5 (2009): 30-6; C.R. Gross et al., "Mindfulness-Based Stress Reduction Versus Pharmacotherapy for Chronic Primary Insomnia," *Explore* 7 (2011): 76-87.

35. F. Li et al., "Tai Chi and Self-Rated Quality of Sleep and Daytime Sleepiness in Older Adults," *Journal of the American Geriatrics Society* 52 (2004): 892-900; M.R. Irwin, R. Olmstead, and S.J. Motivala, "Improving Sleep Quality in Older Adults with Moderate Sleep Complaints," *Sleep* 31 (2008): 1001-8.

36. Amy E. Beddoe, "Mindfulness-Based Yoga During Pregnancy" (PhD diss., University of California, 2007); L. Cohen et al., "Psychological Adjustment and Sleep Quality in a Randomized Trial of the Effects of a Tibetan Yoga Intervention," *Cancer* 100 (2004): 2253-60; S. Telles, K.V. Naveen, and M. Dash, "Yoga Reduces Symptoms of Distress in Tsunami Survivors in the Andaman Islands," *Evidence-based Complementary and Alternative Medicine* 4 (2007): 503-9; N.K.

Manjunath and S. Telles, "Influence of Yoga and Ayurveda on Self-Rated Sleep in a Geriatric Population," *Indian Journal of Medical Research* 121 (2005): 683-90; R.F. Afonso et al., "Yoga Decreases Insomnia in Postmenopausal Women," *Menopause* 19 (2012): 186-93.

37.   S.B. Khalsa, "Treatment of Chronic Insomnia with Yoga," *Applied Psychophysiology and Biofeedback* 29 (2004): 269-78; S.B. Khalsa, "Yoga as an Intervention for Chronic Primary Insomnia," paper presented at the annual meeting for the Associated Professional Sleep Societies, Seattle, Washington, June 6-11, 2009; e-mail exchange, April, 2010.

38.   Paul McKenna, *I Can Make You Sleep*, ed. Hugh Willbourn (New York: Sterling, 2009), 50; Peter Hauri, *No More Sleepless Nights* (New York: J. Wiley, 1991), 129.

39.   H.S. Driver and S.R. Taylor, "Exercise and Sleep," *Sleep Medicine Reviews* 4 (2000): 387-402; S.D. Youngstedt, "Effects of Exercise on Sleep," *Clinics in Sports Medicine* 24 (2005): 355-65.

40.   Youngstedt, "Effects of Exercise," 357-8.

41.   Driver and Taylor, "Exercise and Sleep," 387-402; National Sleep Foundation, *2013 Sleep in America Poll* (Washington, DC: National Sleep Foundation, 2013), 11-22.

42.   See, for example, C. Guilleminault et al., "Nondrug Treatment Trials in Psychophysiologic Insomnia," *Archives of Internal Medicine* 155 (1995): 838-44. Subjects in a four-week experiment involving brisk walking for forty-five minutes a day showed modest but significant improvements in sleep in comparison to controls. See also S.S. Tworoger et al., "Effects of a Yearlong Moderate-Intensity Exercise and a Stretching Intervention on Sleep Quality in Postmenopausal Women," *Sleep* 26 (2003): 830-6. Among the postmenopausal, overweight, sedentary subjects in this study (a demographic prone to insomnia), participants in a yearlong, five-day-a-week aerobic exercise program significantly increased the maximum volume of oxygen they could consume compared to women in a stretching program. Subjects who increased their maximum volume of oxygen by at least 10 percent by the end of the year had longer and better sleep, and used fewer sleeping pills.

43.   G.S. Passos et al., "Effects of Moderate Aerobic Exercise Training on Chronic Primary Insomnia," *Sleep Medicine* 12 (2011): 1018-27; A.C. King et al., "Moderate-Intensity Exercise and Self-Rated Quality of Sleep in Older Adults," *Journal of the American Medical Association* 277 (1997): 32-7; K.J. Reid et al., "Aerobic Exercise Improves Self-Reported Sleep and Quality of Life in Older Adults with Insomnia," *Sleep Medicine* 11 (2010): 934-40.

44.   P. Ekkekakis and S.J. Petruzzello, "Acute Aerobic Exercise and Affect," *Sports Medicine* 28 (1999): 337-74; R.H. Cox et al., "Effects of Acute 60 and 80% VO2max Bouts of Aerobic Exercise on State Anxiety of Women of Different Age Groups Across Time," *Research Quarterly for Exercise and Sport* 75 (2004): 165-75; M.P. Herring et al., "Feasibility of Exercise Training for the Short-Term Treatment of Generalized Anxiety Disorder," *Psychotherapy and Psychosomatics* 81 (2012): 21-8; N.A. Singh, K.M. Clements, and M.A. Fiatarone, "A Randomized Controlled Trial of the Effect of Exercise on Sleep,"

Sleep 20 (1997): 95-101. In this study, researchers found that a ten-week weight training treatment three times a week for older depressed adults decreased their depression and improved their sleep quality and daytime functioning, in comparison to controls. K. Daley and V. Gil-Rivas, "Exercise-Based Cognitive Therapy as a Novel Treatment for Insomnia and Depression, *Sleep* 33, abstract supplement (2010): A223. In this study involving an exercise-based cognitive therapy program for people with insomnia and depression, researchers found that subjects experienced significant reductions in anxiety, depression, perceived stress, and the time it took to fall asleep.

45. G.S. Passos et al., "Effect of Acute Physical Exercise on Patients with Chronic Primary Insomnia," *Journal of Clinical Sleep Medicine* 6 (2010): 270-5.

46. J.A. Horne and L.H. Staff, "Exercise and Sleep: Body-Heating Effects," *Sleep* 6 (1983): 36-46; J.A. Horne and V.J. Moore, "Sleep EEG Effects of Exercise With and Without Additional Body Cooling," *Electroencephalography and Clinical Neurophysiology* 60 (1985): 33-8; D.E. Bunnell et al., "Passive Body Heating and Sleep," *Sleep* 11 (1988): 210-9.

47. Driver and Taylor, "Exercise and Sleep," 387-402; S.D. Youngstedt, D.F. Kripke, and J.A. Elliott, "Is Sleep Disturbed by Vigorous Late-Night Exercise?" *Medicine and Science in Sports and Exercise* 31 (1999): 864-9; H.Yoshida et al., "Effects of Timing of Exercise on the Night Sleep," *Psychiatry and Clinical Neurosciences* 52 (1998): 139-40.

48. O. Van Reeth et al., ""Nocturnal Exercise Phase Delays Circadian Rhythms of Melatonin and Thyrotropin Secretion," *American Journal of Physiology* 266 (1994): E964-74; L.K. Barger et al., "Daily Exercise Facilitates Phase Delays of Circadian Melatonin Rhythm in Very Dim Light," *American Journal of Physiology. Regulatory, Integrative, and Comparative Physiology* 286 (2004): R1077-84.

Chapter 10: Perils of the Pill

1. National Sleep Foundation, *2009 Sleep in America Poll* (Washington, DC: National Sleep Foundation, 2009), 53; Sabrina Tavernise, "Drug Agency Recommends Lower Doses of Sleep Aids for Women," *The New York Times*, January 10, 2013; Roni Caryn Rabin, "Sleeping Pills Rising in Popularity Among Young Adults," *The New York Times*, January 15, 2009.

2. Moloney et al., "The Medicalization of Sleeplessness," 1430; D.J. Buysse, "Insomnia State of the Science: An Evolutionary, Evidence-Based Assessment," *Sleep* 28 (2005): 1045-6.

3. Douglas Moul et al., "Treatments for Insomnia and Restless Legs Syndrome," *A Guide to Treatments That Work*, ed. Peter Nathan and Jack Gorman (New York: Oxford University Press, 2007).

4. Jean K. Haddad, "The Pharmaceutical Industry's Influence on Physician Behavior and Health Care Costs," San Francisco Medical Society, October 9, 2009, http://www.zoominfo.com/#!search/profile/person?personId=12429193 99&targetid=profile; Mary Ebeling, "Beyond Advertising: The Pharmaceutical Industry's Hidden Marketing Tactics," February 21, 2008, http://www.prwatch.

org; "The U.S. Sleep Market," Marketdata Enterprises, June 1, 2008, http://www.marketresearch.com/Marketdata-Enterprises-Inc-v416/Sleep-1788286/; Moloney et al., "The Medicalization of Sleeplessness," 1431.

5. Moloney et al., "The Medicalization of Sleeplessness," 1430.

6. "World Sleep Disorders Market Analysis 2009-2024," accessed June 2009, http://www.piribo.com.

7. D.F. Kripke, R.D. Langer, and L.E. Kline, "Hypnotics' Association With Mortality or Cancer," *BMJ Open* 2 (2012): 1-8.

8. Bill Hayes, *Sleep Demons: An Insomniac's Memoir* (New York: Pocket Books, 2001), 235-6.

9. Two papers that touch on the subject are E. Estivill, "Behaviour of Insomniacs and Implication for Their Management," *Sleep Medicine Reviews* 6, supplement 1 (2002): S3-6; and J. Hislop and S. Arber, "Understanding Women's Sleep Management," *Sociology of Health and Illness* 25 (2003): 815-37.

10. "The Use of Medicines in the United States: Review of 2010," IMS Institute for Healthcare Informatics, April 2011, http://www.imshealth.com/deployedfiles/imshealth/Global/Content/IMS%20Institute/Static%20File/IHII_UseOfMed_report.pdf; Andrea Petersen, "Dawn of a New Sleep Drug?" July 19, 2011, http://www.wsj.com/article/SB10001424052702304567604576454102061138630.html; R. Mojtabai and M. Olfson, "Proportion of Antidepressants Prescribed Without a Psychiatric Diagnosis Is Growing," *Health Affairs (Millwood)* 30 (2011): 1434-42.

11. Thomas Roth and Michael Perlis, "Hypnotic Induced Sleep Is as Good as Natural Sleep: A Pro/Con Debate," presentation at the annual meeting for the Associated Professional Sleep Societies, Minneapolis, Minnesota, June 11-15, 2011.

12. Perlis et al., "Intermittent and Long-Term Use," 3456-7.

13. Wallace Mendelson, "Long-Term Use of Hypnotic Medications," in *Insomnia: Principles and Management*, ed. Martin P. Szuba, Jacqueline D. Kloss, and David F. Dinges (New York: Cambridge University Press, 2003), 115-21.

14. At sleep onset, neurons in the ventrolateral preoptic area (the VLPO) become active, releasing galanin and GABA. GABA then binds to receptors on adjacent nerve cells, fitting like a key in a lock and enabling the opening of special cellular channels. Chloride ions then rush into the cells and render them inert, putting the brain to sleep.

15. Daniel Buysse, "When You Have a Hammer, Everything Looks Like a Nail," paper presented at the annual meeting for the Associated Professional Sleep Societies, Seattle, Washington, June 6-11, 2009.

16. Perlis et al., "Intermittent and Long-Term Use," 3456.

17. H. Wayne Morgan, *Drugs in America: A Social History, 1800-1980* (Syracuse: Syracuse University Press, 1981), 2-3.

18. D.W. Cathell, *The Physician Himself*, 9th edition (Baltimore: Cushings and Bailey, 1889), 180.

19. Horace B. Day, *The Opium Habit* (New York: Harper and Bros., 1868), 232-9.

20. Morgan, *Drugs in America*, 29-30.

21. William A. Hammond, "The Therapeutics of Wakefulness," *Scientific American*, February 20, 1869; F.D. Pierce, "Sleep and Insomnia or Wakefulness,"

The Physicians' and Surgeons' Investigator, August 15, 1881; Hartmann, *The Sleeping Pill*, 11; F. Lopez-Munoz, R. Ucha-Udabe, and C. Alamo, "The History of Barbiturates a Century after Their Clinical Introduction," *Neuropsychiatric Disease and Treatment* 1 (2005): 329-43.

22. "Hydrate of Chloral," *Chicago Tribune*, January 16, 1870; "Poisonous Sleep Producers," *Scientific American*, May 10, 1884; "How Drugs Are Abused," *The Washington Post*, April 30, 1891; William Rosser Cobbe, *Doctor Judas: A Portrayal of the Opium Habit* (Chicago: S.C. Griggs and Co., 1895), 135.

23. "Sleeplessness," *Scientific American*, November 24, 1883; H.H. Kane, "The Opium Habit Among American Women," *Harper's Bazaar*, October 27, 1883.

24. "An Infallible Insomnia Cure," *The Washington Post*, July 26, 1903; Adam Doble, Ian L. Martin, and David Nutt, *Calming the Brain: Benzodiazepines and Related Drugs from Laboratory to Clinic* (New York: Martin Dunitz, 2004), 1-2; R.D. Gillespie, *Sleep and the Treatment of Its Disorders* (New York: William Wood and Co., 1930), 149-52.

25. William S. Burroughs, *Naked Lunch* (New York: Grove Press, 1959), 225.

26. James Harvey Young, *The Medical Messiahs* (Princeton: Princeton University Press, 1992), 260-81; Dimitri Cozanitis, "One Hundred Years of Barbiturates and Their Saint," *Journal of the Royal Society of Medicine* 97 (2004): 594-8.

27. Lois Mattox Miller, "Dangerous Lullabies," *Hygeia*, July 1938; Vera Connolly, "Lethal Lullaby," *Colliers*, October 19, 1946; "Sleeping Pills Dangerous," *Hygeia*, July 1946; William Engle, "Sleeping Pills: Doorway to Doom," *Coronet*, January 1951; Mort Weisinger, "Sleeping Pills Are Worse Than Dope," *Coronet*, January 1955; Ralph Bass, "The Menace of the Sleeping Pill Habit," *Coronet*, March 1958.

28. "Judy Garland's Death Ascribed to Long Use of Sleeping Drugs," *Los Angeles Times*, June 26, 1969; "Finds Hendrix Took Nine Times Normal Pills," *Chicago Tribune*, September 29, 1970.

29. Paul H. Fluck, "So You Can't Sleep?" *Today's Health*, April 1950; Maxine Davis, "Some people find it hard to sleep," *Good Housekeeping*, February 1951; "Insomnia, Part Two," *Consumer Reports*, May 1952; "How To Cure Insomnia," *Science Digest*, January 1952; Donald A. Laird, "Sleeplessness and what to do about it," *Today's Health*, August 1957; T.F. James, "How Much Sleep Do You Really Need?" *Cosmopolitan*, April 1959.

30. A.D. Clift, "Factors Leading to Dependence on Hypnotic Drugs," *British Medical Journal* 3 (1972): 614-7; "Barbiturate Abuse in the United States," (Washington, DC: U.S. Government Printing Office, 1972), 523-4.

31. Cozanitis, "One Hundred Years of Barbiturates," 597.

32. The Insight Team of The Sunday Times of London, *Suffer the Children: The Story of Thalidomide* (New York: Viking Press, 1979).

33. Morton Mintz, "Thalidomide Incident Smacked of Profiteering," *The Washington Post*, Sept. 17, 1962; Robert C. Toth, "U.S. Cites Maker of Thalidomide," *The New York Times*, Feb. 23, 1963; *Suffer the Children*, 72.

34. *Suffer the Children*, 73; Herbert Lawson, "Dangers in Drugs: Government, Industry Aim to Improve Safety," *Wall Street Journal*, August 1, 1962.

35. Lawson, "Dangers in Drugs"; "Dr. Kelsey's Predecessor Told Senators of Drug Perils in 1960," *The New York Times*, August 10, 1962.

36. William M. Freeman, "Sales of Tranquilizers Decrease in Wariness Over Thalidomide," *The New York Times*, August 3, 1962.

37. WHO Review Group, "Use and Abuse of Benzodiazepines," *Bulletin of the World Health Organization* 61 (1983): 551-62.

38. Donald F. Klein and John M. Davis, *Diagnosis and Drug Treatment of Psychiatric Disorders* (Baltimore: Williams and Wilkins, 1969); Donald R. Wesson and David E. Smith, "The Use and Abuse of Barbiturates: Statement for the Senate Health Committee" (Washington, DC: U.S. Government Printing Office, 1973), 147-52; Lawrence Mayer, "That Confounding Enemy of Sleep," *Fortune*, June 1975; Carol Kahn, "Do You Dream Perchance of Sleeping," *Family Health*, September 1977; "Insomnia Remedies: Which Ones Work Best?" *Consumer Reports*, October 1977.

39. A.J. Bond and M.H. Lader, "The Residual Effects of Flurazepam," *Psychopharmacologia* 32 (1973): 223-35; R.G. Borland and A.N. Nicholson, "Comparison of the Residual Effects of Two Benzodiazepines," *British Journal of Clinical Pharmacology* 2 (1974): 9-17.

40. Peter Ritson, *Alive and Kicking* (Liverpool: Casa Publishing, 1989).

41. Douglas Colligan, *Creative Insomnia* (New York: Franklin Watts, 1978), 90; Malcolm Lader, "Dependence on Benzodiazepines," *Journal of Clinical Psychiatry* 44 (1983): 121-7; Eve Bargmann et al., *Stopping Valium* (New York: Warner Books, 1983).

42. A. Kales, M.B. Scharf, and J.D. Kales, "Rebound Insomnia: A New Clinical Syndrome," *Science* 201 (1978): 1039-41; A. Kales et al., "Rebound Insomnia," *Journal of the American Medical Association* 241 (1979): 1692-5.

43. A. Kales et al., "Hypnotic Efficacy of Triazolam," *Journal of Clinical Pharmacology* 16 (1976): 399-406; E.O. Bixler et al., "Effectiveness of Temazepam with Short-Intermediate-, and Long-Term Use," *Journal of Clinical Pharmacology* 18 (1978): 110-8; C.R. Soldatos et al., "Tolerance and Rebound Insomnia With Rapidly Eliminated Hypnotics," *International Clinical Psychopharmacology* 14 (1999): 287-303; A. Kales et al., "Rebound Insomnia and Rebound Anxiety," *Pharmacology* 26 (1983): 121-37; Louis Lasagna, "The Halcion Story: Trial by Media," *The Lancet* (1980): 815-6.

44. Cindy Ehrlich, "Halcion Nightmare," *California,* September 1988; Cindy Ehrlich, "Halcion: Prescription for Trouble?" *California,* October 1988.

45. William Styron, *Darkness Visible: A Memoir of Madness* (New York: Random House, 1990).

46. M.N. Graham Dukes and Barbara Swartz, *Responsibility for Drug-Induced Injury* (New York, Elsevier, 1998), 381.

47. Jacqueline Mitchell, "Upjohn's U.S. Halcion Sales Fall 55%," *Wall Street Journal*, November 16, 1992; Malcolm Gladwell, "There May Be Nothing Unsafe in the Numbers About Halcion," *The Washington Post,* June 15, 1992.

48. "Halcion: Sweet Dreams or Nightmare?" *Newsweek*, August 19, 1991; "Does Halcion Spur Aggression?" *ABA Journal,* November 1991.

49. Liz Hunt, "Data on Sleeping Pill's Effects Were Incomplete, Upjohn Says," *The Washington Post,* August 28, 1991; Gina Kolata, "Maker of Sleeping Pill Hid Data," *The New York Times,* January 20, 1992.

50. Philip J. Hilts, "FDA Opens Inquiry on Upjohn's Handling of Data on Sleeping Pill," *The New York Times*, April 26, 1994; John Schwartz, "Halcion's Effects Hidden, FDA Investigators Claim," *The Washington Post*, April 26, 1994; John Schwartz, "Abrupt Cutoff of FDA Halcion Probe Suggests a Coverup," *The Washington Post*, October 28, 1994; Ron Stodghill and Seanna Browder, "How the FDA Let Halcion Slip Through," *Business Week*, June 17, 1996; Malcolm Gladwell, "Why the FDA Cleared Halcion," *The Washington Post*, June 2, 1992.

51. Nora Underwood, "The Halcion Debate," *Maclean's*, February 17, 1992.

52. J.K. Walsh and P.K. Schweitzer, "Ten-Year Trends in the Pharmacological Treatment of Insomnia," *Sleep* 22 (1999): 371-5.

53. Ibid.; J.K. Walsh, "Drugs Used to Treat Insomnia in 2002," *Sleep* 27 (2004), 1441-2.

54. I. Montgomery et al., "Trazodone Enhances Sleep in Subjective Quality but Not in Objective Duration," *British Journal of Clinical Pharmacology* 16 (1983): 139-44; Michael H. Wiegand, "Antidepressants for the Treatment of Insomnia," *Drugs*, 68 (2008): 2411-7; Walsh, "Drugs Used to Treat Insomnia," 1441-2.

55. N.A. DeMartinis and A. Winokur, "Effects of Psychiatric Medications on Sleep and Sleep Disorders," *CNS and Neurological Disorders Drug Targets* 6 (2007): 17-29; S.J. Aton et al., "The Sedating Antidepressant Trazodone Impairs Sleep-Dependent Cortical Plasticity," *PLoS ONE* 4 (2009): 1-10.

56. See, for example, A.J. Roth, W.V. McCall, and A. Liguori, "Cognitive, Psycho-motor and Polysomnmographic Effects of Trazodone in Primary Insomniacs," *Journal of Sleep Research* 20 (2011): 552-8. In this study, trazodone was associated with fewer nighttime awakenings, fewer minutes of stage 1 (light) sleep, and fewer self-reports of difficulty sleeping. See also Wiegand, "Antidepressants for Insomnia," 2411-7.

57. Kripke et al., "Hypnotics' Association With Mortality," 1-8.

58. D.F. Kripke, "Who Should Sponsor Sleep Disorders Pharmaceutical Trials?" *Journal of Clinical Sleep Medicine* 3 (2007): 671-3.

59. N. Buscemi et al., "The Efficacy and Safety of Drug Treatments for Chronic Insomnia," *Journal of General Internal Medicine* 22 (2007): 1335-50.

60. Jim Giles, "Stacking the Deck," *Nature* (2006): 270-2.

61. Ibid., J.E. Bekelman, Y. Li, and C.P. Gross, "Scope and Impact of Financial Conflicts of Interest in Biomedical Research," *Journal of the American Medical Association* 289 (2003): 454-65; Marcia Angell, *The Truth About the Drug Companies* (New York: Random House, 2005), 98.

62. Kripke, "Who Should Sponsor Trials?" 671-3.

63. Giles, "Stacking the Deck," 270-2.

Chapter 11: The Insomniac's Pharmacopeia

1. Abdul Rahman Al-Rashed, "Interview with Colin Powell," *Asharq Al-Awsat*, November 5, 2003.

2. Sabrina Tavernise, "Drug Agency Recommends Lower Doses of Sleep Aids for Women," *The New York Times*, January 10, 2013.

3. Hans Mohler et al., "GABA(A) Receptor Subtypes: A New Pharmacology," *Current Opinion in Pharmacology* 1 (2001): 22-5; A.D. Krystal, "In Vivo Evidence of the Specificity of Effects of GABA(A) Receptor Modulating Medications," *Sleep* 33 (2010): 859-60.

4. Malcolm Lader, "Rebound Insomnia and Newer Hypnotics," *Psychopharmacology* 108 (1992): 248-55; D. Wheatley, "Prescribing Short-Acting Hypnosedatives," *Drug Safety* 7 (1992): 106-15; M.B. Scharf et al., "A Multicenter, Placebo-Controlled Study Evaluating Zopidem in the Treatment of Chronic Insomnia," *The Journal of Clinical Psychiatry* 55 (1994): 192-9; J.M. Monti et al., "Sleep in Patients with Chronic Primary Insomnia During Long-Term Zolpidem Administration," *International Clinical Psychopharmacology* 11 (1996): 255-63; L. Parrino and M.G. Terzano, "Polysomnographic Effects of Hypnotic Drugs," *Psychopharmacology* 126 (1996): 1-16; J.M. Monti, F. Alvariño, and D. Monti, "Conventional and Power Spectrum Analysis of the Effects of Zolpidem on Sleep EEG," *Sleep* 23 (2000): 1075-84.

5. "U.S. Pharmaceutical Sales," Drugs.com, accessed February 18, 2013, http://www.drugs.com/stats/top100/.

6. D.P. Brunner et al., "Effect of Zolpidem on Sleep and Sleep EEG Spectra in Healthy Young Men," *Psychopharmacology* 104 (1991): 1-5; H.P. Landolt et al., "Zolpidem and Sleep Deprivation: Different Effect on EEG Power Spectra," *Journal of Sleep Research* 9 (2000): 175-83; I. Feinberg, T. Maloney, and I.G. Campbell, "Effects of Hypnotics on the Sleep EEG of Healthy Young Adults," *Journal of Psychiatric Research* 34 (2000): 423-38; Scharf et al., "A Multicenter, Placebo-Controlled Study," 192-9; M. Lancel, "Role of GABA(A) Receptors in the Regulation of Sleep," *Sleep* 22 (1999): 33-42; P.T. Morgan et al., "Retrograde Effects of Triazolam and Zolpidem on Sleep-Dependent Motor Learning in Humans," *Journal of Sleep Research* 19 (2010): 157-64.

7. Morgan et al., "Retrograde Effects," 157-64; J. Seibt et al., "The Non-Benzodiazepine Hypnotic Zolpidem Impairs Sleep-Dependent Cortical Plasticity," *Sleep* 31 (2008): 1381-91.

8. E. Ganzoni et al., "Zolpidem in Insomnia: A 3-Year Post-Marketing Surveillance Study in Switzerland," *Journal of International Medical Research* 23 (1995): 61-73; J.P. Sauvanet et al., "Open Long-Term Trials with Zolpidem in Insomnia," in *Imidazopyridines in Sleep Disorders*, ed. J.P. Sauvanet, S.Z. Langer, and P.L. Morselli, (New York: Raven Press, 1988); C.R. Dolder and M.H. Nelson, "Hypnosedative-Induced Complex Behaviors," *CNS Drugs* 22 (2008): 1021-36.

9. Tavernise, "Lower Doses of Sleep Aids for Women"; A. Vermeeren, "Residual Effects of Hypnotics: Epidemiology and Clinical Implications," *CNS Drugs* 18 (2004): 297-328.

10. Dolder and Nelson, "Hypnosedative-Induced Complex Behaviors," 1021-36; R. Hoque and A.L. Chesson, "Zolpidem-Induced Sleepwalking, Sleep Related Eating Disorder, and Sleep Driving," *Journal of Clinical Sleep Medicine* 5 (2009): 471-6.

11. "The DAWN Report," Substance Abuse and Mental Health Services Administration, May 1, 2013, http://www. samhsa.gov/data/2k13/DAWN079/sr079-Zolpidem.htm.

12. J.K. Walsh et al., "Eight Weeks of Non-Nightly Use of Zolpidem for Primary Insomnia," *Sleep* 23 (2000): 1087-96; M.L. Perlis et al., "Long-Term, Non-Nightly Administration of Zolpidem in the Treatment of Patients with Primary Insomnia," *Journal of Clinical Psychiatry* 65 (2004): 1128-37; A.D. Krystal et al., "Long-Term Efficacy and Safety of Zolpidem Extended-Release 12.5 mg," *Sleep* 31 (2008): 79-90.

13. C.R. Soldatos et al., "Tolerance and Rebound Insomnia," 287-303; U. Voder-holzer et al., "A Double-Blind, Randomized and Placebo-Controlled Study on the Polysomnographic Withdrawal Effects of Zopiclone, Zolpidem and Triazolam," *European Archives of Psychiatry and Clinical Neuroscience* 251 (2001): 117-23; R.C. Voshaar, A.J. van Balkom, and F.G. Zitman, "Zolpidem Is Not Superior to Temazepam with Respect to Rebound Insomnia," *European Neuropsychopharmacology* 14 (2004): 301-6; T. Roth et al., "Efficacy and Safety of Zolpidem-MR," *Sleep Medicine* 7 (2006): 397-406; Krystal et al., "Long-Term Efficacy," 79-90.

14. T.A. Roehrs et al., "Twelve Months of Nightly Zolpidem Does Not Lead to Rebound Insomnia or Withdrawal Symptoms," *Journal of Psychopharmacology* 26 (2011): 1088-95.

15. G. Hajak et al., "Abuse and Dependence Potential for the Non-Benzodiazepine Hypnotics Zolpidem and Zopiclone," *Addiction* 98 (2003): 1371-8; C. Victorri-Vigneau et al., "Evidence of Zolpidem Abuse and Dependence," *British Journal of Clinical Pharmacology* 64 (2007): 198-209; G. Zammit, "Comparative Tolerability of Newer Agents for Insomnia," *Drug Safety* 32 (2009): 735-48; M. Soyka, R. Bottlender, and H.J. Möller, "Epidemiological Evidence for a Low Abuse Potential of Zolpidem," *Pharmacopsychiatry* 33 (2000): 138-41.

16. S. Ancoli-Israel et al., "Zaleplon, a Novel Nonbenzodiazepine Hypnotic, Effec-tively Treats Insomnia in Elderly Patients," *Primary Care Companion to the Journal of Clinical Psychiatry* 1 (1999): 114-20; R. Elie et al., "Sleep Latency Is Shortened During 4 Weeks of Treatment with Zaleplon," *Journal of Clinical Psychiatry* 60 (1999): 536-44; Vermeeren, "Residual Effects of Hypnotics," 297-328; S. Ancoli-Israel et al., "Long-Term Use of Sedative Hypnotics in Older Patients with Insomnia," *Sleep Medicine* 6 (2005): 107-13; J. Barbera and C. Shapiro, "Benefit-Risk Assessment of Zaleplon in the Treatment of Insomnia," *Drug Safety* 28 (2005): 301-18; Zammit, "Comparative Tolerability," 735-48.

17. J.K. Walsh et al., "A Five Week, Polysomnographic Assessment of Zaleplon 10 mg for the Treatment of Primary Insomnia," *Sleep Medicine* 1 (2000): 41-9; Y. Dündar et al., "Comparative Efficacy of Newer Hypnotic Drugs for the Short-Term Management of Insomnia," *Human Psychopharmacology* 19 (2004): 305-22; Zammit, "Comparative Tolerability," 735-48; D.J. Nutt and S.M. Stahl, "Searching for the Perfect Sleep," *Journal of Psychopharmacology* 24 (2010): 1601-12.

18. H. Allain et al., "Preference of Insomniac Patients Between a Single Dose of Zolpidem 10 mg Versus Zaleplon 10 mg," *Human Psychopharmacology* 18 (2003): 369-74.

19. A.D. Krystal et al., "Sustained Efficacy of Eszopiclone Over 6 Months of Nightly Treatment," *Sleep* 26 (2003): 793-9.

20. "U.S. Pharmaceutical Sales," Drugs.com, accessed February 18, 2013, http://www.drugs.com/stats/top100/.

21. R. Rosenberg et al., "An Assessment of the Efficacy and Safety of Eszopiclone in the Treatment of Transient Insomnia," *Sleep Medicine* 6 (2005): 15-22; G.K. Zammit et al, "Efficacy and Safety of Eszopiclone Across 6 Weeks of Treatment for Primary Insomnia," *Current Medical Research and Opinion* 20 (2004): 1979-91; M.K. Erman et al., " A Polysomnographic Placebo-Controlled Evaluation of the Efficacy and Safety of Eszopiclone," *Journal of Clinical Sleep Medicine* 4 (2008): 229-34; Nutt and Stahl, "Searching for the Perfect Sleep," 1601-12; H. Joffe et al., "Eszopiclone Improves Insomnia and Depressive and Anxious Symptoms in Perimenopausal and Postmenopausal Women with Hot Flashes," *American Journal of Obstetrics and Gynecology* 202: (2010): 171.e1-171.e11.

22. See Nutt and Stahl, "Searching for the Perfect Sleep," 1602-5. While zopiclone appears to have its greatest effect via the alpha-1 and –5 receptors, eszopiclone (Lunesta) acts mainly through the alpha-2 and –3 receptors (and alpha-1 to a lesser extent).

23. J.M. Monti and S.R. Pandi-Perumal, "Eszopiclone: Its Use in the Treatment of Insomnia," *Neuropsychiatric Disease and Treatment* 3 (2007): 441-53; J. Boyle et al., "Next-Day Cognition, Psychomotor Function, and Driving-Related Skills Following Nighttime Administration of Eszopiclone," *Human Psychopharmacology* 23 (2008): 385-97; Nutt and Stahl, "Searching for the Perfect Sleep," 1601-12; Krystal et al., "Sustained Efficacy of Eszopiclone," 793-9; Rosenberg et al., "Efficacy and Safety of Eszopiclone," 15-22; T. Roth et al., "An Evaluation of the Efficacy and Safety of Eszopiclone over 12 Months in Patients with Primary Insomnia," *Sleep Medicine* 6 (2005): 487-95; J.K. Walsh et al., "Nightly Treatment of Primary Insomnia with Eszopiclone for Six Months," *Sleep* 30 (2007): 959-68; Zammit et al., "Efficacy and Safety of Eszopiclone," 1979-91.

24. F.L. Joya et al., "Meta-Analyses of Hypnotics and Infections: Eszopiclone, Ramelteon, Zaleplon, and Zolpidem," *Journal of Clinical Sleep Medicine* 5 (2009): 377-83.

25. D.F. Kripke, "Greater Incidence of Depression with Hypnotic Use Than with Placebo," *BMC Psychiatry* 7 (2007): 42.

26. Kripke et al., "Hypnotics' Association With Mortality," 1-8.

27. Daniel J. DeNoon, "Sleeping Pills Called 'as Risky as Cigarettes,'" WebMD Health News, February 27, 2012, http://www.webmd.com/sleep-disorders/news/20120227/sleeping-pills-called-as-risky-as-cigarettes.

28. D.F. Kripke et al., "Mortality Hazard Associated with Prescription Hypnotics," *Biological Psychiatry* 43 (1998): 687-93; L. Mallon, J.E. Broman, and J. Hetta, "Is Usage of Hypnotics Associated with Mortality?" *Sleep Medicine* 10 (2009): 279-86; G. Belleville, "Mortality Hazard Associated with Anxiolytic and Hypnotic Drug Use," *Canadian Journal of Psychiatry* 55 (2010): 558-67.

29. A.N. Vgontzas et al., "Insomnia with Short Sleep Duration and Mortality," *Sleep* 33 (2010): 1159-64; K.L. Chien et al., "Habitual Sleep Duration and Insomnia and the Risk of Cardiovascular Events and All-Cause Death," *Sleep* 33 (2010): 177-84; C. Hublin et al., "Heritability and Mortality Risk of Insomnia-Related

Symptoms," *Sleep* 34 (2011): 957-64; J.H. Bjorngaard et al., "Sleeping Problems and Suicide in 75,000 Norwegian Adults," *Sleep* 34 (2011): 1155-9.

30. Kripke, "Hypnotics' Association with Mortality, 7.

31. S.R. Pandi-Perumal et al., "Ramelteon: A Review of Its Therapeutic Potential in Sleep Disorders," *Advances in Therapy* 26 (2009): 613-26.

32. M.J. Sateia, P. Kirby-Long, and J.L. Taylor, "Efficacy and Safety of Ramelteon," *Sleep Medicine Reviews* 12 (2008): 319-32; G. Mayer et al., "Efficacy and Safety of 6-month Nightly Ramelteon Administration in Adults with Chronic Primary Insomnia," *Sleep* 32 (2009): 351-60.

33. D.N. Neubauer, "A Review of Ramelteon in the Treatment of Sleep Disorders," *Neuropsychiatric Disease and Treatment* 4 (2008): 69-79.

34. Ibid., 74-5.

35. R.R. Markwald et al., "Effects of the Melatonin MT-1/MT-2 Agonist Ramelteon on Daytime Body Temperature and Sleep," *Sleep* 33 (2010): 825-31.

36. G. Hajak et al., "Doxepin in the Treatment of Primary Insomnia," *Journal of Clinical Psychiatry* 62 (2001): 453-63; T. Roth et al., "Efficacy and Safety of Doxepin 1 mg, 3 mg, and 6 mg in Adults with Primary Insomnia," *Sleep* 30 (2007): 1555-61; M. Scharf et al., "Efficacy and Safety of Doxepin 1 mg, 3 mg, and 6 mg in Elderly Patients with Primary Insomnia," *Journal of Clinical Psychiatry* 69 (2008): 1557-64; A.D. Krystal et al., "Efficacy and Safety of Doxepin 1 mg and 3 mg in a 12-Week Sleep Laboratory and Outpatient Trial of Elderly Subjects with Chronic Primary Insomnia," *Sleep* 33 (2010): 1553-61; A.D. Krystal et al., "Efficacy and Safety of Doxepin 3 and 6 mg in a 35-Day Sleep Laboratory Trial in Adults with Chronic Primary Insomnia, *Sleep* 34 (2011): 1433-42.

37. J. Weber et al., "Low-Dose Doxepin: In the Treatment of Insomnia," *CNS Drugs* 24 (2010): 713-20; Krystal et al, "35-Day Sleep Laboratory Trial," 1433-42; Krystal, "Sleep Laboratory and Outpatient Trial," 1553-61.

38. Stephen M. Stahl, "Selective Histamine H(1) Antagonism," *CNS Spectrums* 13 (2008): 1027-38.

39. M. Mamelak et al., "A Pilot Study on the Effects of Sodium Oxybate on Sleep Architecture and Daytime Alertness in Narcolepsy," *Sleep* 27 (2004): 1327-34; J. Black et al., "The Nightly Administration of Sodium Oxybate Results in Significant Reduction in the Nocturnal Sleep Disruption of Patients with Narcolepsy," *Sleep Medicine* 10 (2009): 829-35.

40. G.P. Galloway et al., "Gamma-Hydroxybutyrate: An Emerging Drug of Abuse," *Addiction* 92 (1997): 89-96.

41. "U.S. Pharmaceutical Sales," Drugs.com, accessed February 18, 2013, http://www.drugs.com/stats/top100/; Anahad O'Connor, "Wakefulness Finds a Powerful Ally," *The New York Times,* June 29, 2004; Evelyn Pringle, "The Rise and Fall of Provigil—Part II," September 21, 2010, http://evelynpringle.blogspot.com/2010/09/rise-and-fall-of-provigil-part-ii.html.

42. M.L. Perlis et al., "The Effects of Modafinil and Cognitive Behavior Therapy on Sleep Continuity in Patients with Primary Insomnia," *Sleep* 27 (2004): 715-25.

43. Jonathan R.L. Schwartz, "Modafinil in the Treatment of Excessive Sleepiness," *Drug Design, Development and Therapy* 2 (2008): 71-85; Perlis et al., "The Effects of Modafinil and Cognitive Behavior Therapy," 722.

44. T. Roth et al., "Evaluation of the Safety of Modafinil for Treatment of Excessive Sleepiness," *Journal of Clinical Sleep Medicine* 3 (2007): 595-602; Schwartz, "Modafinil in the Treatment of Excessive Sleepiness," 80.

45. H. Myrick et al., "Modafinil: Preclinical, Clinical, and Post-Marketing Surveillance," *Annals of Clinical Psychiatry* 16 (2004): 101-9; N.D. Volkow et al., "Effects of Modafinil on Dopamine and Dopamine Transporters in the Male Human Brain," *Journal of the American Medical Association* 301 (2009): 1148-54.

46. Saper et al., "Hypothalamic Regulation of Sleep," 1260.

47. Francois Jenck, "The Dual Hypocretin/Orexin Receptor Antagonist Almorexant," paper presented at the annual meeting for the Associated Professional Sleep Societies, San Antonio, Texas, June 5-9, 2010; D.N. Neubauer, "Almorexant, a Dual Orexin Receptor Antagonist for the Treatment of Insomnia," *Current Opinion in Investigational Drugs* 11 (2010): 101-10.

48. T. Sakurai et al., "Orexins and Orexin Receptors: A Family of Hypothalamic Neuropeptides and G Protein-Coupled Receptors That Regulate Feeding Behavior," *Cell* 92 (1998): 573-85; L. de Lecea et al., "The Hypocretins: Hypothalamus-Specific Peptides with Neuroexcitatory Activity," *Proceedings of the National Academy of Sciences of the United States of America* 95 (1998): 322-7.

49. L. Lin et al., "The Sleep Disorder Canine Narcolepsy Is Caused by a Mutation in the Hypocretin Receptor 2 Gene," *Cell* 98 (1999): 365-76; R.M. Chemelli et al., "Narcolepsy in Orexin Knockout Mice," *Cell* 98 (1999): 437-51; T.C. Thannickal et al., "Reduced Number of Hypocretin Neurons in Human Narcolepsy," *Neuron* 27 (2000): 469-74; C. Peyron et al., "A Mutation in a Case of Early Onset Narcolepsy," *Nature Medicine* 6 (2000): 991-7.

50. Buscemi et al., "Efficacy and Safety of Drug Treatments," 1335-50.

51. Perlis et al., "Intermittent and Long-Term Use," 3464.

Chapter 12: Destination Sleep

1. M.M. Ohayon, "Prevalence and Comorbidity of Sleep Disorders in General Population," *La Revue du praticien* 57 (2007): abstract.

2. "NIH Estimates of Funding for Various Research, Condition and Disease Categories," accessed September 2012, http://www.report.nih.gov/categorical_spending.aspx.

3. "Big Pharma Spends More on Advertising Than Research and Development," *ScienceDaily,* January 5, 2008, http://www.sciencedaily.com/releases/2008/01/080105140107.htm; Matthew Herper, "The Truly Staggering Cost of Inventing New Drugs," *Forbes,* February 10, 2012, http://www.forbes.com/sites/matthewherper/2012/02/10/the-truly-staggering-cost-of-inventing-new-drugs/.

4. Riemann et al., "The Hyperarousal Model of Insomnia," 19-31.

5. E. Fortier-Brochu et al., "Insomnia and Daytime Cognitive Performance," *Sleep Medicine Reviews* 16 (2012): 83-94; E. Fortier-Brochu and C. Morin, "Memory Complaints and Objective Performance in Individuals with Insomnia," *Sleep* 35, abstract supplement (2012): A230-1.

6. Saper et al., "Hypothalamic Regulation of Sleep," 1259.

7. Michael Perlis et al., "Neurobiologic Mechanisms in Chronic Insomnia," *Sleep Medicine Clinics*, in press.

8. Winkelman et al., "Reduced Brain GABA," 1499-506; Plante et al., "Reduced GABA in Cingulate Cortices," 1548-57.

9. Pigeon and Perlis, "Birds of a Feather," 82-91; T. Roth, M. Franklin, and T.J. Bramley, "The State of Insomnia and Emerging Trends," *The American Journal of Managed Care* 13 (2007): S117-20; Bonnet and Arand, "Hyperarousal and Insomnia," 10; Perlis et al., "Neurobiologic Mechanisms in Chronic Insomnia," in press.

10. D. Riemann et al., "REM Sleep Instability—A New Pathway for Insomnia?" *Pharmacopsychiatry* 45 (2012): 167-76.

11. Morgan et al., "Retrograde Effects of Triazolam and Zolpidem," 157-64; M. Erman et al., Zolpidem Extended-Release 12.5 mg Associated with Improvements in Work Performance," *Sleep* 31 (2008): 1371-8; Nutt and Stahl, "Searching for the Perfect Sleep," 1601-12; I. Gustavsen et al., "Road Traffic Accident Risk Related to Prescriptions of the Hypnotics Zopiclone, Zolpidem, Flunitrazepam, and Nitrazepam," *Sleep Medicine* 9 (2008): 818-22; Walsh et al., "Treatment of Primary Insomnia with Eszopiclone," 959-68.

12. Sanchez-Ortuno et al., "Effects of Insomnia Treatment on Daytime Measures," A252; Castronovo et al., "Clinical Outcomes of Group Cognitive-Behavioral Therapy," A254; Altena et al., "Prefrontal Hypoactivation and Recovery," 1271-6. These previously cited studies suggest that CBT ameliorates some of the daytime symptoms of insomnia.

13. A. Germain et al., "Effects of a Brief Behavioral Treatment for Late-Life Insomnia," *Journal of Clinical Sleep Medicine* 2 (2006): 403-6; D.J. Buysse et al., "Efficacy of Brief Behavioral Treatment for Chronic Insomnia in Older Adults," *Archives of Internal Medicine* 171 (2011): 887-95.

14. J. Harris et al., "Intensive Sleep Retraining Treatment for Chronic Primary Insomnia," *Journal of Sleep Research* 16 (2007): 276-84; J. Harris et al., "A Randomized Controlled Trial of Intensive Sleep Retraining (ISR)," *Sleep* 35 (2012): 49-60.

15. E.A. Nofzinger and D.J. Buysse, "Frontal Cerebral Thermal Transfer as a Treatment for Insomnia: A Dose-Ranging Study," *Sleep* 34, abstract supplement (2011): A183.

16. D. Riemann et al., "Chronic Insomnia: Clinical and Research Challenges," *Pharmacopsychiatry* 44 (2011): 1-14.

17. F. Scott Fitzgerald, "Sleeping and Waking," *The Crack-up,* ed. Edmund Wilson (New York: New Directions, 1956), 113-7.

18. P. Meerlo et al., "New Neurons in the Adult Brain," *Sleep Medicine Reviews* 13 (2009): 187-94.

19. G. Tononi and C. Cirelli, "Sleep Function and Synaptic Homeostasis," *Sleep Medicine Reviews* 10 (2006): 49-62.